Nutrition and Vulnerable Groups

Nutrition and Vulnerable Groups

Special Issue Editors

Amanda Devine

Tanya Lawlis

MDPI • Basel • Beijing • Wuhan • Barcelona • Belgrade

Special Issue Editors
Amanda Devine
Edith Cowan Univerity
School of Medical and Health Sciences
Australia

Tanya Lawlis
University of Canberra
School of Clinical Sciences
Australia

Editorial Office
MDPI
St. Alban-Anlage 66
4052 Basel, Switzerland

This is a reprint of articles from the Special Issue published online in the open access journal *Nutrients* (ISSN 2072-6643) from 2018 to 2019 (available at: https://www.mdpi.com/journal/nutrients/special_issues/Nutrition_Vulnerable)

For citation purposes, cite each article independently as indicated on the article page online and as indicated below:

LastName, A.A.; LastName, B.B.; LastName, C.C. Article Title. *Journal Name* **Year**, *Article Number*, Page Range.

ISBN 978-3-03921-120-3 (Pbk)
ISBN 978-3-03921-121-0 (PDF)

Contents

About the Special Issue Editors

Amanda Devine is the Professor of Public Health and Nutrition and Director of Public Health at the School of Medical and Health Sciences, Edith Cowan University and an Adjunct Associate Professor, at the Faculty of Health and Medical Sciences, University of Western Australia. During her career, Devine's research has focused on high-quality randomised controlled trials to better understand how diet affects bone and vascular health. In collaboration with others, she has conducted longitudinal observational epidemiological studies to provide insights into the impacts of nutrition on chronic disease. Her current nutrition research areas include statewide food literacy in adults and children, system changes to improve food security, and the influence of plant-based diets on vascular, gestational diabetes, ulcerative colitis, gut, and mental health. Devine's research output includes co-authorship of >116 publications, community-based food literacy programs with relevant sectors, as well as the development websites and, through their implementation, communities of practice have formed to extend nutritional education for children from K-10, Early Years Education and Care Services, and dietitians.

Tanya Lawlis is an Associate Professor and Program Director in the Faculty of Health, University of Canberra. She is an inaugural Fellow of UC CELTS, a Fellow of the UK Higher Education Academy (HEA) and has been awarded three Vice Chancellor's Awards (2015) (Teaching Excellence, Citations for Outstanding Contributions to Student Learning, and USS Recognition). Lawlis has a PhD in interprofessional tertiary education, and her research interests include nutrition science competency development, interprofessional learning, work-integrated learning of food literacy, and household food insecurity. Lawlis has led a national review of nutrition science competencies, and currently leads the national working party to promote and develop resources to assist with the translation of the competencies to tertiary curriculum. Lawlis is particularly interested in the nexus between academic learning, practice, and the workplace, and brings together her research to develop work-integrated learning programs for students enrolled in non-clinical health programs.

nutrients

MDPI

Editorial

Nutrition and Vulnerable Groups

Amanda Devine [1,*] and Tanya Lawlis [2]

[1] School of Medical and Health Sciences, Edith Cowan University, Joondalup, Perth WA 6027, Australia
[2] Discipline Nutrition and Dietetics, University of Canberra, Canberra, ACT 2601, Australia; Tanya.Lawlis@canberra.edu.au
* Correspondence: a.devine@ecu.edu.au; Tel.: +61-8-6304-5527

Received: 9 May 2019; Accepted: 13 May 2019; Published: 14 May 2019

Food insecurity is a complex 'wicked' problem that results from a range of unstable and uncertain physical, social, cultural, and economic factors that limit access to nutritious food. Globally, 800 million people are undernourished, around 1.9 billion are overweight/obese, and 2 billion have micronutrient deficiency [1]. This, in part, is explained by changes in food production and manufacturing and their impacts on climate change [2], the retraction in economic climates, increases in food prices, and, in some regions, reduced food availability and access [3,4]. Vulnerable groups include, but are not limited to, migrant populations, Indigenous peoples, elderly populations, pregnant women, those with disabilities, homelessness people, young children, and youth. Poor nutrition during significant periods of growth and development and throughout life impacts long-term health outcomes; increases non-communicable disease prevalence, healthcare costs, and disease burden; and negatively impacts economic and human productivity [5]. This special edition has brought together a variety of articles, some positioned in developing countries where disease burden is high and food insecurity issues impact the growth and development of young children while also negatively affecting adults, specifically their mental and physical health. This issue, Nutrition and Vulnerable Groups, reports novel strategies to address individual, household, and community food security, and draws together quantitative and qualitative research that has attempted to address the challenges of food security while considering the complexity of the problem, the need for locally-driven and scalable solutions, and policy implications.

The double burden of disease exists in many countries, especially in developing countries and those transitioning to Western-style diets. Factors influencing infant feeding practices in Haitian children have been examined, and despite a high prevalence of malnutrition and poor adherence to the World Health Organization's recommendations exacerbating malnutrition, factors including low maternal education and greater family size have been negatively associated with infant nutritional status [6]. Households that experience child stunting have simultaneous issues with overweight and obese parents, the odds of which relate to the level of food insecurity and appear to be greater in those with mild food insecurity [7]. This may be explained by marginally greater access to food, but food of poor nutritional quality, explaining the juxtaposition of the disease burden. Other vulnerable food insecure groups, such as refugees, are experiencing additional impacts of increased obesity including metabolic syndrome. An increased likelihood of this condition has been related to older age, synonymous to years of exposure, as well as younger marital age [8]. Author recommendations suggest large-scale community intervention programs to tackle obesity as well as cultural change to increase age at marriage.

In both developing and developed countries, socioeconomic status is a known driver of food insecurity and the association with increased Body Mass Index (BMI) in children and adults is clear. This issue examines children who have experienced abandonment and are being supported by the welfare state, and how sociodemographic factors negatively impact children's body size and body shape satisfaction [9]. Authors recommend body image awareness as a consideration in obesity prevention programs. Moreover, poor academic performance in low socioeconomic adolescents has been related to greater body size and fatness, alone or in combination with diet and exercise patterns, and seems more likely to occur in males than females [10]. Poor food choice or limited access to nourishing food, such as fruit and vegetables, is associated with food insecure populations [11,12], especially youth, and is explained by a lack of economic means, education, food availability, access, and other socioeconomic factors. Support mechanisms, including programs to increase access to healthy food, are paramount for vulnerable communities, and this issue provides evidence of the importance of food pantries [13], as well as school and university settings [14,15]. However, in some countries popular restaurants that support low income families and provide cheap, energy-dense foods to support the cultural aspects of the traditional food supply simultaneously increase the risk of chronic disease [16].

Similarly to developing countries, cities and neighborhoods in developed countries are experiencing a greater emergence of vulnerable populations, thus requiring an informed workforce to support these communities. This workforce needs to identify modifiable factors that can be incorporated into future schemes and food security interventions in order to efficiently manage food shortages and address drivers in the immediate and broader geographical locations [17,18]. A greater understanding from the workforce is required, as evidence suggests a divergence in views between those who address the problem and those with the lived experience of food insecurity [19]. Therefore, more engagement and attention to those with the lived experience is required to inform interventions. Strategies outlined in this issue to influence nutritional intake include greater access to local food pantries [13], educational interventions for children and adults [20,21], and increased local food production and livestock keeping [22].

Food literacy is among the key components required to improve food security, as evidence in this issue highlights the lack of understanding by food-insecure households about food labelling, product attributes, and food choice [12]. Authors in this issue outline a framework that builds the capacity and capability of the charitable food organization workforce, through the inclusion of the university or higher education sector, to support their training needs in food literacy [15].

To better understand the practice and policy environment of the broader food system, barriers and enablers have been examined [17]. This issue has outlined novel applications of a Systemic Innovation Lab, which capture initiatives within a defined local geographical area that support community food security [18]. This innovative system examines systems change. Initiatives that had a greater number of characteristics to reinforce a better way of working to address food insecurity or had strategies and systems to implement place-based change were identified. Those without these characteristics were identified, and strategies were co-designed by the community to improve the initiative to more comprehensively address food security. Community and government buy-in, relationship building, and education were among the strategies required to improve systems change.

The diverse articles in this special issue highlight the complexity and extent to which nutrition-related issues may impact vulnerable and marginalized groups. The impact of over- and undernutrition is not specific to one group or area, as similar problems have been identified in developing and developed countries and between rural and urban areas. As seen by the various findings and recommendations, not only is more work in this area required but the translation of this work to practice and policy is imperative if we are to address the issues impacting upon the nutrition and health of those experiencing vulnerability.

Author Contributions: A.D. and T.L. wrote the editorial.

Funding: This research received no external funding.

Conflicts of Interest: The authors declare no conflict of interest.

References

1. Global Panel on Agriculture and Food Systems for Nutrition. *Food Systems and Diets: Facing the Challenges of the 21st Century*; Global Panel on Agriculture and Food Systems for Nutrition: London, UK, 2016.

2. Willett, W.; Rockstrom, J.; Loken, B.; Springmann, M.; Lang, T.; Vermeulen, S.; Garnett, T.; Tilman, D.; DeClerck, F.; Wood, A.; et al. Food in the Anthropocene: The EAT-Lancet Commission on healthy diets from sustainable food systems. *Lancet* **2019**, *393*, 447–492. [CrossRef]
3. Springmann, M.; Clark, M.; Mason-D'Croz, D.; Wiebe, K.; Bodirsky, B.L.; Lassaletta, L.; de Vries, W.; Vermeulen, S.J.; Herrero, M.; Carlson, K.M.; et al. Options for keeping the food system within environmental limits. *Nature* **2018**, *562*, 519–525. [CrossRef] [PubMed]
4. Global Panel. *Improving Nutrition through Enhanced Food Environments*; Global Panel on Agriculture and Food Systems for Nutrition: London, UK, 2017.
5. GBD Diet Collaborators. Health effects of dietary risks in 195 countries, 1990–2017: A systematic analysis for the Global Burden of Disease Study 2017. *Lancet* **2019**, *393*, 1916–1918. [CrossRef]
6. Irarrazaval, B.; Barja, S.; Bustos, E.; Doirsaint, R.; Senethmm, G.; Guzman, M.P.; Uauy, R. Influence of Feeding Practices on Malnutrition in Haitian Infants and Young Children. *Nutrients* **2018**, *10*. [CrossRef] [PubMed]
7. Mahmudiono, T.; Nindya, T.S.; Andrias, D.R.; Megatsari, H.; Rosenkranz, R.R. Household Food Insecurity as a Predictor of Stunted Children and Overweight/Obese Mothers (SCOWT) in Urban Indonesia. *Nutrients* **2018**, *10*. [CrossRef] [PubMed]
8. Massad, S.G.; Khalili, M.; Karmally, W.; Abdalla, M.; Khammash, U.; Mehari, G.M.; Deckelbaum, R.J. Metabolic Syndrome among Refugee Women from the West Bank, Palestine: A Cross-Sectional Study. *Nutrients* **2018**, *10*. [CrossRef] [PubMed]
9. Rahim, N.N.; Chin, Y.S.; Sulaiman, N. Socio-Demographic Factors and Body Image Perception Are Associated with BMI-For-Age among Children Living in Welfare Homes in Selangor, Malaysia. *Nutrients* **2019**, *11*. [CrossRef] [PubMed]
10. Correa-Burrows, P.; Rodriguez, Y.; Blanco, E.; Gahagan, S.; Burrows, R. Increased Adiposity as a Potential Risk Factor for Lower Academic Performance: A Cross-Sectional Study in Chilean Adolescents from Low-to-Middle Socioeconomic Background. *Nutrients* **2018**, *10*. [CrossRef] [PubMed]
11. Godrich, S.L.; Loewen, O.K.; Blanchet, R.; Willows, N.; Veugelers, P. Canadian Children from Food Insecure Households Experience Low Self-Esteem and Self-Efficacy for Healthy Lifestyle Choices. *Nutrients* **2019**, *11*. [CrossRef] [PubMed]
12. Butcher, L.M.; Ryan, M.M.; O'Sullivan, T.A.; Lo, J.; Devine, A. Food-Insecure Household's Self-Reported Perceptions of Food Labels, Product Attributes and Consumption Behaviours. *Nutrients* **2019**, *11*. [CrossRef] [PubMed]
13. Wright, B.N.; Bailey, R.L.; Craig, B.A.; Mattes, R.D.; McCormack, L.; Stluka, S.; Franzen-Castle, L.; Henne, B.; Mehrle, D.; Remley, D.; et al. Daily Dietary Intake Patterns Improve after Visiting a Food Pantry among Food-Insecure Rural Midwestern Adults. *Nutrients* **2018**, *10*. [CrossRef] [PubMed]
14. Godrich, S.L.; Davies, C.R.; Darby, J.; Devine, A. Strategies to Address the Complex Challenge of Improving Regional and Remote Children's Fruit and Vegetable Consumption. *Nutrients* **2018**, *10*. [CrossRef] [PubMed]
15. Lawlis, T.; Sambell, R.; Douglas-Watson, A.; Belton, S.; Devine, A. The Food Literacy Action Logic Model: A Tertiary Education Sector Innovative Strategy to Support the Charitable Food Sectors Need for Food Literacy Training. *Nutrients* **2019**, *11*. [CrossRef] [PubMed]
16. Carrijo, A.P.; Botelho, R.B.A.; Akutsu, R.; Zandonadi, R.P. Is What Low-Income Brazilians Are Eating in Popular Restaurants Contributing to Promote Their Health? *Nutrients* **2018**, *10*. [CrossRef]
17. Haynes-Maslow, L.; Osborne, I.; Jilcott Pitts, S.B. Best Practices and Innovative Solutions to Overcome Barriers to Delivering Policy, Systems and Environmental Changes in Rural Communities. *Nutrients* **2018**, *10*. [CrossRef] [PubMed]
18. Godrich, S.L.; Payet, J.; Brealey, D.; Edmunds, M.; Stoneham, M.; Devine, A. South West Food Community: A Place-Based Pilot Study to Understand the Food Security System. *Nutrients* **2019**, *11*. [CrossRef] [PubMed]
19. Butcher, L.M.; Ryan, M.M.; O'Sullivan, T.A.; Lo, J.; Devine, A. What Drives Food Insecurity in Western Australia? How the Perceptions of People at Risk Differ to Those of Stakeholders. *Nutrients* **2018**, *10*. [CrossRef] [PubMed]
20. El Harake, M.D.; Kharroubi, S.; Hamadeh, S.K.; Jomaa, L. Impact of a Pilot School-Based Nutrition Intervention on Dietary Knowledge, Attitudes, Behavior and Nutritional Status of Syrian Refugee Children in the Bekaa, Lebanon. *Nutrients* **2018**, *10*. [CrossRef] [PubMed]

21. Law, L.S.; Norhasmah, S.; Gan, W.Y.; Siti NurAsyura, A.; Mohd Nasir, M.T. The Identification of the Factors Related to Household Food Insecurity among Indigenous People (Orang Asli) in Peninsular Malaysia under Traditional Food Systems. *Nutrients* **2018**, *10*. [CrossRef] [PubMed]
22. de Bruyn, J.; Thomson, P.C.; Darnton-Hill, I.; Bagnol, B.; Maulaga, W.; Alders, R.G. Does Village Chicken-Keeping Contribute to Young Children's Diets and Growth? A Longitudinal Observational Study in Rural Tanzania. *Nutrients* **2018**, *10*. [CrossRef] [PubMed]

nutrients

Article

Influence of Feeding Practices on Malnutrition in Haitian Infants and Young Children

Belén Irarrázaval [1], Salesa Barja [2,*], Edson Bustos [3], Romel Doirsaint [4], Gloria Senethmm [4], María Paz Guzmán [5] and Ricardo Uauy [1]

1 Division of Pediatrics, School of Medicine, Pontificia Universidad Católica de Chile, Santiago 8330023, Chile; belen.irarrazaval@gmail.com (B.I.); ruauy@med.puc.cl (R.U.)
2 Department of Pediatric Gastroenterology and Nutrition, Division of Pediatrics, School of Medicine, Pontificia Universidad Católica de Chile, Hospital Josefina Martínez, Santiago 8330023, Chile
3 Department of Health Sciences (Nutrition and Dietetics), School of Medicine, Pontificia Universidad Católica de Chile, Hospital Josefina Martínez, Santiago 8330023, Chile; edsonbustos@gmail.com
4 Klinik Saint Espri Health Center, Port Au Prince, HT 6311, Haiti; romeldorsaint@yahoo.fr (R.D.); gloriaasenethmm@yahoo.es (G.S.)
5 Fundación América Solidaria, Santiago 7500776, Chile; mariapazguzman@gmail.com
* Correspondence: sbarja@uc.cl; Tel.: +56-22-354-3887

Received: 7 January 2018; Accepted: 9 March 2018; Published: 20 March 2018

Abstract: Infant malnutrition remains an important cause of death and disability, and Haiti has the highest prevalence in the Americas. Therefore, preventive strategies are needed. Our aims were (1) To assess the prevalence of malnutrition among young children seen at a health center in Haiti; (2) Examine adherence to infant feeding practices recommended by the World Health Organization (WHO) and the association to nutritional status. This cross-sectional study recruited children from the Saint Espri Health Center in Port Au Prince in 2014. We recorded feeding practices, socio-demographic data, and anthropometric measurements (WHO-2006). We evaluated 278 infants and children younger than two years old, aged 8.08 ± 6.5 months, 53.2% female. 18.35% were underweight (weight/age <−2 SD); 13.31% stunted (length/age <−2 SD), and 13.67% had moderate or severe wasting (weight/length <−2 SD). Malnutrition was associated with male gender, older age, lower maternal education level, and greater numbers of siblings (Chi^2, $p < 0.05$). Adherence to recommended breastfeeding practices was 11.8–97.9%, and to complementary feeding practices was 9.7–90.3%. Adherence was associated with a lower prevalence of malnutrition. Conclusion: Prevalence of infant and young child malnutrition in this population is high. Adherence to WHO-recommended feeding practices was associated with a better nutritional status.

Keywords: breastfeeding; feeding practices; infant feeding; nutrition; malnutrition; pediatrics; primary health care

1. Introduction

The Ministry of Health and various international organizations performed several health surveys in Haiti between 2006 and 2012 [1–3]. In 2012, infant mortality in Haiti was 59–73 per 1000 live births, and under-five mortality was 88 per 1000 live births [4,5], the highest in the WHO region [4]. Although the prevalence of wasting has decreased to 4.1% (weight/height <−2 SD), great vulnerability and nutritional risk persists [6]. The prevalence of stunting (height/age <−2 SD) is 23.4% in children <6 years of age [1]. Infant feeding depends on cultures and customs, which can vary regionally and locally. The only study of infant feeding practices in Haiti [6] to date did not evaluate the association between such practices and the nutritional status of children.

Klinik Saint Espri Health Center is located in the Croix de Bouquetes commune, near Port Au Prince. This center opened in 2001 and is run by the American non-governmental organization (NGO) Haiti Medical Missions of Memphis [7]. Malnutrition is a frequent cause of consults and treatment program referrals at this center, but the magnitude of the issue is unknown. Low-cost evaluation methods using local staff and resources are needed to gather relevant data at the community level. This information could enhance planning, resource utilization, and intervention strategies. Studying and improving feeding practices is one important strategy [8].

The objectives of the present study were to assess the prevalence of malnutrition among infants and young children visiting the Klinik Saint Espri Health Center, to measure adherence to WHO-recommended feeding practices [9,10], and to evaluate the association between feeding practices and nutritional status.

2. Materials and Methods

We conducted a cross-sectional study at the Klinik Saint Espri Health Center in September 2014, using a convenience sample of infants and young children seen for acute morbidity, health check of newborns and infants, vaccination, or malnutrition within the Child Health Programs. We aimed to reach a sample of 200 children, based on a previous estimate of 323 visits per month. Recruitment was carried out by general and individual invitation in the waiting room. Children younger than two years old whose parents agreed to participate and who signed the informed consent form were included. Children who required immediate care due to severe disease or with clinical dehydration were excluded; excluded children were similar in age and sex to the final sample.

We developed a survey for the purposes of this study, translated into Haitian Creole by medical staff. The instrument was pilot-tested by two interviewers, and then final adaptations of the format and language were applied (Appendix A). The pilot instrument was administered to 20 children recruited from the waiting room, 2 months before the beginning of the definitive study. The survey evaluated five areas: (1) Identification and general characteristics of the patient (birth date was verified in the clinical records); (2) Brief social evaluation (maternal education, work, number of siblings); (3) 24-h dietary recall, collected once per participant by personal interview with each caregiver; to assess portion size, we used common plates and glasses obtained from local businesses and made models of common foods with painted plastic foam (Appendix B). For breastfed infants, it was not possible to estimate the volume of milk consumed, due to the variety of breastfeeding practices; (4) Use of nutritional supplements during the last week; and (5) Additional breastfeeding-related questions, including age at first breastfeeding, duration of exclusive breastfeeding, age at introduction to solid foods, and age at weaning from breastfeeding. The survey was conducted privately in an individual room by one of five trained interviewers; two were center staff and three were volunteers; all spoke fluent Haitian Creole. After the survey was completed, standardized anthropometry was performed, and the nutritional diagnosis was communicated to the child's guardian. Children with wasting were immediately referred to the center's malnutrition program. Daily reviews of the surveys were carried out to detect duplications and mistakes. Based on the information reported in the survey, specifically the 24-h dietary recall, indicators of feeding practices were calculated based on the methodology proposed by the WHO [6].

Anthropometry: Children were weighed without clothing, using a ADE non-digital infant scale, calibrated daily. A handmade wooden infantometer was used to measure supine length, with the head supported at one end, the torso and lower limbs extended, and feet flexed to 90° and supported by the lower-end stopper, to the nearest 0.1 cm. Head circumference (HC) was measured with a non-elastic measuring tape, fixed on the occiput and passing around the head and above the supraorbital ridges, as a marker of chronic undernutrition. Mid-brachial arm circumference was loosely measured at the mid-point between the acromion and the olecranon with the same non-elastic tape. Measurements were performed twice, rated, and repeated if inconsistencies were identified. Most of the measurements were performed by the first author (BI). The first author also trained the health center team (3 nurses and 1 paramedic) during a 4-h session and supervised in the application of the questionnaires (initially for the duration of the entire interview, and subsequently via intermittent daily observations). We excluded five subjects with incomplete data or inconsistent measurements who were not available for a new measurement.

The 2006 WHO Child Growth Standard was used; z-scores were calculated using the Anthro® program [11,12]: for weight/age (zW/A), length/age (zL/A), weight/length (zW/L), head circumference/age (zHC/A), and mid-brachial circumference/age (zBC/A) [13]. The presence of edema was recorded. We used the 2006 WHO classifications for nutritional status [14]. A zBC/A value <−2 SD or measurement <125 mm was considered suggestive of malnutrition.

Adherence to feeding practice indicators: After applying the survey and before defining the nutritional status, the principal investigator (BI) calculated the indicator scores according to the WHO 2010 criteria for the child's age [6].

Statistical analyses: Descriptive statistics of numerical variables were performed; distributions were verified using the Anderson-Darling test. Variables were expressed as mean (±SD) or median (range). Parametric (Student's *t*-test) or non-parametric (Mann-Whitney) tests were used to compare results. Prevalence by sex and age were calculated (chi-squared test), and univariate correlation analyses were carried out to evaluate for associations. We evaluated the association between adherence to recommended feeding practices and nutritional status using the chi-squared test. The MINITAB-17® program was used for statistical analyses. $p < 0.05$ was considered significant.

Ethics: The Research Ethics Committee of the Faculty of Medicine, Pontificia Universidad Católica de Chile; the medical directors of the Klinik Saint Espri Health Center; and the Haitian ambassador in Chile approved this study. All parents or guardians signed a written informed consent form, written in Creole. If the guardian was illiterate, a trusted person read the consent form (Ethics approval code 14-003).

3. Results

We assessed 278 infants, aged 8.08 ± 6.5 months (range: 13 days to 24 months); 41% were younger than six months, 31% were 6–12 months, and 28% were 13–25 months. Overall, 53.2% were female. There was no difference in age between girls and boys: 7.89 ± 6.05 and 8.31 ± 6.97 months, respectively (Mann–Whitney test, $p = 0.59$). Table 1 shows the characteristics and living conditions of the families. Most caregivers reported living near the Health Center, and the remaining came mainly from areas where the camps of the displaced populations following the 2010 earthquake are concentrated. Only 17.9% reported living in camps and/or housing made from lightweight materials. Parental employment was 34.5%, mostly small-scale trade jobs.

Table 1. General sociodemographic information in in 278 infants that attended the Klinik Saint Espri Health Center, Port au Prince, Haiti (August to September 2014).

Sociodemographic Characteristics		Percentage
Housing	Located in Croix de Bouquetes	70.77%
	Lightweight material houses or camp	17.9%
Parental work	Any kind of work: formal/informal	34.5%
Parental education	Completed primary education	43.5%
	Illiterate	15.35%
	Never attended to school	6.5%
Number of children	One child	35.7%
	Two or three children	41.8%
	Four or more children	22.5%

Median maternal age was 28 years range: (16–46 years). 43.5% of surveyed mothers had completed primary education, and 6.5% had no schooling. 15.35% of caregivers were unable to sign their names upon request (classified as illiterate). 35.7% of mothers reported having one child, 41.8% two or three children, and 22.5% four or more.

3.1. Prevalence of Malnutrition

Table 2 shows the prevalence of malnutrition according to various indices: 18.35% were underweight (weight/age <−2 SD); 13.31% had stunting (length/age <−2 SD); and 13.67% had moderate or severe wasting (weight/length <−2 SD). It is noteworthy that 10.8% had microcephaly and only 4.67% had low brachial perimeter.

The curves for the anthropometric indices were displaced to the left relative to the WHO standard, both globally and by age and sex (Figures 1 and 2). Importantly, only 30.6% of the infants with zW/L <−2 SD (acute malnutrition or wasting) were enrolled in the Malnutrition Program of the Health Center. None of the children had edema.

Table 2. Nutritional status in 278 infants seen at the Klinik Saint Espri Health Center, Port au Prince, Haiti (August to September 2014).

Anthropometric Index	Nutritional Diagnosis	Degree	z-Score (WHO 2006)	Prevalence (%)
Weight/Age	Underweight	Severe	z W/A ≤ −3	6.12
		Moderate	z W/A −2 to −3	12.23
	Normal		z W/A −2 to +2	80.22
	Overweight		z W/A ≥ +2	1.44
Weight/Length	Wasting	Severe	z W/L < −3	3.60
		Moderate	z W/L −2 to −3	10.07
	Normal		z W/L −2 to +2	84.9
	Overweight and obesity		z W/L > +2	1.80
Length/Age	Stunting		z L/A < −2	13.31
	Normal		z L/A −2 to +2	85.25
	Tall		z L/A > +2	1.44
Head circumference/Age	Microcephaly		z HC/A < −2	10.80
	Normal		z HC/A −2 to +2	86.68
	Macrocephaly		z HC/A > +2	2.52
Brachial Circumference/Age	Low		z BC/A < −2	4.67
	Normal		z BC/A > −2	95.33

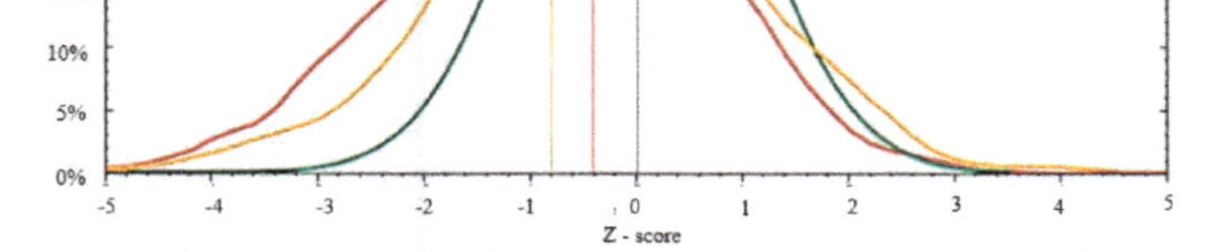

Gender	n	zL/A	SD	95% CI
Female	148	-0.44	1.33	(-0.655 -0.226)
Male	130	-0.79	1.32	(-1.020 -0.562)

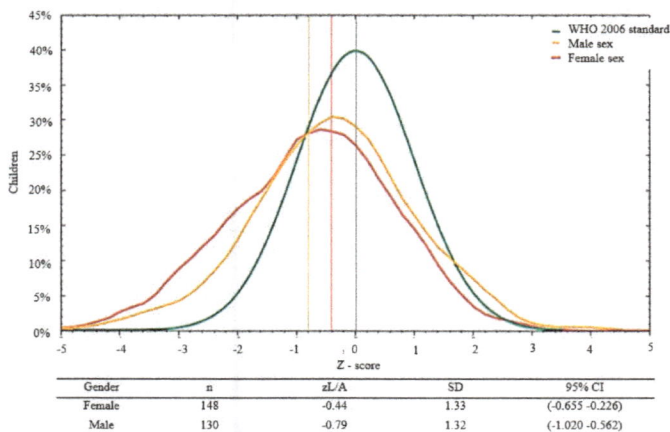

Figure 1. Distribution of L/A *z*-scores by sex* in 278 infants and young children seen at the Klinik Saint Espri Health Center, Port au Prince, Haiti (August 2014). Footnote: The green line indicates the WHO 2006 standard; the yellow line represents males and the red line females. * ANOVA, $p = 0.029$.

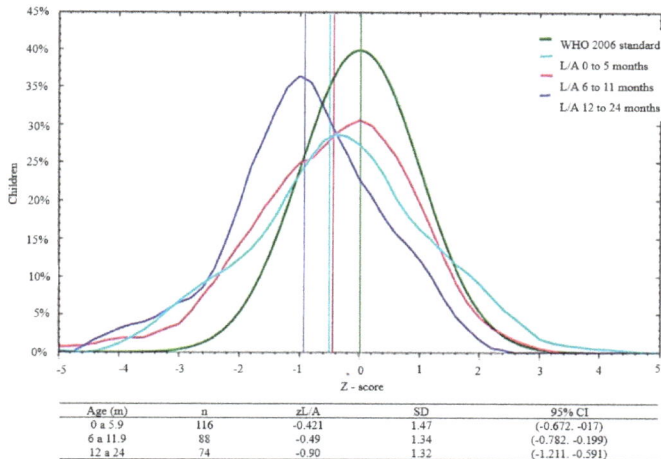

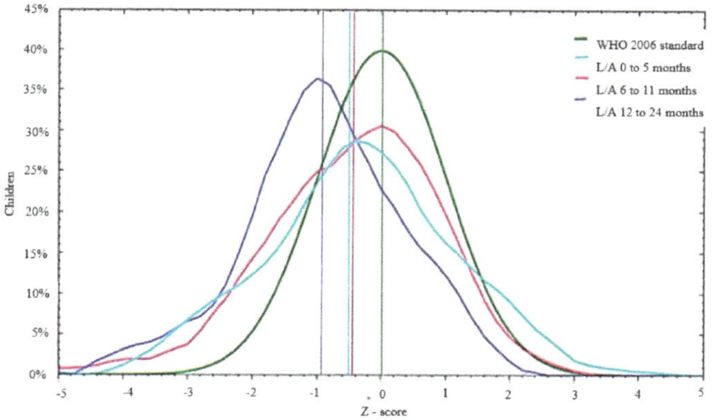

Age (m)	n	zL/A	SD	95% CI
0 a 5.9	116	-0.421	1.47	(-0.672. -017)
6 a 11.9	88	-0.49	1.34	(-0.782. -0.199)
12 a 24	74	-0.90	1.32	(-1.211. -0.591)

Figure 2. Distribution of L/A z-scores by gender* in 278 infants and young children who attended the Klinik Saint Espri Health Center, Port au Prince, Haiti (August 2014). Footnote: The green line indicates the WHO 2006 standard; the light blue line represents children between 0 and 6 months, the lilac children between 6 and 11 months, and the blue children between 12 and 24 months (* ANOVA, $p = 0.038$).

3.2. Malnutrition by Sex and Age

We found a non-significant trend of lower zW/A in male versus female infants, at -1.01 ± 1.44 versus -0.716 ± 1.29, respectively (Student's t-test, $p = 0.07$). We also observed a non-significant trend of lower z W/A in older infants: 0–5 months: -0.69 ± 1.46, 6–11 months: -0.85 ± 1.32, and 12–24 months: -1.1 ± 1.25, respectively (ANOVA, $p = 0.13$). Male infants had a significative lower z L/A compared to females (Figure 1), and older infants had a lower z L/A than younger infants (Figure 2). There was a non-significant trend for lower z W/L in male versus female infants: -0.61 ± 1.15 versus -0.73 ± 1.38, respectively (Student's t-test, $p = 0.42$). Finally, there was a tendency towards higher z W/L in younger infants: -0.55 ± 1.39 (0–5 months), -0.70 ± 1.14 (6–11 months), and -1.80 ± 1.20 (12–24 months) (ANOVA, $p = 0.38$).

3.3. Malnutrition According to Family Characteristics

Children of mothers lacking formal education had significantly lower z W/A, z L/A, z HC/A, and z BC/A scores than those of mothers with primary or secondary education (Figure 3), with a non-significant trend for z W/L. There was no difference between children of mothers with primary versus secondary education.

Children from older mothers had lower z W/L: -0.31 ± 1.38 (mothers <20 years of age), -0.55 ± 1.20 (mothers 20–29), and -0.89 ± 1.11 (mothers $\geq$30 years old) (ANOVA, $p = 0.015$). There was an inverse correlation between maternal age and z W/L (adjusted R^2: 1.9, $p = 0.013$).

We observed lower anthropometric z-scores in families with more children; z W/A scores were -0.62 ± 1.19 in one-child families, -0.94 ± 1.30 in families with 2 or 3 children, and -1.14 ± 1.50 in families with 4 or more children (ANOVA, $p = 0.04$). The mean z BC/A were: -0.40 ± 0.96, -0.42 ± 1.09, and -0.90 ± 1.29, respectively, for the same groups (ANOVA, $p = 0.05$). There were no significant differences based on place of living or paternal employment.

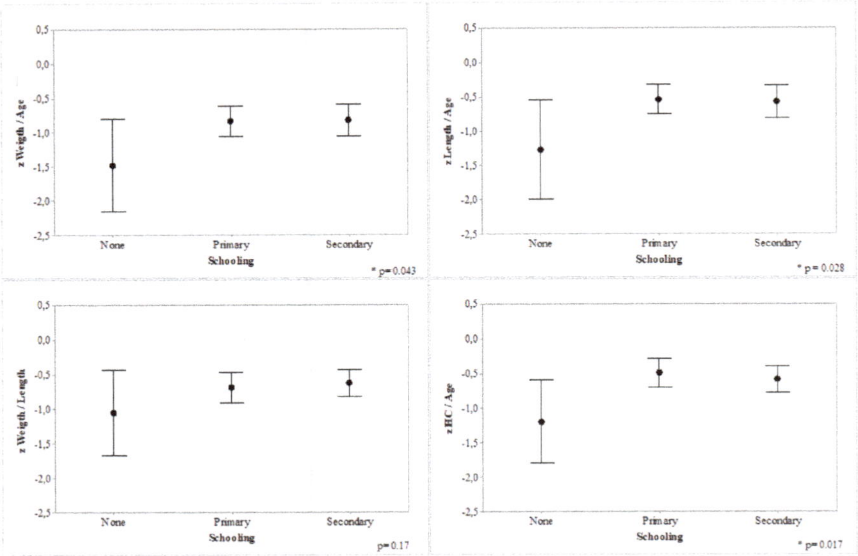

Figure 3. *z*-score of anthropometric indices according to maternal education, in 278 infants seen at the Klinik Saint Espri Health Center, Port au Prince, Haiti (August 2014). Footnote: 95% Confidence Interval, medians represented by black circles. * $p < 0.05$, ANOVA. Comparing children from mothers lacking formal education with those with mothers having primary or secondary education.

3.4. Feeding Practices

The number of cases used to calculate each feeding practice indicator was heterogeneous, given the different sizes of groups by age. Overall adherence was between 98.21% (children ever breastfed) and 3.1% (consumption of iron-rich foods). Adherence to complementary feeding practices was lower than adherence to recommended breastfeeding practices (Figures 4 and 5). Malnourished children were less likely than healthy children to have met recommendations for breastfeeding practices. The differences were significant for: exclusive breastfeeding at 6 months ($p = 0.032$) and age-appropriate breastfeeding ($p = 0.029$). We defined age-appropriate breastfeeding according to the following feeding practice indicators [6]: Infants 0–5 months of age who received only breast milk during the previous day and children 6–23 months of age who received breast milk as well as solid, semi-solid, or soft foods during the previous day, according to the 24-h dietary recall. Adherence to complementary feeding indicators was higher among healthy than malnourished children, although the difference was only significant for "Milk feeding frequency for non-breastfed children".

The association between adherence indicators and malnutrition is shown in Table 3; more breastfeeding practice indicators than complementary feeding practice indicators were associated with malnutrition. Adherence to many of the recommended feeding practices was significantly lower in children with wasting, stunting, and malnutrition than in healthy children.

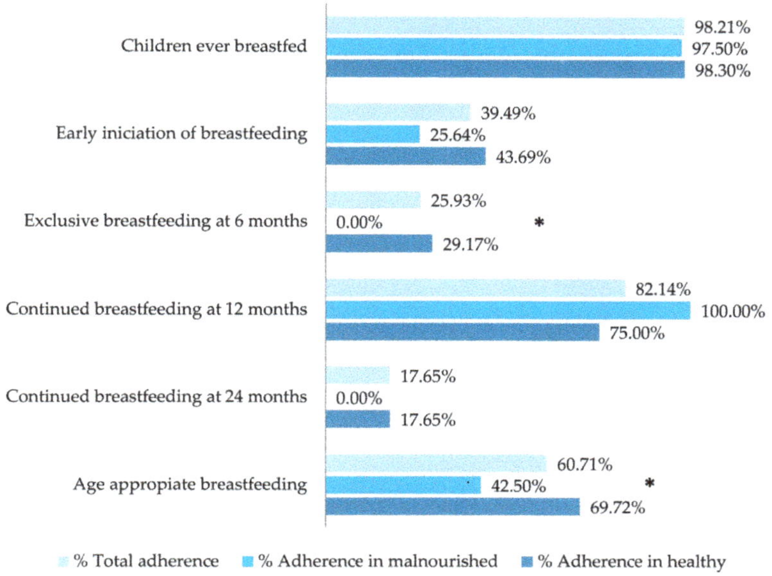

Figure 4. Indicators of breastfeeding practices recommended by WHO in 278 infants seen at the Klinik Saint Espri Health Center, Port au Prince, Haiti (August 2014): Percent adherence in the total group, children with wasting, and healthy children. Footnote: Wasting is defined as W/L <−2 SD according to the WHO 2006 standard. * $p < 0.05$, Chi^2 test.

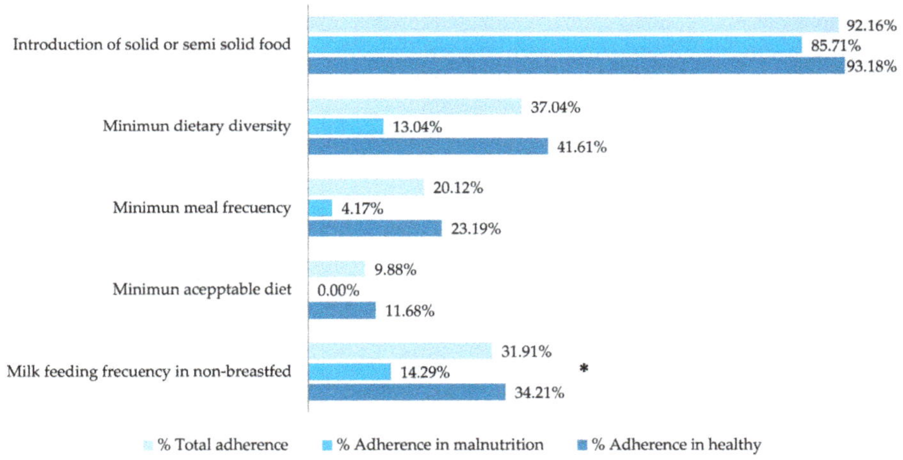

Figure 5. Indicators of adherence to complementary feeding practices (WHO 2008): prevalence in the total group, in children with wasting, and in healthy children. Footnote: Wasting is defined as W/L <−2 SD according to the WHO 2006 standard. * $p < 0.05$ test Chi^2 test.

Table 3. Association between breastfeeding or complementary feeding indicators (WHO, 2010) and malnutrition, in 278 infants and young children seen at the Klinik Saint Espri Health Center, Port au Prince, Haiti (August 2014).

Indicator	Nutritional Status # (p)		
	Wasting	Underweight	Stunting
1. Children ever breastfed	0.92	0.59	0.13
2. Early initiation of breastfeeding	0.21	0.002 *	0.04 *
3. Exclusive breastfeeding under 6 months	0.09	0.32	0.59
4. Predominant breastfeeding under 6 months	0.97	0.000 *	0.02 *
5. Exclusive breastfeeding at 6 months	0.03 *	0.003 *	0.54
6. Continued breastfeeding at 12 months	0.73	0.82	1.00
7. Continued breastfeeding at 24 months	0.16	0.54	nv
8. Age-appropriate breastfeeding	0.03 *	0.20	0.20
9. Introduction of complementary foods	0.83	0.97	0.34
10. Minimum dietary diversity	0.10	0.11	0.90
11. Minimum meal frequency	0.75	0.70	0.90
12. Minimum acceptable diet	0.21	0.049 *	0.35
13. Milk feeding frequency for non-breastfed children	0.02 *	0.06	0.23
14. Consumption of iron rich foods	nv	nv	nv

Malnutrition was defined according to z-scores <−2 SD (WHO 2006 reference). * Chi^2 test for comparisons against children with normal nutritional status (z-scores −2 to +2). $p < 0.05$ was considered significant.

4. Discussion

The present study shows a high prevalence of malnutrition among Haitian infants and young children seen at an outpatient health center near Port Au Prince. Malnutrition rates were related to several maternal and child characteristics. Associations between malnutrition and adherence to the WHO's recommended feeding practices varied, with a possible protective effect of breastfeeding. This is the first study exploring this association in a pediatric Haitian population.

This sample of 278 children represented approximately 80% of the children in this age group seen at the Klinik Saint Espri Health Center during the one-month study period. Patients at this health center mainly live in the nearest commune, Croix de Bouquetes [15]. While assessment over a short period may under- or overestimate malnutrition due to seasonal variations in food access, this urban sample is less susceptible to this issue than other populations.

The prevalence of underweight (18.35%) and wasting (13.67%) was higher than in a 2012 national survey [1]: 11.6% and 5.2%, respectively, but stunting was lower: 13.31% vs. 21.90%

Despite changes from the reference standards used in studies since 2010 [16], an observed historical trend [1] reflects a general improvement of nutritional indices in Haiti. Our results are most consistent with data obtained in the most recent studies. The principal differences between our study and others may be attributed to the lower age of our sample: younger than 2 years versus up to 5 years in the national studies cited [1–3,5,17]. Previous reports in Haitian children found that that 18.5% were underweight, 10.3% had wasting, and 29.7% had stunting [1,2,5]. Our results were similar except for a higher rate of stunting in the previous study, likely due to the different historical period, the use of the 2006 WHO standard [16], and the inclusion of older children, as stunting is usually a consequence of long-term malnutrition [18,19]. It is also important to consider that children with acute malnutrition are more likely to visit the health services due to more frequent illness or a referral to the Malnutrition Program.

The higher prevalence of wasting in males differs from other international [18] and Latin American reports [20] but is consistent with other from Haiti [3]. Cultural practices that might explain this trend include a higher milk-formula feeding and an earlier introduction to solid foods in male. In addition, higher nutritional impairment in older children is expected [19]. Higher maternal age and larger number of children per family were associated with malnutrition possibly due to progressive poverty in larger families. These risk factors are possibly modifiable by early-life educative interventions and support [21,22]. Maternal education influences the ability to provide adequate food, stimulation and a cleaner environment for the child [23,24]. In the present study, few mothers reported no access to education, a probable underestimation because 15.3% were illiterate and their children had smaller head circumference, indicator of poorer future cognitive function [11,24]. We found association between maternal education and not only of cranial perimeter, but also of H/A, W/A and PB/A, reflecting its importance.

Indicators of adherence to feeding practices in the present study were similar to those reported in a 2005–2006 WHO study [6]; however, that study was conducted nationwide and did not explore the association between malnutrition and feeding practices. There are no data available for comparison at the local level. We found a lower adherence to recommendations regarding continued breastfeeding at two years, age-appropriate breastfeeding, minimum meal frequency, and minimum acceptable diet than the older study. On the other hand, we observed a greater adherence to exclusive breastfeeding until 6 months, predominant breastfeeding until six months, and minimum dietary diversity. An aggressive program to educate and follow up mothers has had a possible positive impact on awareness of the importance of breastfeeding up to six months of age. However, a lack of promotion of continued breastfeeding may have increased the use of breastfeeding substitutes, as shown by the low values for indicators of breastfeeding in infants older than 12 months and age-appropriate breastfeeding. The most specific indicator to assess breastfeeding is exclusive breastfeeding at six months; it shows the greatest in nutritional impact, whereas the other results are mixed. This result is logical, as there is a drop in weight indices at around six months of age, and this indicator groups the children who have managed to continue exclusively breastfeeding until the end of the 0–6-month period. The impact of early initiation of breastfeeding may be reflected in more successful long-term breastfeeding; suggesting an opportunity for an intervention with potential impact at the population level [21,25].

We found a lower prevalence of wasting in children who met feeding recommendations, especially some of the breastfeeding practices. Although some trends were not statistically significant for all complementary feeding practice indicators, it should be noted that improving the diet with currently-available local foods may have a protective effect; such cultural issues must be recognized in designing an intervention [21,22,24–32]. However, WHO recommendations [9,10] refer only to food frequency or food groups, not to portions; therefore, real intake may vary according to context, customs, and food availability.

One limitation of our study, with implications for the analysis of the impact of breastfeeding practices, was the difficulty to obtain records for birth weight, gestational age or prematurity. Undernutrition during the first months of life could therefore be overestimated. Since our study was conducted in a limited area within a homogeneous population, we used a convenience sample, prioritizing the recruitment of as many children as possible. Although we compared our results with the reference data available from national surveys of the general population [2–5], our target population consisted of children seen at a local primary health center [15].

The size of the sample in the present study is lower than other studies in Haiti, but large in relation to the center's consulting population. These aspects limit partially the application to the general Haitian population.

The reasons for the health center visits were mainly preventive and were not included in this analysis. We did record children who were enrolled in the child malnutrition program, to detect potential biases associated with this variable. This result is not reported in detail, and no additional analyses were performed, as only a small percentage of the sample was enrolled in the program. Exclusion criteria included referral to urgent care, serious illness, and/or clinical dehydration, as these conditions can temporarily lower weight, thereby leading to a false positive diagnosis of malnutrition.

Finally, although the health center is low-complexity, the study population is at greater risk than the general population given the younger age range and the need to visit a health center. This is a relevant analysis at the local level, especially for planning activities designed to prevent and manage malnutrition. The practical implication for the health center is that any child visiting the center is at elevated risk for undernourishment as compared to the national population; and in agreement with other studies [19], the peak of acute malnutrition (and the possibility of timely treatment) occurs before 2 years of age, and more specifically between six and 24 months. By analyzing the association of nutritional status with feeding and lactation practices, we contribute more precise information that can be used locally to develop possible strategies.

As a strength of the study, we developed and administered our own survey after considering studies from other developing countries, selecting items that could better describe this population and contribute to guiding future interventions. The center´s staff participated in and assessed the survey, so the local relevance of the study is strong; however, these findings can also be extrapolated to similar settings. A major difficulty for health centers in developing countries is planning actions beyond everyday contingencies and global recommendations, in a context of limited resources [31–34]. In the present study, we implemented a simple methodology with low technological and technical support requirements, which allowed us to obtain relevant data from the target population [32].

5. Conclusions

In conclusion, we found a significant prevalence of child malnutrition, especially among males and older infants. Maternal illiteracy, older maternal age, and larger numbers of children per family were associated with higher rates of malnutrition. We found that low adherence to WHO-recommended feeding practices was also associated with malnutrition; good breastfeeding practices may be an important protective strategy.

According to evidence-based practices currently recommended by the WHO [21,22,30,33–35], our results indicate that the principal recommendations for improving nutritional status in this population are early initiation of breastfeeding, exclusive breastfeeding for infants under six months, continued breastfeeding to two years of age, and complementary feeding beginning at six months and no later. We also recommend strengthening the existing malnutrition program to target the groups of children at the highest risk of malnutrition identified in this study. We hope that our study will contribute to increased awareness in the target population of the Klinik Saint Espri and other health centers and guide child nutrition interventions, using the strengths and resources available in the health center and the community.

Acknowledgments: We thank the Klinik Saint Espri Health Center, the children who participated in the study, and their families. This project was supported by the Vice-rectory of Investigation (VRI) of the Pontificia Universidad Católica de Chile through an Agreement of Academic Collaboration with the Fundación América Solidaria. The funder, Pontificia Universidad Católica de Chile, had no role in the design, analysis, or writing of this article. We will receive funds for publishing, from: the Josefina Martínez de Ferrari Foundation, the School of Medicine of Pontificia Universidad Católica de Chile and from the authors.

Author Contributions: B.I. and S.B. (instrument questions and design). B.I., M.P.G., R.D., and G.S. (field development and instrument adjustment). B.I., S.B., and E.B. (data analysis). B.I. and S.B. (article writing). S.B. and R.U. (article revision).

Conflicts of Interest: The authors declare no conflict of interest.

Appendix A

Survey used in the study, in Haitian Créole and in English:

1. Identification and general characteristics of the patient
2. Brief social evaluation
3. Nutritional information
    3.1. 24-h dietary recall
    3.2. Use of nutritional supplements
    3.3. Additional breastfeeding questions
4. Anthropometry

Additional page: calculation of individual indicators of feeding practices (WHO 2003).

Patient Record «Influence of Feeding Practices on Malnutrition in Haitian Infants and Young Children»

Date	
Survey Number	

1. Identification of the child								
1.1 Birthdate	Day	Month	Year	Age in months	Do you know the date of birth well?			
					Yes		No	
1.2 Gender	Female		Male					
1.3 Place of residence	Do you live in a camp?		Yes		No		Zone	

2. Socio demographic data			
2.1 Maternal age How old is the mother ?			
2.2 Maternal Education What was the last year of school you completed?	Never attended school	Primary education	Secondary education
2.3 Number of children of the mother How many children do you have ?	1 child	2 or 3 children	4 or more children
2.4 Parents income What parents do for a living?	Regular work	Sporadic work	No job or beggar
2.5 What do you think about your child's health?			
2.6 Do you think you can give your child all the food he needs?	Yes	No	

3. Feeding: Reminder food consumed last 24 hours

Record all the food and drinks the child took, including breastfeeding; write down the amounts and approximate time.
Put all the foods and drinks to take the baby, including breastfeeding; Write the amount and approximate time. Number according to the guide, record amount corresponding to what the child actually ate from the serving. Remember everything the children eat and drink the day before: * If the child is breastfeeding specifying how often.

Time	Type of food	Amount
Morning meal		
Midday meal		
Food of the afternoon		

4. Consumption of food supplements (times per week)			
Multivitamínico En pastilla o jarabe	Iron	Peannut butter food supplement Like "mamba" or "plumpy nut"	Fortified cereal type food supplement As "baby blend"

5.Breastfeeding			
5.1 When the child born, after how much time his mother breast feed him?	Hours of life	Never breastfeed	
5.2 Until what age was the child fed only with breastmilk? That is, he took only breastmilk and no other type of food or drink	Hours of life	Months	Currently breastfeeding
5.3 At what age did the child eat solid foods for the first time? That is, he ate porridge or puree with a spoon	Hours of life	Months	Currently breastfeeding
5.4 Until what age did you breastfeed him? At what age did the child stop receiving breastmilk?	Hours of life	Months	Currently breastfeeding

6.1 Anthropometry	
6.1.1 Weight Weigh the naked child, balance at zero, measurement in kilos and grams	(Kg)
6.1.2 Size Measure the child lying on the pedometer, in centimeters and millimeters	(cm)
6.1.3 Head circunference Circumference measured between occipital protuberance passing through ciliary rim	(cm)
6.1.4 Brachial Perimeter Circumference measured at the midpoint of the arm between acromion and elbow with the arm hanging, at rest.	(mm)

6.2 Nutritional Diagnosis		**Nutritional Diagnosis**
6.2.1 Weight / age		
6.2.2 Height/ age		
6.2.3 Cranial perimeter / age		
6.2.4 Brachial Perimeter / age		
6.2.5 Weigth / Height		

Figure A1. Patient Record <<Influence of Feeding Practices on Malnutrition in Haitian Infants and Young Children>>.

Calculation indicators of feeding practices (Not asked, this sheet is attached later)

6.1 Breastfeeding			
6.1.1 Child 0 to 23 months who started breastfeeding in 1st hour of life Applies to all children between 0 and 23 months	Yes	No	
6.1.2 Child between 0 and 5 months who only feeds on breastfeeding Applies only to children under 6 months	Yes	No	Does not apply
6.1.3 Child between 4 and 5 months who only feeds on breastfeeding Applies only to children of 4 and 5 months	Yes	No	Does not apply
6.1.4 Child between 12 and 15 months who took breastmilk the previous day Applies only to children between 12 and 15 months	Yes	No	Does not apply
6.2 Complementary feeding			
6.2.1 Child between 6 and 8 years old who received solid food the previous day Applies only to children between 6 and 8 months	Yes	No	Does not apply
6.2.2 Child between 6 and 23 months who received food from at least 4 different groups the previous day Applies only to children between 6 and 23 months	Yes	No	Does not apply
6.2.3 Child between 6 and 8 months who ate 2 or more times the day before, besides breastmilk Applies only to children between 6 and 8 months who also took breastmilk	Yes	No	Does not apply
6.2.4 Child between 9 and 23 months who ate 3 or more times the previous day, besides breastmilk Applies only to children between 9 and 23 months who also took maternal breast	Yes	No	Does not apply
6.2.5 Child between 6 and 23 months who ate 4 or more times the day before, that aren´t breastfeed Applies only to children between 9 and 23 months who don´t take breastmilk	Yes	No	Does not apply
6.2.6 Child between 6 and 23 months who took milk 2 or more times a day previous and does not take breastmilk Applies only to children between 9 and 23 months who do not take breastmilk	Yes	No	Does not apply
6.3 Additional Indicators			
6.3.1 Child who whas ever breast fed Applies to all children between 0 and 23 months	Yes	No	
6.3.2 Child between 20 and 23 months who took breastmilk the previous day Applies only to children between 20 and 23 months	Yes	No	Does not apply

Figure A2. Calculation Indicators of Feeding Practices (Not asked, this sheet is attached later).

Appendix B

Example of common plates and glasses obtained from local businesses and models of common foods with painted plastic foam used for assessing portion size in 24-h dietary recall.

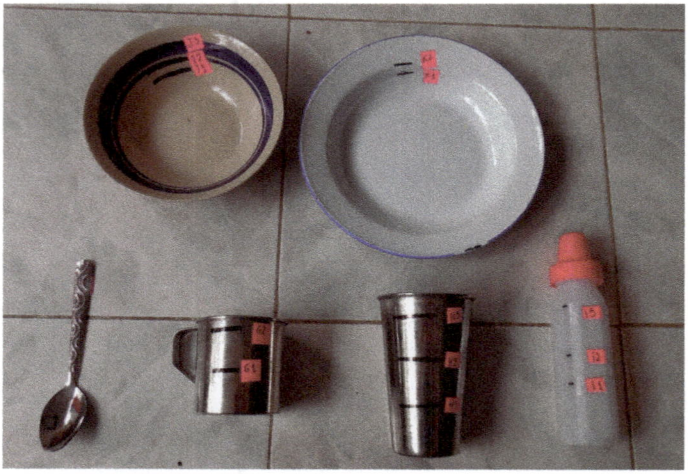

Figure A3. Pictures of plates and glasses from local businesses used for assessing portion size. The plates were code labeled and corresponding volume was mesured.

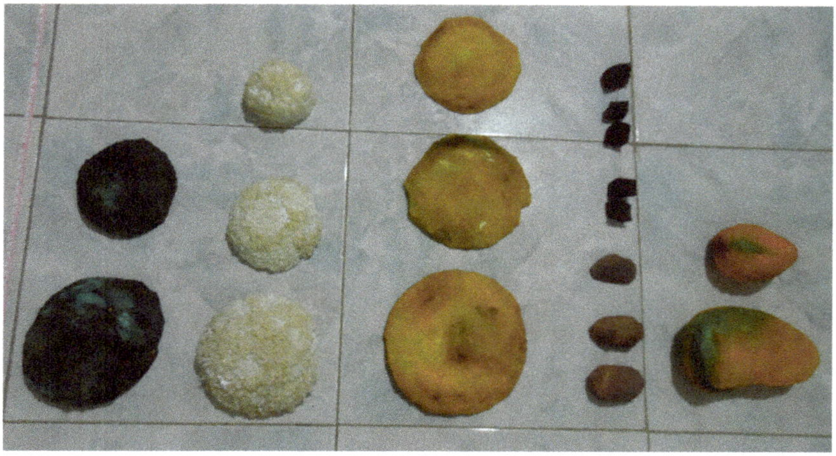

Figure A4. Picture of foam models used to assess portion size, they mimic most common food choices for children in different servings. Models were code labeled.

References

1. Ministry of health and population Haiti. Rapport de l'enquete Nutritionnelle Nationale Avec la Methodologie SMART. 2012. Available online: http://mspp.gouv.ht/site/downloads/SMART.pdf (accessed on 10 April 2016).
2. Ministère de la Santé Publique et de la Population. *Enquete Mortalite, Morbidite et Utilisation des Services EMMUS–IV Haiti 2005–2006*; Institut Haïtien de l'Enfance Pétion-Ville, Haïti y Macro International Inc.: Calverton, MD, USA, 2007. Available online: https://dhsprogram.com/pubs/pdf/FR192/FR192.pdf (accessed on 10 April 2016).
3. Ministère de la Santé Publique et de la Population. *Enquete Mortalite, Morbidite et Utilisation des Services EMMUS–V Haiti 2012*; Institut Haïtien de l'Enfance Pétion-Ville: Borno, Haiti, 2012. Available online: http://unfpahaiti.org/pdf/JMP2013_Rapport_de_synthEse_Haiti.pdf (accessed on 10 April 2016).
4. World Health Organization (WHO) Country profiles. Haiti Country Profile. 2012. Available online: http://www.who.int/countries/hti/en/ (accessed on 18 January 2016).
5. Ministry of Public Health and Population. [le Ministère de la Santé Publique and de la Population] (MSPP), Haitian Childhood Institute [l'Institut Haïtien de l'Enfance] (IHE) and ICF International. *2012 Haïti Mortality, Morbidity, and Service Utilization Survey: Key Findings*; Ministry of Public Health and Population: Port-au-Prince, Haiti; MSPP, IHE, and ICF International: Calverton, MD, USA, 2013; p. 8. Available online: http://procurement-notices.undp.org/view_file.cfm?doc_id=17735 (accessed on 10 April 2016).
6. World Health Organization. *Indicators for Assessing Infant and Young Child Feeding Practices, Country profiles, Part I Definitions. Maternal, Newborn, Child and Adolescent Health*; World Health Organization: Geneva, Switzerland, 2010; ISBN 9789241596664. Available online: http://www.who.int/maternal_child_adolescent/documents/9789241596664/en/ (accessed on 10 April 2016).
7. Dependent on the Church of the Holy Spirit Catholic Church in Memphis, Tenesse. Available online: http://www.hspirit.com/ (accessed on 10 April 2016).
8. Sunguya, B.F.; Poudel, K.C.; Mlunde, L.B.; Shakya, P.; Urassa, D.P.; Jimba, M.; Yasuoka, J. Effectiveness of nutrition training of health workers toward improving caregivers' feeding practices for children aged six months to two years: A systematic review. *Nutr. J.* **2013**, *12*, 66–80. [CrossRef] [PubMed]
9. Panamerican Health Organization. *Guiding Principles for Complementary Feeding of the Breastfed Child*; Nutrition Unit, Family Health and community Panamerican Health Organization: Washington, DC, USA, 2003; ISBN 9275324603. Available online: http://iris.paho.org/xmlui/handle/123456789/752 (accessed on 10 April 2016).

10. World Health Organization. *Guiding Principles for Feeding Non-Breastfed Children 6–24 Months of Age*; World Health Organization: Geneva, Switzerland, 2005; ISBN 9789275327951. Available online: http://www.who.int/maternal_child_adolescent/documents/9241593431/en/ (accessed on 10 April 2016).
11. World Health Organization. *WHO Growth Standards for 0–5 Years*; World Health Organization: Geneva, Switzerland, 2006; Available online: http://www.who.int/childgrowth/standards/en/ (accessed on 18 January 2016).
12. Department of Nutrition, World Health Organization. *WHO Anthro: Software for Assessing Growth and Development of the World's Children*; World Health Organization: Geneva, Switzerland, 2011.
13. De Onis, M.; Yip, R.; Mei, Z. The development of MUAC-for age reference data recommended by a WHO Expert Committee. *Bull. World Health Organ.* **1997**, *75*, 11–18. [PubMed]
14. De Onis, M.; Blössner, M. *WHO Global Database on Child Growth and Malnutrition*; World Health Organization: Geneva, Switzerland, 1997; pp. 45–47.
15. *Report of Monthly Patient Care Statistics*; Klinik Saint Esprit: Port Au Prince, Haiti, 2014.
16. WHO Multicentre Growth Reference Study Group. *WHO Child Growth Standards: Length/Height-for-Age, Weight-for-Age, Weight-for-Length, Weight-for-Height and Body Mass Index-for-Age: Methods and Development*; World Health Organization, Child Growth Standards: Geneva, Switzerland, 2016.
17. Black, R.E.; Allen, L.H.; Bhutta, Z.A.; Caulfield, L.E.; de Onis, M.; Ezzati, M.; Mathers, C.; Rivera, J. Maternal and Child Undernutrition Study Group. Maternal and child undernutrition: Global and regional exposures and health consequences. *Lancet* **2004**, *371*, 243–260. [CrossRef]
18. Lozano, R.; Naghavi, M.; Foreman, K.; Lim, S.; Shibuya, K.; Aboyans, V.; Abraham, J.; Adair, T.; Aggarwal, R.; Ahn, S.Y.; et al. Global and regional mortality from 235 causes of death for 20 age groups in 1990 and 2010: A systematic analysis for the Global Burden of Disease Study 2010. *Lancet* **2012**, *380*, 2095–2128. [CrossRef]
19. Victora, C.G.; de Onis, M.; Hallal, P.C.; Blössner, M.; Shrimpton, R. Worldwide timing of growth faltering: Revisiting implications for interventions. *Pediatrics* **2010**, *125*, 473–480. [CrossRef] [PubMed]
20. Kac, G.; Alvear, J.L.G. Malnutrition in Latin America Network Program of Science and Technology for Development. Epidemiology of malnutrition in Latin America: Current situation. *Nutr. Hosp.* **2010**, *25* (Suppl. 3), 50–56.
21. Haroon, S.; Das, J.K.; Salam, R.A.; Imdad, A.; Bhutta, Z.A. Breastfeeding promotion interventions and breastfeeding practices: A systematic review. *BMC Public Health* **2013**, *13* (Suppl. 3), S20. [CrossRef] [PubMed]
22. Dewey, K.G.; Adu-Afarwuah, S. Systematic review of the efficacy and effectiveness of complementary feeding interventions in developing countries. *Matern. Child Nutr.* **2008**, *4* (Suppl. 1), 24–85. [CrossRef] [PubMed]
23. Prado, E.L.; Dewey, K.G. Nutrition and brain development in early life. *Nutr. Rev.* **2014**, *72*, 267–284. [CrossRef] [PubMed]
24. Imdad, A.; Yakoob, M.Y.; Bhutta, Z.A. Impact of maternal education about complementary feeding and provision of complementary foods on child growth in developing countries. *BMC Public Health* **2011**, *13*, S25. [CrossRef] [PubMed]
25. Renfrew, M.J.; McCormick, F.M.; Wade, A.; Quinn, B.; Dowswell, T. Support for healthy breastfeeding mothers with healthy term babies. *Cochrane Database Syst. Rev.* **2012**, CD001141. [CrossRef]
26. Heckert, J.; Boatemaa, S.; Altman, C.E. Migrant youth's emerging dietary patterns in Haiti: The role of peer social engagement. *Public Health Nutr.* **2014**, *18*, 1262–1271. [CrossRef] [PubMed]
27. Diop El, H.I.; Dossou, N.I.; Ndour, N.M.; Briend, A.; Wade, S. Comparison of the efficacy of a solid ready-to-use food and a liquid, milk-based diet for the rehabilitation of severely malnourished children: A randomized trial. *Am. J. Clin. Nutr.* **2003**, *78*, 302–307. [CrossRef] [PubMed]
28. Ciliberto, M.A.; Sandige, H.; Ndekha, M.J.; Ashorn, P.; Briend, A.; Ciliberto, H.M.; Manary, M.J. Comparison of home-based therapy with ready-to-use therapeutic food with standard therapy in the treatment of malnourished Malawian children: A controlled, clinical effectiveness trial. *Am. J. Clin. Nutr.* **2005**, *81*, 864–870. [CrossRef] [PubMed]
29. Bisits Bullen, B.A. The positive deviance/hearth approach to reducing child malnutrition: Systematic review. *Trop. Med. Int. Health* **2011**, *16*, 1354–1366. [CrossRef] [PubMed]

30. Picot, J.; Hartwell, D.; Harris, P.; Mendes, D.; Clegg, A.J.; Takeda, A. The effectiveness of interventions to treat severe acute malnutrition in young children: A systematic review. *Health Technol. Assess.* **2012**, *16*, 1–316. [CrossRef] [PubMed]
31. Uauy, R. Undernutrition is undernourished. *Public Health Nutr.* **2008**, *11*, 647–649. [CrossRef] [PubMed]
32. Pridmore, P.; Carr-Hill, R. Tackling the drivers of child undernutrition in developing countries: What works and how should interventions be designed? *Public Health Nutr.* **2011**, *14*, 688–693. [CrossRef] [PubMed]
33. World Health Organization and UNICEF. *Global Strategy for Infant and Young Child Feeding*; WHO: Geneva, Switzerland, 2003; ISBN 924356221. Available online: http://www.who.int/nutrition/publications/infantfeeding/9241562218/en/ (accessed on 10 April 2016).
34. World Health Organization. *Essential Nutrition Actions: Improving Maternal, Newborn, Infant and Young Child Health and Nutrition*; WHO: Geneva, Switzerland, 2013; ISBN 9789241505550. Available online: http://www.who.int/nutrition/publications/infantfeeding/essential_nutrition_actions/en/ (accessed on 10 April 2016).
35. Ward, K.N.; Byrne, J.P. A critical review of the impact of continuing breastfeeding education provided to nurses and midwives. *J. Hum. Lact.* **2011**, *27*, 381–393. [CrossRef] [PubMed]

nutrients

MDPI

Article

Is What Low-Income Brazilians Are Eating in Popular Restaurants Contributing to Promote Their Health?

Alinne de Paula Carrijo, Raquel Braz Assunção Botelho, Rita de Cássia Coelho de Almeida Akutsu and Renata Puppin Zandonadi *

Research Group in Nutritional and Nourishment Quality, Department of Nutrition, University of Brasilia, Brasilia DF 70910-900, Brazil; alinnecarrijo@yahoo.com.br (A.d.P.C.); raquelbabotelho@gmail.com (R.B.A.B.); rita.akutsu@gmail.com (R.d.C.C.d.A.A.); renatapz@yahoo.com.br (R.P.Z.)

* Correspondence: raquelbotelho@terra.com.br; Tel.: +55-61-3307-2510; Fax: +55-61-3273-3676

Received: 22 January 2018; Accepted: 5 March 2018; Published: 27 March 2018

Abstract: This study evaluates the healthfulness of the meals offered to and consumed by low-income Brazilians in Popular Restaurants (PR). It is a cross-sectional, exploratory study. The final sample includes 36 PRs, respecting the stratification criteria for each of the five Brazilian regions. To identify the quantity and quality of food consumption, consumers' meals are evaluated. The sample calculation uses a minimum of 41 consumers in each PR. Consumption evaluation is carried out by weighing and direct observation of the meal that each consumer served to his plate. Each dish of the meals had its Technical preparation files (TPF) developed by observing the production and weighing all the ingredients. Evaluations of Energy density (ED), meal's weight components and sodium composition are conducted. Plate's composition is compared to "My plate" guidelines United States Department of Agriculture (USDA). The final sample includes 1771 low-income Brazilians consumers. The plate of PRs consumers is adequate only for the "protein group" in comparison to "My plate". Rice and beans compose more than 50% of the plate's weight, as expected, since it is a Brazilian habit of consumption at lunch. Thus, grains are the major group consumed by PRs consumers. The average ED for all PRs is 1.34 kcal/g. Regarding sodium content, rice and main courses presented the highest values and are classified as high, according to Food and Drug Administration (FDA). Concerning sodium, PRs are putting Brazilian low-income population at risk for chronic diseases. However, in general, PRs are good choices because they promote access to cheap and quality traditional Brazilian foods.

Keywords: low-income population; popular restaurant; lunch; energy density; nutrition

1. Introduction

Popular Restaurants (PR) is an assistance program created by the Brazilian Government and it is characterized as food service units that offer inexpensive and healthy meals to low-income population in Brazil [1,2]. The purpose of this program is to guarantee the social rights of feeding, consolidated by the Universal Declaration of Human Rights [3]. It is also to improve health of low-income population, since food access and choices have a substantial impact on prevention and treatment of several diseases [4–6].

In the last decades, globalization and modernization have been changing feeding habits. A consumption increase of fatty and sugary industrialized foods, with high energy density (ED) and low fiber content can be verified. Further, people have no time to prepare meals and they are frequently eating out. In Brazil, eating out represents, to low-income population, an access to snacks that are cheap, easy and fast to intake. Usually, they have inadequate nutrients and poor sanitary conditions [2,7,8]. This situation results an increase of chronic and foodborne diseases that are very common in low-income population in developing countries such as Brazil [4–6]. Besides this panorama, we have many people that do not have access to food, or to good quality meals to guarantee survival and health.

Despite the need of eating out and knowing the difficulties to access healthy food, the Brazilian government provides more than 120,000 daily meals through the PRs. In this plan, PRs have to offer access to healthy and cheap meals as well as improve cultural food habits to low-income population [2].

However, there is no report about evaluation of this social program as a tool to promote health and to guarantee food access to low-income population in the literature. Then, the aim of this study is to evaluate the healthfulness of the meals offered to and consumed by low-income Brazilians in Popular Restaurants (PR).

2. Materials and Methods

This research is transversal and exploratory based on direct documentation. The Research Ethics Committee (Protocol No. 0372/10) approved it.

2.1. Sampling

To select PRs, we used the following inclusion criteria: (i) a food service belonging to the Popular Restaurants program of the Brazilian Federal Government; (ii) signature of the Institutional Acknowledgement Agreement by the dietitian responsible for the food service; (iii) open during lunch; and (iv) service of more than 500 meals daily. Given the inclusion criteria, 65 PRs were eligible to be part of the study. From the selected population (N), the sampling plan was calculated considering an error (e) of a daily meal and a level of significance (α) of 5% [9]. A simple random sample was estimated through the procedure "survey select" of the SAS 9.1.3 program. The final sample included 36 PRs, respecting the stratification criteria for each of the five Brazilian geographical regions.

To identify the quantity and quality of food consumption, consumers' meals were evaluated. A minimum sample of 41 consumers in each PR was necessary. The inclusion criteria were: be a frequent consumer (more than 3 times a week) and be over 18 years old. The excluding group from the sample was pregnant women because of different nutritional needs. The individuals' selection occurred while they were waiting in line to serve their meal at lunchtime (self-service). Invitations to participate occurred to the first person in line, then the 15th person, and this pattern was used until sample was completed. Participants signed the acknowledgement and agreement term and evaluation occurred during 4 days at the PRs. On the first day, participants were recruited and, on the other 3 days, their meals were weighed and evaluated. After recruitment, the same participant continued evaluation for the rest of the study. For this study, participants had to complete the three days of consumption evaluation to be qualified. Social demographic variables, sex and age groups (<21 years old, 21–30, 31–40, 41–50, 51–59 and $\geq$60 years old) were used to qualify the analyzed variables of this study.

The analyzed variables were: (i) the weight of the meal (g) of each component of the meal, e.g., main course (protein preparation offered on the menu, usually of animal origin and decisive for the selection of other items), garnish (menu item accompanying the main course, which may have as main ingredients vegetables, pasta, tubers, and cassava flour dishes), side dishes (items such as rice and beans, culturally daily consumed by the Brazilian population), salad and dessert (fruit or sweets) [10]; (ii) the portion of each component on the plate; (iii) the consumption of fruit and vegetables; (iv) the composition of garnish (pasta or vegetable) and desserts (sweets or fruits); and (v) the energy density of the meal.

2.2. Consumption Evaluation

The consumption evaluation was carried out by weighing and direct observation of the meal that each consumer served in his or her plate, according to the procedures proposed by Savio, Costa, Miazaki and Schmitz [11]. The meal weight was measured to relate the percentage of each dish preparation in the meal composition. It was important to check the meal weight on a scale to evaluate whether the observed portions of each dish were correctly described.

To evaluate the nutritional composition of the meals, we developed technical preparation files (TPF) according to the protocol proposed by Camargo and Botelho [12]. Based on the data recorded in the TPFs, the nutritional value was calculated using the information available in the Brazilian Food Composition Table [13]. When this information did not exist, we used scientific publications and labels on processed food products and then entered the information into the system database (DietWin®, Porto Alegre, Brazil).

The nutritional analysis was carried out considering the Total Energy Value (TEV) (2000 kcal/day) [1] as a benchmark, following the Brazilian guideline recommendation. The Brazilian Surveillance agency uses 2000 kcal as the energy parameter for nutrition labeling in the Brazilian products. We considered that the lunch meal should provide 40% of TEV [1]. After the calculation of the energy values of each preparation in 100 g of food, we calculated ED expressed in kcal/g of food. According to the Centers for Disease Control and Prevention [14], the preparations were classified as: high energy density (4 to 9 kcal/g), medium energy density (1.5 to 4 kcal/g), low energy density (0.7 to 1.5 kcal/g) and very low energy density (0 to 0.6 kcal/g). The results of these analyses helped to evaluate if the PR program is promoting access to quality food and health.

For sodium evaluation, we compared the results to the Food and Drug Administration standards for sodium content of foods [15]. They considered a general rule of 5% daily value (DV) or less of sodium per serving is low; 20% DV or more is high. Additionally, FDA settles that 140 mg of sodium or less per serving is "low sodium"; 35 mg of sodium or less per serving is "very low sodium".

In some PRs, Salt sachets were available to consumers who could add salt to their plate before consumption. This salt addition was not measured, and this could be a possible bias of this research. Therefore, sodium results might be underestimated.

2.3. Statistical Analysis

Descriptive analysis was carried out by SPSS 20® software. The amount of dietary preparations' intake (in grams) and the consumption of fruits and vegetables were adjusted considering intrapersonal variability to estimate the usual consumption of individuals through MSM® software (2012).

T-test was used for comparisons between sexes and ANOVA for comparisons among age group and sexes. It was established that $p < 0.05$ was statistically significant.

3. Results and Discussions

The final sample included 1771 low-income Brazilians consumers (60% male and 40% female; age range 45 ± 17.39 years) distributed proportionally among the PRs of the five regions of Brazil.

Healthy eating is a mix of many factors, including stage of life, preference, access to food, culture, and traditions. The PRs were created to promote access to food respecting habits and meal quality. In Brazil, lunch is the main meal and PRs are open for it from 11:00 a.m. to 2:00 p.m. to guarantee access to a greater number of consumers. Menu is the same from the time the PR opens until it closes.

According to Brazilians food habits, PR menus should include the following preparations: rice (grains), beans, main course (protein), garnish (pasta, some cooked vegetables or other carbohydrate dishes such as couscous and "farofa" (manioc flour dish)), salad and dessert [2]. It is important to highlight that all PRs offer a fixed meal composed of one protein dish (main course), one garnish, one type of rice, one type of beans, a mixed salad, and one type of dessert. Therefore, consumers only have one menu option each day they eat at the PR. Energetic value and sodium intake are related to the mean portions consumed by the population of the whole study. PRs are located in different regions, but since they are part of a governmental program, all of them have to offer an equal fixed number of dishes. They may vary the type of protein, garnish, salads and desserts, but not the number of options.

Figure 1 represents the composition of the main plate (percentage of weight) consumed by low-income Brazilians in PRs and the distribution according to recommend groups of "My plate" (USDA). According to "My plate"—United States Department of Agriculture (USDA) food guide—the plate should have the composition of 20% protein group; 30% grains group; 30% vegetables group;

and 20% fruit. "My plate" illustrates (proportionally in the plate) groups of foods that should be present and consumed for a healthy diet.

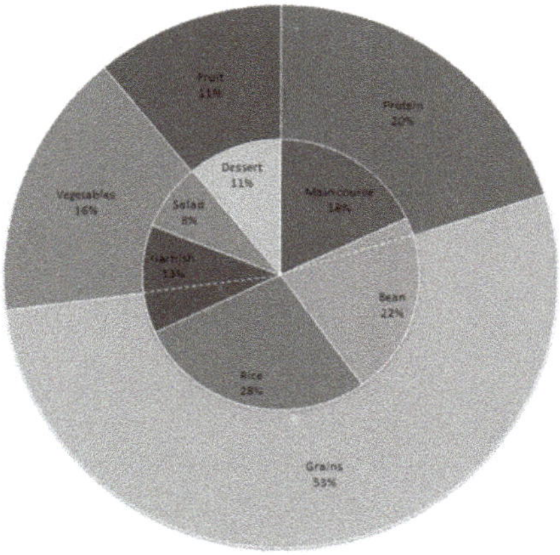

Figure 1. Plate composition by type of preparation consumed by low-income Brazilians in Popular Restaurants and distribution according to recommend groups of "My plate" United States Department of Agriculture (USDA) groups.

The PR consumers' plate is adequate only for the "protein group" in comparison to "My plate". In the USDA guide, all foods made from meat, poultry, seafood, beans, peas, eggs, and soy products are in the "protein group", which recommends 5–6 portions daily. Thus, PRs should provide 2.0–2.5 portions (40%) of this group. In our study, PRs consumers ate about 117.88 g $\pm$ 21.76 of the main course (protein group) and 139.67 g $\pm$ 48.52 of beans. According to "My plate", beans are part of the "grains group" and "protein group". In Brazil, we consume beans with 50% broth and 50% beans, so we have an average amount of 70 g of beans. Considering that beans have about 5% protein (according to the Brazilian composition table) [13], we considered this percentage as part of "protein group" and added the remaining percentage to "grains group". Therefore, at lunch, low-income Brazilians consumed about 2.5 portions of the protein group. It is important to highlight that protein/meat is the most expensive group of foods in Brazil. Probably, low-income population would not buy these products to eat at home. Thus, the highest consumption of this group at PRs is important to guarantee protein access and to promote a balanced and healthy diet during the day.

Evaluating protein group consumption, there was no statistical difference between males and females ($p = 0.063$). However, there was a significant difference among age groups: females over 60 and less than 21 years old ate less protein than the other age groups ($p < 0.00$), while males over 51 years and younger than 21 years ate less protein ($p < 0.00$).

We highlight that in our study rice and beans comprise more than 50% of the weight of the plate, which was expected since it is a Brazilian habit of consumption at lunch. Thus, grains are the major group (53%) consumed by PRs consumers. It is almost 2$\times$ greater than "My plate" recommendation for this group. Comparing to this food guide, people need to consume 6–7 portions of grains (rice is included) daily. In Brazil, we consider that the lunch meal should provide 40% of TEV [1], so we have to guarantee 2.4–2.8 portions of grains (about 230 g) at lunch. In our study, the average rice portion was 181.93 g $\pm$ 74.93 (Table 1) and pasta consumption (as a type of garnish) was 79.42 $\pm$ 39.35. We also have to include part of the beans' weight. Therefore, the grains group amount consumed at lunch in PRs was about 330 g, more than the USDA recommendation. Table 1 shows TEV and the average consumption of meals, ED and sodium density (SD) of each preparation that compose the plate (in grams).

Table 1. Average and standard deviation (SD) of consumption (grams), total energetic value (TEV) Energy density (ED) and Sodium content of meals and preparations by low-income Brazilians in popular restaurants.

	Average in Brazil	Rice	Bean	Main Course	Garnish	Salad	Dessert
Meal weight ± SD (g)	648.34 ± 133.08	181.93 ± 74.93	139.67 ± 48.52	117.88 ± 21.76	86.56 ± 23.44	51.70 ± 20.47	70.50 ± 37.76
Energetic value ± SD (kcal)	881 ± 222.02	147.93 ± 60.3	108.80 ± 61.20	213.25 ± 92.54	151.85 ± 133.01	35.02 ± 20.94	68.60 ± 46.90
Energy Density ± SD (kcal/g)	1.34 ± 0.25	1.48 ± 0.60	1.09 ± 0.61	2.13 ± 0.93	1.52 ± 1.33	0.35 ± 0.21	0.97 ± 1.32
Sodium content (mg/portion)	2362.87	795.03	445.54	749.72	241.50	118.39	12.69
Sodium Percent Daily Value (% DV)	98.45	33.13	18.56	31.24	10.06	4.93	0.53

The consumption of rice and beans (together) is a Brazilian habit at lunch. Barbosa [16] evaluated Brazilians food habits (2136 participants) and 94% of Brazilian's meals showed the combination of rice and beans in their study. The amino acids combination of these two groups represents the major part of Brazilian's protein intake [17].

Despite the recommendation from the Brazilian Food Guide (BFG), [18], we observe that the consumption of rice and beans at home has been declining over time [19]. The explanation could be the reduced time to prepare food at home. Therefore, the PRs are contributing to this consumption within low-income Brazilians with low cost.

The adequate consumption of fruits and vegetables is associated to the reduction of chronic and cardiovascular diseases [20]. According to WHO/FAO, the individual recommendation of fruits and vegetables intake is about 400 g/day. In our study, we verified the consumption of 122.44 g ± 33.04 of fruits and vegetables, which represents about 30% of the daily recommendation, not the expected 40%. In comparison with "My plate", fruit and vegetables should compose 50% of the graphic representation of the plate, while only 27% of this group were on the PRs plates. Men consumed more salads and vegetables than women ($p = 0.000$; $p = 0.003$). When comparing groups by age, the population over 60 years and the ones younger than 21 are statistically different from the groups between 21 and 40 years ($p = 0.000$), eating less salads.

Corroborating with our data, Levy, Claro, Mondini, Sichieri and Monteiro [21] showed that the availability and the consumption of fruits and vegetables at home in Brazil is under the recommendation, contributing only 2.8% of daily TEV per person. Fruits and vegetables are very perishable and demand frequent shop and adequate storage. Therefore, it is improbable that low-income Brazilians consume large amount of these products outside of PRs to compensate low consumption there. Besides, "My plate" USDA guide recommends the plate's composition be 50% fruits and vegetables, which does not occur in meals consumed by low-income Brazilians in PRs. In this viewpoint, PRs are not providing all the needs for fruits and vegetables to promote health.

The consumption of fruits (68.05 g ± 47.68) in PRs is 2.5× higher than the offer of sweet desserts (24.40 g ± 30.25). When comparing fruit consumption between male and female, there were statistical differences with higher consumption on the male group (69.18 g, $p = 0.026$). Statistical differences among age groups were not observed ($p = 0.451$, female; $p = 0.805$, male). It is important to highlight that the sweet desserts offered in PRs were made from fruits with sugar (such as guava paste, banana candy paste, and coconut candy). It is a very important data showing that PRs are not providing the total amount of fruits, but they are careful on planning more fruits than sweets for desserts to avoid health damage. Another relevant aspect is that in Brazil we consume higher amounts of fruits for breakfast and snack meals. Since we evaluated only lunch, it is not possible to guarantee that the fruit consumption during the day is under recommendation.

In general, the average energy intake for low-income Brazilians in PRs lunch was 881 kcal (±222.02). There were no statistical differences among sex ($p = 0.145$). It is higher than recommended by the Brazilian Worker Food Program (WFP) of 800 kcal [1] to guarantee adequate energy intake to maintain the organism. If the energy intake was the single parameter to guarantee health, the PRs program would be reaching its goal. However, PRs should guarantee food quality access.

The ratio of the energetic value and the weight of the meal is estimated by ED which is one of the coefficients that increases obesity and overweight or underweight on population, and foods ED affects population health [22].

The average of ED for all PRs, in this study, was 1.34 kcal/g ($\pm$0.25). This value is higher than the American Institute for Cancer Research's [23] recommendation (1.25 kcal/g). The EDs shown in our study were smaller than the EDs presented by Stella [24] (1.98 kcal/g) and Canella [25] (1.43 kcal/g). The first one evaluated the ED consumption of 710 consumers in São Paulo/Brazil. Canella [25] evaluated the ED of menus offered by 21 food service in São Paulo/Brazil. ED varied among the five regions, being higher in the north (1.51 kcal/g $\pm$ 0.16) and lower in the south (1.15 kcal/g $\pm$ 0.12). Differences were not observed between the center-west region and the southeast region ($p = 0.701$). All other comparisons of ED were statistically different (all p values = 0.000).

Energy density as a measurement of overall diet has been the focus of many recent studies. The high-ED foods or meals are known as an "obesity-inducing dietary pattern". High ED diets are rich in fat and energy, but low in fiber, fruits and vegetables. Moreover, higher ED is inversely related to diet quality, which may encourage weight gain, increase the risk of metabolic syndrome and diabetes [26–28].

In this study, 78.1% were low ED (and 21.9% were medium ED). Although most meals presented low ED, the average TEV is in accordance with WFP recommendation. It could be explained by the portions size of the food offered by PRs, especially rice and beans that presented low mean ED. Main courses had higher EDs. These data show that the PRs are offering meals with expected ED adequacy, contributing to prevent overweight, obesity and other chronic diseases associated to high ED food consumption. However, it is important to encourage the population to consume more fruits and vegetables for better micronutrients intake.

The Institute of Medicine has alerted to reduce salty foods [29], and the FDA set standards for the sodium content of foods [15]. They considered a general rule of 5% DV or less of sodium per serving is low; 20% DV or more is high. Additionally, FDA settles that 140 mg of sodium or less per serving is "low sodium"; 35 mg of sodium or less per serving is "very low sodium".

Regarding sodium content, rice and main courses presented the highest values and according to FDA are high in sodium [15]. Rice presented the highest value because it represents the biggest portion on the plate. Main courses did not represent big portions, but PRs generally use pork sausages, hot dog sausages and jerked beef that are cheap, but present high sodium content. All others are classified as medium Sodium Density, except salads and desserts groups which presented low sodium and very low sodium, respectively. It is important to emphasize that the mean sodium content at lunch meal (considering all the preparations and respective portion of the day) was about 2400 mg. This sodium amount in only one meal represents the total sodium expected for an entire day. Furthermore, the total meal sodium content might be underestimated, since the salt sachet was not considered.

4. Conclusions

These data are alarming, and PRs need to review their TPF to lower sodium contribution and highlight the importance of increasing the consumption of vegetables and fruits. It is also important to increase the offer of low ED foods. In some PRs, the sodium intake could be even worse if consumers added extra salt to their plates.

Concerning sodium, PRs are putting Brazilian low-income population at risk for chronic diseases, mainly cardiovascular diseases [29,30]. A better menu planning is necessary in these restaurants to guarantee sodium reduction throughout time, so the population can adjust without rejecting the new preparations. However, in general, the PRs are good choices for low income Brazilians because they promote access to cheap and quality Brazilian traditional foods. Better menu planning to increase fruit and vegetables offer in place of grains group is necessary. Fruits should be the only option for desserts in PRs and educational strategies are necessary to encourage more salad intake. Protein offer is adequate and it is important for this population because of its high cost. However, the negative aspect is that this protein offer is often achieved with high fat and high sodium meat sources. Low cost better option should be encouraged.

PRs contribute to promote health in low-income Brazilians overall (energy intake and macronutrients distribution). This program is a big step to guarantee Brazilians the universal right to food. However, in general, since the purpose of the program is to offer healthy food for low-income population, menu planning should be the focus of the program. PRs are good choices for low-income Brazilians because they promote access to cheap and traditional Brazilian foods, but better protein quality, more vegetable and fruits and lower sodium content are major challenges to this program.

Further studies can be developed to evaluate this population after a longer period of consumption at the PRs. Other variables such as lunch's contribution on the daily intake and the type of food acquired at home may bring new data to evaluate the program's importance to these consumers.

Author Contributions: A.d.P.C., R.B.A.B. and R.d.C.C.d.A.A. conceived and designed the experiments; A.d.P.C., R.B.A.B. and R.d.C.C.d.A.A. performed the experiments; A.d.P.C., R.B.A.B., R.P.Z. and R.d.C.C.d.A.A. analyzed the data; and A.d.P.C., R.B.A.B., R.P.Z. and R.d.C.C.d.A.A. wrote the paper.

Conflicts of Interest: The authors declare no conflict of interest. The founding sponsors had no role in the design of the study; in the collection, analyses, or interpretation of data; in the writing of the manuscript, and in the decision to publish the results.

References

1. Programa de Alimentação do Trabalhador. *Portaria Interministerial n°. 66, de 25 de Agosto de 2006*; Diário Oficial da União: Rio de Janeiro, Brazil. Publicada no DOU de 25 de Agosto de 2006.
2. Ministério do Desenvolvimento Social. *Manual Programa Restaurantes Populares*; Ministério do Desenvolvimento Social: Brasilia, Brazil, 2004.
3. General Assembly of the United Nations. *Universal Declaration of Human Rights*; General Assembly of the United Nations: New York, NY, USA, 1948.
4. Diez Garcia, R.W. Reflexos da globalização na cultura alimentar: Considerações sobre as mudanças na alimentação urbana. *Rev. Nutr.* **2003**, *16*, 483–492. [CrossRef]
5. Popkin, B.M.; Adair, L.S.; Ng, S.W. Global nutrition transition and the pandemic of obesity in developing countries. *Nutr. Rev.* **2012**, *70*, 3–21. [CrossRef] [PubMed]
6. Huneault, L.; Mathieu, M.È.; Tremblay, A. Globalization and modernization: An obesogenic combination. *Obes. Rev.* **2011**, *12*, e64–e72. [CrossRef] [PubMed]
7. Bezerra, I.N.; Sichieri, R. Características e gastos com alimentação fora do domicílio no Brasil. *Rev. Saude Publica* **2010**, *44*, 221–229. [CrossRef] [PubMed]
8. Lachat, C.; Nago, E.; Verstraeten, R.; Roberfroid, D.; Van Camp, J.; Kolsteren, P. Eating out of home and its association with dietary intake: A systematic review of the evidence. *Obes. Rev.* **2012**, *13*, 329–346. [CrossRef] [PubMed]
9. Cochran, W.G. *Sampling Techniques*; John Wiley & Sons: Hoboken, NJ, USA, 2007.
10. Domene, S.M.Á. *Técnica Dietética: Teoria e Aplicações*; Guanabara Koogan: Rio de Janeiro, Brazil, 2011.
11. Savio, K.E.O.; Costa, T.H.M.D.; Miazaki, E.; Schmitz, B.D.A.S. Avaliação do almoço servido a participantes do programa de alimentação do trabalhador. *Rev. Saúde Pública* **2005**, *39*, 148–155. [CrossRef] [PubMed]
12. Camargo, E.; Botelho, R.A. *Técnica Dietética: Seleção e Preparo de Alimentos–Manual de Laboratório*; Atheneu: São Paulo, Brazil, 2012.
13. Lima, D. *Tabela Brasileira de Composição de Alimentos-TACO*; NEPA-UNICAMP: Campinas, Brazil, 2006.
14. Centers for Disease Control and Prevention. *Can Eating Fruits and Vegetables Help People to Manage Their Weight?* Centers for Disease Control and Prevention: Atlanta, GA, USA, 2012.
15. Lichtenstein, A.H.; Appel, L.J.; Brands, M.; Carnethon, M.; Daniels, S.; Franch, H.A.; Franklin, B.; Kris-Etherton, P.; Harris, W.S.; Howard, B.; et al. Diet and lifestyle recommendations revision 2006: A scientific statement from the American Heart Association nutrition committee. *Circulation* **2016**, *114*, 82–96. [CrossRef] [PubMed]

16. Barbosa, L. Feijão com arroz e arroz com feijão: O Brasil no prato dos brasileiros. *Horizontes Antropológicos* **2007**, *13*, 87–116. [CrossRef]
17. Instituto Brasileiro de Geografia e Estatística. *Pesquisa de Orçamentos Familiares 2008-2009: Antropometria e Estado Nutricional de Crianças, Adolescentes e Adultos no Brasil*; Instituto Brasileiro de Geografia e Estatística: Rio de Janeiro, Brazil, 2010.
18. Ministério da Saúde. *Guia Alimentar Para a População Brasileira: Promovendo a Alimentação Saudável*; Ministério da Saúde: Brasília, Brazil, 2014.
19. Levy, R.B.; Claro, R.M.; Mondini, L.; Sichieri, R.; Monteiro, C.A. Distribuição regional e socioeconômica da disponibilidade domiciliar de alimentos no Brasil em 2008–2009. *Rev. Saude Publica* **2012**, *46*, 6–15. [CrossRef] [PubMed]
20. World Health Organization. *Fruit and Vegetables for Health: Report of a Joint FAO/WHO Workshop, 1–3 September, 2004, Kobe, Japan*; World Health Organization: Geneva, Switzerland, 2005.
21. Levy, R.B.; Claro, R.M.; Bandoni, D.H.; Mondini, L.; Monteiro, C.A. Availability of added sugars in Brazil: Distribution, food sources and time trends. *Revista Brasileira de Epidemiologia* **2012**, *15*, 3–12. [CrossRef] [PubMed]
22. Duffey, K.J.; Popkin, B.M. Energy density, portion size, and eating occasions: Contributions to increased energy intake in the United States, 1977–2006. *PLoS Med.* **2011**, *8*, e1001050. [CrossRef] [PubMed]
23. World Cancer Research Fund; American Institute for Cancer Research. *Food, Nutrition, Physical Activity, and the Prevention of Cancer: A Global Perspective*; American Institute for Cancer Research: Washington, DC, USA, 2007.
24. Stella, R.H. Densidade Energética: Relação com Variáveis Demográficas, de Estilo de Vida, Nutricionais e Socioeconômicas em Amostra Representativa da População Adulta do Município de São Paulo. Ph.D. Thesis, Universidade de São Paulo, São Paulo, Brazil, 2008.
25. Canella, D.S.; Bandoni, D.H.; Jaime, P.C. Densidade energética de refeições oferecidas em empresas inscritas no programa de alimentação do Trabalhador no município de São Paulo. *Rev. Nutr.* **2011**, *24*, 715–724. [CrossRef]
26. Rouhani, M.H.; Haghighatdoost, F.; Surkan, P.J.; Azadbakht, L. Associations between dietary energy density and obesity: A systematic review and meta-analysis of observational studies. *Nutrition* **2016**, *32*, 1037–1047. [CrossRef] [PubMed]
27. Mendoza, J.A.; Drewnowski, A.; Christakis, D.A. Dietary energy density is associated with obesity and the metabolic syndrome in US adults. *Diabetes Care* **2007**, *30*, 974–979. [CrossRef] [PubMed]
28. Wang, J.; Luben, R.; Khaw, K.-T.; Bingham, S.; Wareham, N.J.; Forouhi, N.G. Dietary energy density predicts the risk of incident type 2 diabetes the European Prospective Investigation of Cancer (EPIC)-Norfolk study. *Diabetes Care* **2008**, *31*, 2120–2125. [CrossRef] [PubMed]
29. Taylor, C.L.; Henry, J.E. *Strategies to Reduce Sodium Intake in the United States*; National Academies Press: Washington, DC, USA, 2010.
30. Zandonadi, R.P.; Botelho, R.B.; Rita de Cássia, C.; de Oliveira Savio, K.E.; Araújo, W.M. Sodium and health: New proposal of distribution for major meals. *Health* **2014**, *6*, 195. [CrossRef]

nutrients

MDPI

Article

Household Food Insecurity as a Predictor of Stunted Children and Overweight/Obese Mothers (SCOWT) in Urban Indonesia

Trias Mahmudiono [1,*], Triska Susila Nindya [1], Dini Ririn Andrias [1], Hario Megatsari [2] and Richard R. Rosenkranz [3]

1. Department of Nutrition, Faculty of Public Health, Universitas Airlangga, Surabaya 60115, East Java, Indonesia; triska.nindya@fkm.unair.ac.id (T.S.N.); dien_ra@yahoo.com (D.R.A.)
2. Department of Health Promotion and Education, Faculty of Public Health, Universitas Airlangga, Surabaya 60115, East Java, Indonesia; hario.megatsari@gmail.com
3. Department of Food, Nutrition, Dietetics and Health, Kansas State University, Manhattan, KS 66506, USA; ricardo@ksu.edu

* Correspondence: trias-m@fkm.unair.ac.id; Tel.: +62-31-596-4808

Received: 9 February 2018; Accepted: 23 April 2018; Published: 26 April 2018

Abstract: (1) Background: The double burden of malnutrition has been increasing in countries experiencing the nutrition transition. This study aimed to determine the relationship between household food insecurity and the double burden of malnutrition, defined as within-household stunted child and an overweight/obese mother (SCOWT). **(2) Methods**: A cross-sectional survey was conducted in the urban city of Surabaya, Indonesia in April and May 2015. **(3) Results**: The prevalence of child stunting in urban Surabaya was 36.4%, maternal overweight/obesity was 70.2%, and SCOWT was 24.7%. Although many households were food secure (42%), there were high proportions of mild (22.9%), moderate (15.3%) and severe (19.7%) food insecurity. In a multivariate logistic regression, the household food insecurity access scale (HFIAS) category significantly correlated with child stunting and SCOWT. Compared to food secure households, mildly food insecure households had the greatest odds of SCOWT (adjusted odds ratio (aOR) = 2.789; 95% confidence interval (CI) = 1.540–5.083), followed by moderately food insecure (aOR = 2.530; 95% CI = 1.286–4.980) and severely food insecure households (aOR = 2.045; 95% CI = 1.087–3.848). **(4) Conclusions**: These results support the hypothesis that the double burden of malnutrition is related to food insecurity, and the HFIAS category is a predictor of SCOWT.

Keywords: food security; HFIAS; double burden of malnutrition; child stunting; Indonesia

1. Introduction

One of the primary public health problems of the 21st century is the obesity epidemic, affecting over half a billion people worldwide [1]. In 2008, an estimated 1.46 billion adults were overweight (body-mass index (BMI) $\geq$ 25 kg/m^2), with 205 million men and 297 million women among them categorized as obese (BMI $\geq$ 30 kg/m^2) [2]. Obesity does not solely affect developed countries; the developing countries of the world have also experienced great increases in prevalence [1]. Data from the World Health Organization (WHO) show that developing countries in Africa and Southeast Asia will soon face the levels of overweight currently prevalent in developed countries such as the USA [3]. In 2013, the prevalence of overweight and obesity among Indonesian males was 20%, while the prevalence among females was already hitting 35% [4].

At the opposite end of the nutritional spectrum, the prevalence of undernutrition remains a major public health problem. Although the United Nations' efforts to combat malnutrition through the

Millennium Development Goals (MDGs) have been progressing toward attainment [5], almost half of all deaths among children under the age of five years are still attributable to undernutrition [6]. The World Health Organization (WHO) recently reported that approximately 45% of all deaths among children under the age of five years were associated with under-nutrition in 2017 [7]. Furthermore, the WHO data showed that 52 million children under age five were suffering from wasting, and 155 million children were stunted in 2016 [7], representing a 10 million decrease from the data in 2011 [8]. In developing nations, the problem of nutrient deficiencies that manifest in undernutrition (underweight, wasting, and stunting) still persist, while the problems of overnutrition, such as overweight and obesity, have increased rapidly. The 2006 Food and Agriculture Organization (FAO) report referred to this phenomenon as a double burden of malnutrition, where under- and overnutrition occur simultaneously among different population subgroups in developing countries [9]. Based on the 2013 National Health Survey, the prevalence of the double burden of malnutrition is around 11% [4] in Indonesia, with some estimates much higher [10].

The double burden of malnutrition has raised public health concerns due to its consequences. The double burden will manifest through the deficiency diseases of undernutrition, while simultaneously leading to increases in the non-communicable diseases (NCDs) of overnutrition, such as obesity, cardiovascular disease, type 2 diabetes mellitus, and hypertension. The present amount of NCDs accounts for 80% of the total burden of disease mortality in developing countries; an estimated US $84 billion of economic production will be lost from heart disease, stroke, and diabetes alone [11]. Hence, the presence of the double burden of malnutrition will continue to burden the already inadequate and overextended health budget in developing countries [12].

Within the peer-reviewed literature, the term "double burden of malnutrition" varies in use among authors. Authors have addressed the double burden of malnutrition at the individual level [13], household level [14–16], and population or country level [17–20]. The double burden occurring within a household, as indicated by high prevalence of child stunting and overweight/obese mothers (SCOWT), has been deemed largely preventable, due to mothers and children sharing the same socioeconomic environment. Moreover, maternal parenting has been portrayed as a key factor to prevent SCOWT, as mothers often control the purchase and distribution of food in the household [21]. A study in Indonesia revealed that in households experiencing the double burden of malnutrition, women were less empowered and less involved in the decision-making process, resulting in higher nutrition and health inequality when compared to normal households [22]. Hence, we hypothesize that empowering women and involving them in the decision-making process for household matters, including food purchasing, could potentially prevent double burden of malnutrition. In this scenario, the role of the mother may be pivotal, but is also based on an assumption that households are not food insecure, limiting access to adequate food, let alone foods enabling a healthy diet.

The evidence shows that food insecurity is one of the risk factors for child stunting, but there is currently little evidence that food insecurity is risk factor for the double burden of malnutrition [5,15]. A cross-sectional study in rural Indonesia demonstrated that higher intakes of animal products was protective against SCOWT [10]. A Guatemalan study revealed that households suffering from SCOWT had the highest per capita animal protein consumption in the third quintile [15] and not in the lowest quintile. The first quintile of per capita consumption indicates that the consumption among households in this group was lowest compared to other households. One might expect that since their per capita consumption was the worst, problems that include stunting only or SCOWT would likely be the highest in this group, as an indication of limited food access. The problem of SCOWT, however, was the highest in the middle (third) quintile group, which has higher per capita consumption than the first quintile group. This was the opposite case to households with child stunting alone, where the per capita food consumption was in the first quintile [15]. Hence, these SCOWT households are believed to have some degree of food security that enables them to be placed in the middle quintile of per capita food consumption. Such evidence has led researchers to hypothesize that food insecurity is not associated with the double burden of malnutrition [15], as it was strongly associated with child stunting [5,15]. In this study, we aimed to determine the relationship between household food insecurity, as measured by the categorization of the household food insecurity access scale (HFIAS) and the prevalence of the double burden of malnutrition, as indicated by household's with a stunted child and an overweight/obese mother (SCOWT).

2. Materials and Methods

This cross-sectional study of food security and the double burden of malnutrition was undertaken with individual assessments administered by trained interviewers in April to May 2015. Urban households were selected using systematic cluster sampling methods from 14 integrated health posts (*"posyandu"*) in Surabaya, Indonesia (Figure A1). Access to the existing secondary data of a monthly child growth monitoring system was given upon approval from the District Health Department in Surabaya, Indonesia. Based on these data, we determined a list of sub-districts in Surabaya City that had high prevalence of child underweight relative to the national prevalence. Sub-districts with a prevalence of child underweight of more than 15% were randomly selected as survey locations. In each sub-district, randomization was performed to select the community health post, so-called *"posyandu"* [23], as the point of anthropometric measurement. Mothers who came for a monthly child health monitoring at the *"posyandu"* were asked to participate in the study and provide informed consent. The inclusion criteria were: informed consent obtained, mother reported no physical disability to walk for minimum 10 min continuously, and mother had a child under five years old.

The power for the study was 82.5% designated to the prevalence of SCOWT, with a 95% confidence interval or 5% alpha level and the population estimate of children under five years old in Surabaya City used 2013 data (n = 181,263 children) [24]. Assuming a 50% response distribution, the minimal sample needed was 662 participants. Accounting for a 5% non-response rate, we surveyed 700 households with mothers and at least one child between two and five years of age. Excluding cases with missing data or extreme values [25], 685 households were analyzed.

A survey questionnaire was administered by a trained research assistant for a one-on-one interview in the mother's house. The interview lasted approximately 30 min. The questionnaire consisted of demographic characteristics; socioeconomic status (based on the Indonesian Basic Health Research Questionnaire/IBHRQ); and food security, using the Household Food Insecurity Access Scale (HFIAS). All questionnaires were translated into the Indonesian language and the survey was delivered in a one-on-one interview using the Indonesian language (Bahasa). The HFIAS score ranged from absolute food security (score = 0) to severely insecure (maximum score = 27). There were four categories of food insecurity status, according to the HFIAS guidelines [26]: "food secure", "mildly food insecure", "moderately food insecure" and "severely food insecure". A reliability analysis was performed to test the internal consistency for the nine HFIAS questions.

Anthropometric measurement was conducted in the *"posyandu"* by a trained research assistant, including maternal weight, maternal height, child weight, and child height/length. Child height and weight were assessed (in light clothing) using a stadiometer SECA 213 (Seca GmbH & Co. Kg, Hamburg, Germany) and a Camry EB6571 digital scale (Camry Electronic Ltd., Guangdong, China) to 0.01 kg for weight. Maternal weight and height were assessed (in light clothing) using a Camry EB6571 digital scale and height rod (stadiometer SECA 213, Seca GmbH & Co. Kg, Hamburg, Germany). Mothers were weighed and measured for height to determine obesity status. Child age in months was assessed using two sources, first from the mother's answers when interviewed, and second based on the date of birth listed on the health monitoring card/registry in *"posyandu"*. If the month did not match, we used the *"posyandu"* registry as the primary source. Child stunting was defined as a z-score less than −2 standard deviations (SD) from the average height for age z-score (HAZ) based on the Multiple Growth Reference Standard (MGRS) of the WHO in 2006 [27]. Quality management of the HAZ data was applied using the cut-off for extreme values recommended by the WHO [25]. Children with a HAZ of more than ±6.0 were excluded from the analysis. Maternal BMI was calculated based on the BMI formula using the appropriate cut-off for an Asian population, with overweight defined as BMI of 23.0 kg/m^2 to 27.4 kg/m^2 and obese as a BMI of $\geq$27.5 kg/m^2 or more. Finally, the double burden of malnutrition, as measured by SCOWT, was defined by the combined occurrence of child stunting and maternal overweight/obesity within one household.

We used a conventional Cronbach's alpha of 0.65 to indicate that the questions in the HFIAS had an acceptable internal consistency [28]. Descriptive statistics were used to illustrate household characteristics and to determine the prevalence of the outcome variables. Potential predictors of child stunting, maternal overweight/obesity and SCOWT were determined by univariate logistic regression, including maternal literacy, maternal education, family type, number of children and number of children under the age of five years in the household, maternal occupation, paternal occupation, household monthly income, household food expenditure, paternal smoking status, and food insecurity status. Prior to the analysis, multicollinearity tests were performed for all independent variables listed above. We employed a variance inflation factor (VIF) of less than 2.5 for all our analyses to determine that multicollinearity was not a problem [29–31]. A Chi-squared test was performed to analyze the differences between household food insecurity status with the number of children under five, paternal occupation, monthly income, and paternal smoking status. Multiple logistic regression was performed to control for confounding factors (the number of children under five, paternal occupation, monthly income, and paternal smoking status) using backward stepwise selection with significance level of 0.2 for removal from the model. The backward stepwise selection was reliable in identifying useful predictors during the exploratory stages of model building. The difference in monthly income between various household food security statuses was tested using analysis of variance (ANOVA).

All data analysis was performed in IBM SPSS Statistics 22 (IBM, Armonk, NY, USA).

This study was approved by the Institutional Review Board (IRB) of Kansas State University, USA (reference or proposal number: 7646). In addition, this study was approved by the Surabaya City Review Board (Bakesbangpol No.: 1366/LIT/2015) in Indonesia. We explained the study objectives and obtained written informed consent during monthly integrated health post meetings (*"posyandu"*), where mothers bring their children under the age of five years for growth monitoring. Participants were free to withdraw from the study at any time without any consequences.

3. Results

The selected characteristics of the samples in this study are presented in Table A1. When we employed the Chi-squared test based on the food insecurity status of the households, significant differences in the household characteristics emerged for maternal literacy ($p = 0.012$) and maternal education ($p < 0.0001$), but not maternal occupation ($p = 0.290$). Most of the households were nuclear families, with 1–2 children and only one child under five years living in the household. Almost all fathers were working and nearly 70% of them were smokers. We obtained a Cronbach's alpha of 0.831, which indicated that the nine questions of the HFIAS for the 685 households had sufficient internal consistency.

Chi-squared tests also showed significant differences in the household's food insecurity status for the number of children under five in the household ($p = 0.046$), paternal occupation ($p < 0.0001$), monthly income ($p < 0.0001$), and paternal smoking status ($p = 0.045$). The ANOVA test showed that compared to the food secure households, households with some level of food insecurity were significantly different in terms of monthly income.

No significant difference, however, was found among households across food insecurity status in father's monthly cigarettes expenses as well as food expenditure. Possession of electricity did not differ between households with different food insecurity statuses.

There were significant differences, however, among households with different food insecurity statuses in the possession of a radio/tape recorder ($p < 0.0001$), television (TV) ($p = 0.013$), telephone/hand phone ($p < 0.0001$), and fridge ($p < 0.0001$). The mean HFIAS score was 4.85 (SD: 5.6), with a range from 0 to 24. Table A2 shows the affirmative responses for the HFIAS items. More than half of the participants were worried about food, and nearly half of households had concerns that they were unable to eat preferred foods (47.4%), ate few kinds of foods (36.4%), and ate foods they really did not want to eat (35.5%).

Approximately 3.2% of the participants stated that in the last four weeks they, or any household member, went a whole day and night without eating anything. The majority of households never experienced a complete lack of food of any kind in the household for the past month (88.5%). Based on the HFIAS guidelines, many households were categorized as food secure (42%), but there were relatively high proportions of mild (22.9%), moderate (15.3%) and severe (19.7%) food insecurity.

The results revealed that when using the cut-off point of a BMI $\geq$ 25 kg/m^2 as overweight, the prevalence of a double burden in the mother–child pair was 21.2%, whereas the prevalence of maternal overweight/obesity was 58.8%. When using the BMI cut-off point for an Asian population with BMI $\geq$ 23 kg/m^2 as defining maternal overweight, the prevalence rose to 70.3%, and the double burden of malnutrition measured as SCOWT was 24.7%, while the prevalence of child stunting was 36.5%. The following results were set to use the cut-off point for overweight recommended for an Asian population.

As seen in Table A3, several variables were significantly associated with a double burden of malnutrition measured as SCOWT when tested using unadjusted logistic regression. They were: maternal height (OR = 0.893; 95% CI = 0.848–0.940), maternal education (OR = 0.565; 95% CI = 0.340–0.937), number of children (OR = 1.852; 95% CI = 1.184–2.898), paternal occupation, and food security. Compared to having their father working with a steady income as a government officer (including army and police), having a father who worked in a job with less steady income, such as in the private sector (OR = 3.963; 95% CI = 1.050–14.961), or in a trade or as an entrepreneur (OR = 4.840; 95% CI = 1.230–19.050), as labor (OR = 5.770; 95% CI = 1.542–21.586), or others (OR = 7.436; 95% CI = 1.871–29.549) increased the risk of SCOWT in the household. Likewise, similar patterns were observed in relation to SCOWT where the risk of SCOWT was increased in mildly food insecure (OR = 2.647; 95% CI = 1.486–4.712), moderately food insecure (OR = 2.254; 95% CI = 1.170–4.342) and severely food insecure households (OR = 2.057; 95% CI = 1.112–3.804) relative to food secure households. Based on the unadjusted model, the strongest predictors of SCOWT was paternal occupation, followed by food insecurity status and number of children. However, after adjustment for potential confounding variables such as maternal height and SES, the stepwise multiple logistic regression model for SCOWT revealed that only food insecurity status served as a significant predictor. Compared to food-secure households, mild food insecurity (aOR = 2.798; 95% CI = 1.540–5.083), moderate food insecurity (aOR = 2.530; 95% CI = 1.286–4.980), and severe food insecurity (aOR = 2.045; 95% CI = 1.087–3.848) increased the likelihood of households experiencing SCOWT.

The results of the univariate logistic regression showed that some variables were protective against stunting, namely maternal height (OR = 0.884; 95% CI = 0.842–0.927), child's gender, maternal education (OR = 0.534; 95% CI = 0.342–0.834), paternal occupation, and food insecurity status. Female children were less likely to be stunted than their male counterparts (OR = 0.612; 95% CI = 0.441–0.849). Maternal education also showed a significant association with stunting; using mothers with low education level as a reference, having an educated mother lessened the likelihood of child stunting (OR = 0.534; 95% CI = 0.342–0.834). Similarly, educated mothers showed a protective effect on SCOWT (OR = 0.565; 95% CI = 0.340–0.937) but not highly educated mothers. For paternal occupation, the risk of child stunting was increased in the households where the father was working in the private sector (OR = 4.914; 95% CI = 1.476–16.360), in trade or as an entrepreneur (OR = 7.274; 95% CI = 2.099–25.208), as labor (OR = 7.196; 95% CI = 2.140–24.201), or others (OR = 11.117; 95% CI = 3.157–39.153), compared to fathers who worked as government officers (including army, police). Using food secure households as a reference, increased likelihood of child stunting was observed in households with mild food insecurity (OR = 1.740; 95% CI = 1.043–2.903), and severe food insecurity (OR = 2.182; 95% CI = 1.280–3.717). The stepwise multiple logistic regression models showed that child gender, maternal education and food insecurity status were significantly associated with child stunting. Factors that were significantly associated with a reduced likelihood of child stunting were child gender (aOR = 1.696; 95% CI = 1.077–2.672), and educated mother (aOR = 0.596; 95% CI = 0.372–0.954). Compared to the food secure households, only households that were severely food insecure increased the likelihood of child stunting (aOR = 2.005; 95% CI = 1.140–3.526). Having 3–4 children, relative to having 1–2 children at home, was associated with an increased likelihood of maternal overweight/obesity (aOR = 1.750; 95% CI = 1.108–2.762).

4. Discussion

The objective of our study was to analyze the relationship between household food insecurity, as measured by the household food insecurity access scale (HFIAS) category, and the double burden of malnutrition, as indicated by household's with a stunted child and an overweight/obese mother (SCOWT). These results support the hypothesis that the double burden of malnutrition is robustly related to food insecurity, and the categorization of the HFIAS as a measure of food insecurity is a predictor of SCOWT. To the best of our knowledge, this is the first published study on the application of this scale within an urban setting in Indonesia.

Our study, based in an urban setting, revealed that the prevalence of the double burden in mother–child pairs was 24.7%, whereas the prevalence of child stunting was 36.4%, and maternal overweight/obesity was 70.2%. This prevalence was higher than that found in a previous study in a rural Indonesian setting that found 11% of the sample consisted of maternal overweight and a stunted child coexisting within the same household [16]. A more recent study in a rural setting of Indonesia reported a higher percentage of double burden, as measured by the coexistence of maternal overweight and child stunting in one household [10]. A staggering 30.6% of the double burden in mother–child pairs was reported in that study [10], where maternal overweight was set at a BMI above 23.5 kg/m^2, while our study used the conventional threshold of above 25.0 kg/m^2 In an Indonesian setting, regional differences were argued to explain the discrepancy in the prevalence of double burden observed in mother–child pairs in urban and rural areas [10,22]. Studies in Nairobi, Kenya showed that the obesogenic environment in an urban setting was characterized by reliance on energy-dense street food and was arguably responsible for the rise of overweight/obesity in this population [32,33]. Unfortunately, we did not collect data on energy-dense street food to be able to make comparisons of our findings with studies from Nairobi, Kenya. Nevertheless, evidence from studies in Indonesia has consistently shown a prevalent problem of the double burden of malnutrition in the form of stunted child and overweight/obese mother pairs across settings and geographical locations. Comparing with previous studies in rural settings, our results from an urban setting have a higher prevalence of the double burden of malnutrition, hence supporting the hypothesis that the double burden of malnutrition is more prevalent in urban areas. These findings have the policy implication that people in urban areas should be educated on the concept of energy balance, improving healthy eating and physical activity through health and nutrition education, as well as environmental conditioning that supports health. On the other hand, the rate of urbanization should be decreased by means of improving the living conditions and employment in rural areas.

Although evidence showing a relationship between food insecurity and child stunting is abundant, there is a scarcity of evidence relating to food insecurity with a double burden of malnutrition. In this study, we found that food insecurity was significantly associated with the double burden of malnutrition, as observed in the coexistence of stunted children and overweight/obese mothers within the same household. Most of the households involved in this study were experiencing some form of food insecurity (58%) as defined by the HFIAS. This is not surprising, as 11% of Indonesia's 252 million people live below the national poverty line of $1 income per day, with an additional 40% hovering marginally above the line. Studies have shown that poverty is closely linked with food insecurity. In a univariate logistic regression, using food secure households as a reference, we revealed that having a mildly food insecure household increased the risk of a double burden by more than three times, having a moderately food insecure household increased the risk by more than three times, and having a severely food insecure household increased the risk by more than two times. This association persisted in the multivariate logistic model; in fact, the likelihood was even stronger. Compared to the food secure households, a mildly food insecure household showed a risk of double burden more than 3.7 times higher. Having a moderately food insecure household increased the risk by 4.5 times, and having a severely food insecure household increased the risk by more than three times.

Our study showed that food insecurity was more robust in predicting the double burden of malnutrition indicated by SCOWT than in predicting child stunting alone. As seen in Table A3, even though four categories of food insecurity were significantly correlated to both SCOWT and child stunting in the univariate logistic regression, only severely food insecure households remained associated with child stunting in the multivariate model, while any form of food insecurity remained significantly associated with SCOWT in the multivariate logistic regression model. We are not aware of any published studies with which to compare our findings that relate food insecurity and the double burden of malnutrition. A study in Indonesia highlighted an association between living in households with a higher socioeconomic status (SES) and an increased risk of the double burden of malnutrition [22]. A study in Guatemala also showed an association between per capita household consumption and SCOWT [15]. Both of these studies revealed that the double burden of malnutrition was related to some form of household access to food, indicated by higher SES and per capita consumption. The fact that our analysis, using levels of food insecurity status, showed a steady association with SCOWT and not with child stunting aligns with this argument. Mildly food insecure and moderately food insecure households were significantly associated with an increased risk of SCOWT, and not significantly correlated with child stunting. This was an indication that lower quality and choice of food as a building block for mildly and moderately food insecure households were sensitive enough to predict SCOWT.

In broader terms, we believe that with minor food insecurity, households may compromise their diet towards cheaper food that is mostly high in energy. Hence, we argue that the double burden of malnutrition exists because the children were stunted due to insufficient availability and intake of growth-promoting and nutrient-dense foods; while mothers were supplied with an abundance of energy-dense foods that promote weight gain. In countries experiencing a nutrition transition, much of the energy-dense food is not nutritionally dense, and hence provides limited support for children's growth [14]. Households that were not facing mild and moderate food insecurity might be able to purchase foods that are more expensive but more nutrient-dense, such as animal-based foods. Animal-based foods are a good source of growth-promoting nutrients, such as protein [34]. A study in rural Indonesia showed that a dietary pattern of "high-animal products" was associated with a decreased likelihood of SCOWT, through a strong inverse correlation with child stunting [10].

The present study's findings also add evidence regarding the relationship between maternal height/stature and the double burden of malnutrition. A similar significant association, however, was seen for maternal height and child stunting alone. Hence, the observed correlation between maternal height and SCOWT might be driven by the association between maternal height and child stunting, even though the adjusted odds was slightly stronger for SCOWT. It is established that maternal height is a genetic predictor for child's height that later defines stunting. For this reason, we believe that compared to food insecurity status as measured by the HFIAS category, maternal height was less robust in predicting SCOWT. Regardless, our study extended the widely-reported association between maternal short stature and child stunting in developing countries such as Bangladesh [16], Brazil [35,36], Indonesia [16] and Mexico [37].

The multivariate logistic regression revealed that households with 3–4 children were more likely to have mothers who were overweight/obese, compared to households with 1–2 children. With less than one-third of mothers exclusively breastfeeding in Indonesia [9,38], it is probable that repeated pregnancy increases the risk for maternal overweight/obesity. Mothers who provide their children with exclusive breastfeeding for three months had four times greater weight loss, compared to mothers who did not exclusively breastfed or who discontinued breastfeeding their child before three months [39]. Household spending of US $100–150 on food per month also increased the risk of maternal overweight/obesity, compared to households with monthly food expenditures of less than US $50. Spending US $50–100 as well as >US $150 was not significantly related to maternal overweight/obesity. This indicates that spending > US $100–150 was the range of monthly food expenses that may contribute to a maternal energy imbalance through the purchase of energy-dense food. However, both variables (number of children and food expenditure) were not significantly correlated with SCOWT.

The strengths of our study were the relatively large sample derived from a fully-powered sample size calculation, random sample, validated food insecurity instrument, and one-on-one interview by trained interviewers to complete questionnaires with the mother. In addition, compared to a recent study on the mother–child double burden in rural Indonesia, this study employed a conventional cut-off point for maternal overweight that was easily comparable to the body of knowledge related to the household-level double burden of malnutrition.

A few limitations should be noted for this study. First, since it was a cross-sectional study, a causal inference for food insecurity status and the double burden of malnutrition as observed in SCOWT cannot be established. An observational cohort study that examines changes in food insecurity over time would add more weight to the evidence for a positive relationship between food insecurity status as measured in the HFIAS category and SCOWT. Second, although the HFIAS was designed for cross-cultural settings, it was possible that some of the local perspectives on food insecurity failed to be captured in the questions. We minimized errors by excluding extreme values according to the recommended cut-off for the height-for-age *z*-score of the WHO [25]. Our results may be limited by reliance on multiple logistic regression with adjustment for the clustering of the samples using a mixed effect model; it is possible that a generalized estimating equation analysis (GEE) might produce more robust results, but it is unlikely that the direction and size of observed relationships would change in meaningful ways. Last, our first attempt to choose the study site by restricting it to only sub-districts with a prevalence of child underweight of more than 15% according to government reports might limit generalization to the general population.

5. Conclusions

In conclusion, one fifth of households in the study site were found to be experiencing the double burden of malnutrition in the form of a stunted child and an overweight/obese mother (SCOWT). The present study supported the hypothesis that the double burden of malnutrition is related to food insecurity. Even though both maternal height and household food insecurity status was significantly associated with the double burden of malnutrition, only the level of food insecurity derived from the HFIAS instrument served as a good predictor of SCOWT in urban Indonesia. Future studies could build on our results using the universally acceptable HFIAS instrument as an early warning indicator for the double burden of malnutrition as defined by the coexistence of maternal overweight/obesity and child stunting. These results should be replicated for different populations and settings to established HFIAS as the common predictor of the double burden of malnutrition and not merely as a food security indicator.

Author Contributions: T.M. was responsible for overall and/or sectional scientific management, formulating the research question, making the concept and design of the study, preparing the draft manuscript, and revisions. T.S.N. led the data collection, coordinated the participants, and set up the ground work for the nutrition education sessions. H.M. developed hands-on activities for the nutrition education sessions and supervised the data collection. D.R.A. was responsible for managing data input and the preliminary cleaning of the data and writing the first draft of the manuscript in Bahasa Indonesia. R.R.R. was responsible for substantial contributions to the design and conception of the study, and was involved in the data analysis and manuscript preparation, providing critique and revision of the manuscript, and supervising the data collection. T.M. gave final approval of the version to be published; and agreed to be accountable for all aspects of the work in ensuring that questions related to the accuracy or integrity of any part of the work are appropriately investigated and resolved. All authors have given approval of the final manuscript.

Funding: This research received no external funding.

Acknowledgments: This study was a self-funded study with no support from external agencies. The costs to publish in open access will be covered by Kansas State University. The authors would like to thank Calista Segalita for initial editing the manuscript.

Conflicts of Interest: We have no conflict of interest to report for this study entitled "Household Food Insecurity as a Predictor of Stunted Children and Overweight/Obese Mothers (SCOWT) in Urban Indonesia".

Appendix A

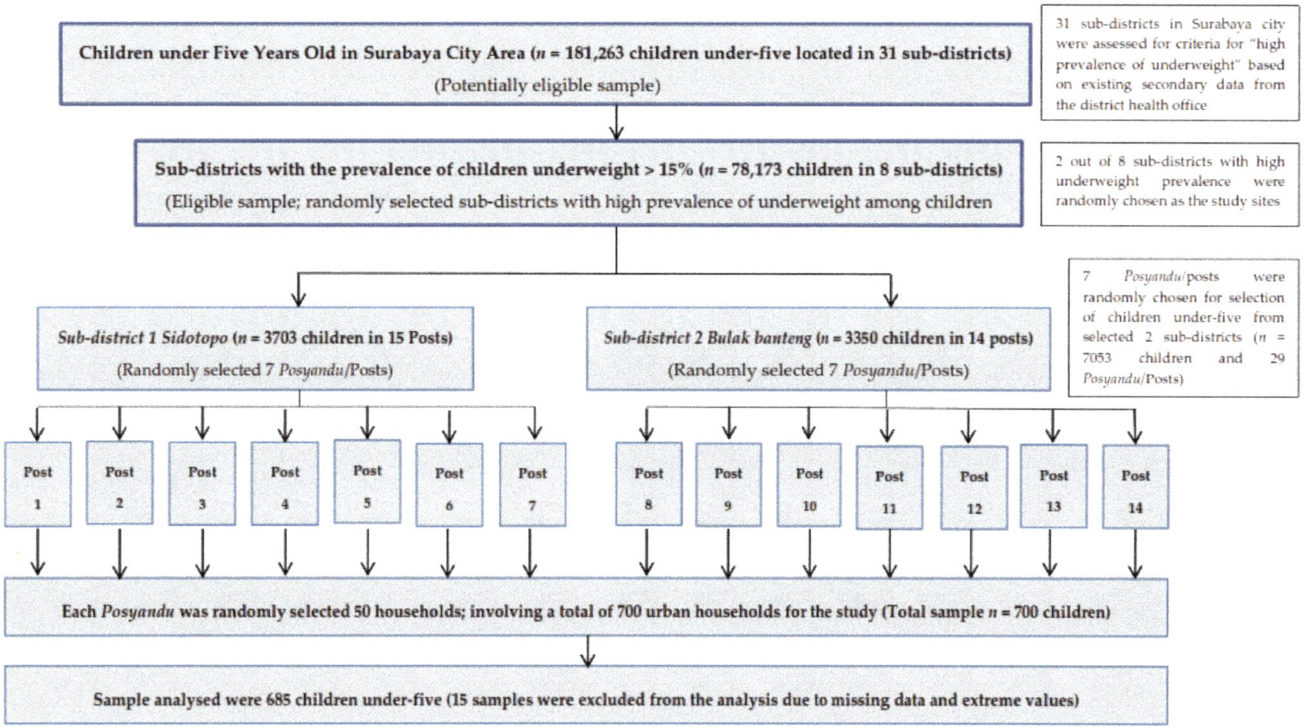
Children under Five Years Old in Surabaya City Area (n = 181,263 children under-five located in 31 sub-districts)
(Potentially eligible sample)
31 sub-districts in Surabaya city were assessed for criteria for "high prevalence of underweight" based on existing secondary data from the district health office
Sub-districts with the prevalence of children underweight > 15% (n = 78,173 children in 8 sub-districts)
(Eligible sample; randomly selected sub-districts with high prevalence of underweight among children
2 out of 8 sub-districts with high underweight prevalence were randomly chosen as the study sites
Sub-district 1 Sidotopo (n = 3703 children in 15 Posts)
(Randomly selected 7 Posyandu/Posts)
Sub-district 2 Bulak banteng (n = 3350 children in 14 posts)
(Randomly selected 7 Posyandu/Posts)
7 Posyandu/posts were randomly chosen for selection of children under-five from selected 2 sub-districts (n = 7053 children and 29 Posyandu/Posts)
Post 1
Post 2
Post 3
Post 4
Post 5
Post 6
Post 7
Post 8
Post 9
Post 10
Post 11
Post 12
Post 13
Post 14
Each Posyandu was randomly selected 50 households; involving a total of 700 urban households for the study (Total sample n = 700 children)
Sample analysed were 685 children under-five (15 samples were excluded from the analysis due to missing data and extreme values)

Figure A1. Systematic cluster sampling methods from 14 different integrated health posts (*posyandu*) involving total of 700 urban households in Surabaya, Indonesia.

Appendix B

Table A1. Characteristics of households with children between 2 and 5 years old from communities with a high risk of underweight children in Surabaya, Indonesia on their food security status.

Variable	Food Security		Mild Insecurity		Moderate Insecurity		Severe Insecurity		Total		p
	n	Row %	n	Row %	n	Row %	n	Row %	n	Column %	
Total	288	42.0	157	22.9	105	15.3	135	19.7	685	100	
Maternal literacy											0.012 *
Illiterate	17	29.8	11	19.3	9	15.8	20	35.1	57	8.3	
Partially literate	32	34.0	20	21.3	19	20.2	23	24.5	94	13.7	
Literate	239	44.8	126	23.6	77	14.4	92	17.2	534	78.0	
Maternal education											<0.001 ***
Low (no schooling or elementary school)	88	27.5	83	25.9	54	16.9	95	29.7	320	46.8	
Medium (junior high school)	62	44.9	32	23.2	27	19.6	17	12.3	138	20.1	
High (senior high school or college/university)	138	460.8	42	18.5	24	10.6	23	10.1	227	33.1	
Number of children under 5 years old in the household											0.046 *
1 child	260	42.1	141	22.9	91	14.8	125	20.3	617	90.1	
2 children	28	43.1	13	20	14	21.5	10	15.4	65	9.5	
Maternal occupation											0.290
Housewife without maid	216	41.5	118	22.7	86	16.5	100	19.2	520	75.9	
Housewife with maid	10	38.5	5	19.2	4	15.4	7	26.9	26	3.8	
Private sector	23	54.8	7	16.7	4	9.5	8	19.1	42	6.1	
Trade and entrepreneur	25	49.0	11	21.6	5	9.8	10	19.6	51	7.5	
Labor/miscellaneous services	11	25.6	16	37.2	6	14.0	10	23.3	43	6.3	
Paternal occupation (n = 650)											<0.001 ***
Government officer (including Army/Police)	56	88.9	4	6.4	2	3.2	1	1.6	63	9.7	
Private sector	93	48.4	49	25.5	24	12.5	26	13.5	192	29.5	
Trade and entrepreneur	44	39.6	26	23.4	28	25.2	13	11.7	111	17.1	
Labor	62	31.5	53	26.9	25	12.7	57	28.9	197	30.3	
Other	23	26.7	18	20.9	22	25.6	23	26.7	86	13.2	
Household's monthly income (n = 508)											<0.001 ***
Low (≤Indonesian Rupiah (IDR) 1,500,000 or≤$150)	74	28.3	71	27.1	48	18.3	69	26.3	262	51.6	
Medium (>IDR 1500,000–2,500,000 or >$150–250)	52	42.6	22	18.0	20	16.4	28	23.0	122	24.0	
High (>IDR 2,500,000 or >$250)	93	75.0	19	15.3	4	3.2	8	6.5	124	22.4	
Paternal smoking status (n = 683)											0.045 *
Non-smoker	102	50	42	20.6	25	12.3	35	17.2	204	29.8	
Smoker	184	38.5	114	23.9	80	16.7	100	20.9	478	69.8	

Variables are significantly associated with food security status: * $p < 0.05$, ** $p < 0.01$, *** $p < 0.001$, p-values obtained with chi-squared tests and Fisher's exact test for small cell sizes (less than 10 participants), n = 685 unless indicated otherwise.

Table A2. Distribution of affirmative responses and mean scores to items on the Household Food Insecurity Access Scale (HFIAS): households (n = 685) in urban Surabaya, Indonesia, May 2015.

HFIAS Questions	**Affirmative Responses**	
(Due to Lack of Food or Limited Resources to Obtain Food, in the Past Four Weeks Did You or Any Household Member . . .)	***n***	**%**
Q1: Worry about food	353	51.5
Q2: Unable to eat preferred foods	325	47.4
Q3: Eat just a few kinds of foods	249	36.4
Q4: Eat foods they really do not want to eat	243	35.5
Q5: Eat small meals a day	199	29.1
Q6: Eat fewer meals in a day	156	22.8
Q7: No food of any kind in the household	79	11.5
Q8: Go to sleep hungry	104	15.2
Q9: Go a whole day and night without eating	22	3.2

HFIAS, Household Food Insecurity Access Scale. Q, question.

Table A3. Odds ratios (ORs) for child stunting, maternal overweight/obesity, and SCOWT using simple and multiple logistic mixed models.

Variable	Child Stunting				Maternal Overweight/Obesity				SCOWT			
	Crude OR	95% CI	Adjusted OR	Adjusted 95% CI	Crude OR	95% CI	Adjusted OR	Adjusted 95% CI	Crude OR	95% CI	Adjusted OR	Adjusted 95% CI
Child Gender												
Male	Ref.		Ref.		Ref.				Ref.			
Female	0.612 **	(0.441–0.849)	1.696 **	(1.077–2.672)	1.16	(0.834–1.614)			0.74	(0.515–1.064)		
Child Age	0.989	(0.969–1.009)			1.014	(0.993–1.036)			0	-		
Maternal Age	0.996	(0.963–1.031)			1.026	(0.99–1.063)			1.02	(0.982–1.06)		
Maternal literacy												
Illiterate	Ref.				Ref.				Ref.			
Partially literate	0.994	(0.47–2.105)			0.897	(0.395–2.037)			1.021	(0.457–2.28)		
Literate	0.702	(0.374–1.316)			0.826	(0.416–1.637)			0.782	(0.396–1.547)		
Maternal education												
Low education	Ref.		Ref.		Ref.				Ref.			
Educated	0.534 **	(0.342–0.834)	0.596 *	(0.372–0.954)	0.814	(0.537–1.235)			0.565 *	(0.34–0.937)		
Highly educated	0.58	(0.213–1.579)	0.735	(0.242–2.23)	0.717	(0.329–1.565)			0.849	(0.294–2.454)		
Family type												
Nuclear family	Ref.				Ref.				Ref.			
Extended family	0.976	(0.663–1.435)			0.901	(0.613–1.324)			1.291	(0.584–1.361)		
Number of child at home												
1–2 children	Ref.				Ref.		Ref.		Ref.			
3–4 children	1.48	(0.978–2.238)			1.75 *	(1.108–2.762)	1.75 *	(1.108–2.762)	1.852 **	(1.184–2.898)		
>4 children	1.381	(0.422–4.525)			0.473	(0.15–1.484)	0.473	(0.15–1.484)	1.229	(0.317–4.766)		
Number of children under 5 years in household												
1 child	Ref.				Ref.				Ref.			
2 children	0.987	(0.524–1.86)			0.745	(0.401–1.384)			1.015	(0.504–2.044)		
3 children	0.877	(0.054–14.25)			0.855	(0.052–13.963)			1.497	(0.091–24.713)		
Maternal occupation												
Housewife without maid	Ref.				Ref.				Ref.			
Housewife with maid	1.472	(0.508–4.267)			2.374	(0.572–9.859)			1.935	(0.653–5.733)		
Private sector	0.435	(0.158–1.198)			1.41	(0.536–3.705)			0.795	(0.286–2.212)		
Trade and entrepreneur	0.772	(0.339–1.756)			0.734	(0.334–1.611)			0.686	(0.262–1.798)		
Labor/miscellaneous	0.719	(0.286–1.807)			1.245	(0.485–3.193)			0.817	(0.294–2.274)		
Paternal occupation												
Government officer	Ref.				Ref.				Ref.			
Private sector	4.914 **	(1.476–16.36)			0.97	(0.441–2.135)			3.963 *	(1.05–14.961)		
Trade and entrepreneur	7.274 ***	(2.099–25.208)			0.904	(0.386–2.12)			4.84 *	(1.23–19.05)		
Labor	7.196***	(2.14–24.201)			1.455	(0.654–3.239)			5.77 **	(1.542–21.586)		
Other	11.117 ***	(3.157–39.153)			0.977	(0.395–2.414)			7.436 **	(1.871–29.549)		
Paternal smoking status												
Non-smoker	Ref.				Ref.				Ref.			
Smoker	0.97	(0.677–1.389)			1.081	(0.756–1.546)			0.973	(0.652–1.451)		
Food insecurity												
Food secure	Ref.		Ref.		Ref.				Ref.		Ref.	
Mildly food insecure	1.74 *	(1.043–2.903)	1.687	(0.985–2.889)	1.286	(0.76–2.176)			2.647 ***	(1.486–4.712)	2.798 ***	(1.54–5.083)
Moderately food insecure	1.514	(0.84–2.729)	1.562	(0.842–2.897)	1.174	(0.646–2.135)			2.254 *	(1.17–4.342)	2.53 **	(1.286–4.98)
Severely food insecure	2.182 **	(1.28–3.717)	2.005 *	(1.14–3.526)	1.111	(0.647–1.91)			2.057 *	(1.112–3.804)	2.045 *	(1.087–3.848)

Households with children between 2 and 5 years old from communities with high risk of underweight children in Surabaya, Indonesia. Odds from those food-secure households.
* $p < 0.05$, ** $p < 0.01$, *** $p < 0.001$; *p*-values and estimated values obtained by fitting a Mixed Effect Model accounting for Posyandu; Adjustment for Multiple Comparisons: Dunnett-Hsu.

References

1. Bhurosy, T.; Jeewon, R. Overweight and obesity epidemic in developing countries: A problem with diet, physical activity, or socioeconomic status? *Sci. World J.* **2014**, *2014*, 964236. [CrossRef] [PubMed]
2. Finucane, M.M.; Stevens, G.A.; Cowan, M.; Lin, J.K.; Paciorek, C.J.; Singh, G.M.; Gutierrez, H.R.; Lu, Y.; Bahalim, A.N.; Farzadfar, F.; et al. National, regional, and global trends in body mass index since 1980: Systematic analysis of health examination surveys and epidemiological studies with 960 country-years and 9.1 million participants. *Lancet* **2011**, *377*, 557–567. [CrossRef]
3. Martorell, R.; Khan, L.K.; Hughes, M.L.; Grummer-Strawn, L.M. Obesity in women from developing countries. *Eur. J. Clin. Nutr.* **2000**, *54*, 247–252. [CrossRef] [PubMed]
4. Riset Kesehatan Dasar Riskesdas 2013. Available online: http://www.depkes.go.id/resources/download/general/Hasil%20Riskesdas%202013.pdf (accessed on 23 March 2018). (In Bahasa Indonesia).
5. Bredenkamp, C.; Buisman, L.R.; van de Poel, E. Persistent inequalities in child undernutrition: Evidence from 80 countries, from 1990 to today. *Int. J. Epidemiol.* **2014**, *43*, 1328–1335. [CrossRef] [PubMed]
6. Restrepo-méndez, M.C.; Barros, A.J.D.; Black, R.E.; Victora, C.G. Time trends in socio-economic inequalities in stunting prevalence: Analyses of repeated national surveys. *Public Health Nutr.* **2015**, *18*, 2097–2104. [CrossRef] [PubMed]
7. United Nations Children's Fund. Improving Child Nutrition. The Achievable Imperative for Global Progress. Available online: https://www.unicef.org/gambia/Improving_Child_Nutrition_-_the_achievable_imperative_for_global_progress.pdf (accessed on 23 March 2018).
8. World Health Organization. Malnutrition. Fact Sheet Updated 2017. Available online: http://www.who.int/mediacentre/factsheets/malnutrition/en/ (accessed on 23 March 2018).
9. Food and Agriculture Organization of the United Nations. The Double Burden of Malnutrition Case Studies from Six Developing Countries. 2006. Available online: http://www.fao.org/tempref/docrep/fao/009/a0442e/a0442e00.pdf (accessed on 23 March 2018).
10. Sekiyama, M.; Jiang, H.W.; Gunawan, B.; Dewanti, L.; Honda, R.; Shimizu-Furuzawa, H.; Abdoellah, O.S.; Watanabe, C. Double burden of malnutrition in rural West Java: Household-level analysis for father-child and mother-child pairs and the association with dietary intake. *Nutrients* **2015**, *7*, 8376–8391. [CrossRef] [PubMed]
11. Abegunde, D.O.; Mathers, C.D.; Adam, T.; Ortegon, M.; Strong, K. The burden and costs of chronic diseases in low-income and middle-income countries. *Lancet* **2015**, *370*, 1929–1939. [CrossRef]
12. Delisle, H.; Agueh, V.; Fayomi, B. Partnership research on nutrition transition and chronic diseases in West Africa—Trends, outcomes and impacts. *BMC Int. Health Hum. Rights* **2011**, *11* (Suppl. 2). [CrossRef] [PubMed]
13. Gartner, A.; El Ati, J.; Traissac, P.; Bour, A.; Berger, J.; Landais, E.; El Hsaini, H.; Ben Rayana, C.; Delpeuch, F. A Double burden of overall or central adiposity and anemia or iron deficiency is prevalent but with little socioeconomic patterning among Moroccan and Tunisian urban women. *J. Nutr.* **2014**, *144*, 87–97. [CrossRef] [PubMed]
14. Dieffenbach, S.; Stein, A.D. Stunted child/overweight mother pairs represent a statistical artifact, not a distinct entity. *J. Nutr.* **2012**, *142*, 771–773. [CrossRef] [PubMed]
15. Lee, J.; Houser, R.F.; Must, A.; de Fulladolsa, P.P.; Bermudez, O.I. Socioeconomic disparities and the familial coexistence of child stunting and maternal overweight in Guatemala. *Econ. Hum. Biol.* **2012**, *10*, 232–241. [CrossRef] [PubMed]
16. Oddo, V.M.; Rah, J.H.; Semba, R.D.; Sun, K.; Akhter, N.; Sari, M.; de Pee, S.; Moench-pfanner, R.; Bloem, M.; Kraemer, K. Predictors of maternal and child double burden of malnutrition in rural Indonesia and Bangladesh. *Am. J. Clin. Nutr.* **2012**, *95*, 951–958. [CrossRef] [PubMed]
17. Nguyen, B.K.L.; Thi, H.L.; Do, V.A.N.; Thuy, N.T.; Huu, C.N.; Do, T.T.; Deurenberg, P.; Khouw, I. Double burden of undernutrition and overnutrition in Vietnam in 2011: Results of the SEANUTS Study in 0·5–11-year-old children. *Br. J. Nutr.* **2013**, *110*, S45–S56. [CrossRef] [PubMed]
18. Rojroongwasinkul, N.; Kijboonchoo, K.; Wimonpeerapattana, W.; Purttiponthanee, S.; Yamborisut, U.; Boonpraderm, A.; Kunapan, P.; Thasanasuwan, W.; Khouw, I. SEANUTS: The nutritional status and dietary intakes of 0.5–12-year-old Thai children. *Br. J. Nutr.* **2013**, *110*, S36–S44. [CrossRef] [PubMed]

19. Sandjaja, S.; Budiman, B.; Harahap, H.; Ernawati, F.; Soekatri, M.; Widodo, Y.; Sumedi, E.; Rustan, E.; Sofia, G.; Syarief, S.N.; et al. Food consumption and nutritional and biochemical status of 0.5–12-year-old Indonesian children: The SEANUTS Study. *Br. J. Nutr.* **2013**, *110*, S11–S20. [CrossRef] [PubMed]
20. Manyanga, T.; El-Sayed, H.; Doku, D.T.; Randall, J.R. The prevalence of underweight, overweight, obesity and associated risk factors among school-going adolescents in seven African countries. *BMC Public Health* **2014**, *14*, 1–11. [CrossRef] [PubMed]
21. Rosenkranz, R.R.; Dzewaltowski, D.A. Model of the home food environment pertaining to childhood obesity. *Nutr. Rev.* **2008**, *66*, 123–140. [CrossRef] [PubMed]
22. Vaezghasemi, M.; Ohman, A.; Eriksson, M.; Hakimi, M.; Weinehall, L.; Kusnanto, H.; Nawi, N. The effect of gender and social capital on the dual burden of malnutrition: A multilevel study in Indonesia. *PLoS ONE* **2014**, *9*. [CrossRef] [PubMed]
23. Mahmudiono, T. Understanding the increased of child height for age index during the decline coverage of posyandu using intrinsic, extrinsic and macro-environmental factors approach: A literature review. *Indones. J. Public Health* **2007**, *4*, 1–7.
24. Kota Surabaya Dalam Angka 2013. Available online: https://surabayakota.bps.go.id/publication/2013/09/13/b42cb3e2d282ce2db333e862/kota-surabaya-dalam-angka-2013.html (accessed on 7 February 2018). (In Bahasa Indonesia).
25. Mei, Z.; Grummer-strawn, L.M. Standard deviation of anthropometric z-scores as a data quality assessment tool using the 2006 WHO growth standards: A cross country analysis. *Bull. World Health Organ.* **2007**, *85*, 441–448. [CrossRef] [PubMed]
26. Coates, J.; Swindale, A.; Bilinsky, P. Household Food Insecurity Access Scale (HFIAS) for Measurement of Food Access: Indicator Guide VERSION 3. 2007. Available online: https://www.fantaproject.org/sites/default/files/resources/HFIAS_ENG_v3_Aug07.pdf (accessed on 23 March 2018).
27. WHO Child Growth Standards: Methods and Development. Available online: http://www.who.int/childgrowth/standards/Technical_report.pdf (accessed on 23 March 2018).
28. Vaske, J.J. *Survey Research and Analysis: Applications in Parks, Recreation and Human Dimensions*; Venture Publishing: State College, PA, USA, 2008.
29. O'Brien, R.M. A Caution regarding rules of thumb for variance inflation factors. *Qual. Quant.* **2007**, *41*, 673–690. [CrossRef]
30. Liao, D.; Valliant, R. Variance inflation factors in the analysis of complex survey data. *Surv. Methodol.* **2012**, *38*, 53–62.
31. Allison, P. When Can You Safely Ignore Multicollinearity? *Statistical Horizons*. Available online: https://statisticalhorizons.com/multicollinearity (accessed on 5 December 2015).
32. Kimani-Murage, E.W.; Schofield, L.; Wekesah, F.; Mohamed, S.; Mberu, B.; Ettarh, R.; Egondi, T.; Kyobutungi, C.; Ezeh, A. Vulnerability to food insecurity in urban slums: Experiences from Nairobi, Kenya. *J. Urban Health* **2014**, *91*, 1098–1113. [CrossRef] [PubMed]
33. Kimani-Murage, E.W.; Muthuri, S.K.; Oti, S.O.; Mutua, M.K.; van de Vijver, S.; Kyobutungi, C. Evidence of a double burden of malnutrition in urban poor settings in Nairobi, Kenya. *PLoS ONE* **2015**, *10*. [CrossRef] [PubMed]
34. Uauy, R.; Kurpad, A.; Tamo-Debrah, K.; Otoo, G.E.; Aaron, G.A.; Toride, Y.; Ghosh, S. Role of protein and amino acids in infant and young child nutrition: Protein and amino acid needs and relationship with child growth. *J. Nutr. Sci. Vitaminol.* **2015**, *61*, S192–S194. [CrossRef] [PubMed]
35. Felisbino-Mendes, M.S.; Villamor, E.; Velasquez-Melendez, G. Association of maternal and child nutritional status in Brazil: A population based cross-sectional study. *PLoS ONE* **2014**, *9*. [CrossRef] [PubMed]
36. Ferreira, H.S.; Moura, F.A.; Cabral Júnior, C.R.; Florêncio, T.M.M.T.; Vieira, R.C.; de Assunção, M.L. Short stature of mothers from an area endemic for undernutrition is associated with obesity, hypertension and stunted children: A population-based study in the semi-arid region of Alagoas, Northeast Brazil. *Br. J. Nutr.* **2009**, *101*, 1239–1245. [CrossRef] [PubMed]
37. Varela-Silva, M.I.; Azcorra, H.; Dickinson, F.; Bogin, B.; Frisancho, A.R. Influence of maternal stature, pregnancy age, and infant birth weight on growth during childhood in Yucatan, Mexico: A test of the intergenerational effects hypothesis. *Am. J. Hum. Biol.* **2009**, *21*, 657–663. [CrossRef] [PubMed]

38. Widodo, Y. Cakupan Pemberian Asi Eksklusif: Akurasi Dan Interpretasi Data Survei Dan Laporan Program. *Gizi Indones.* **2011**, *34*, 101–108. (In Bahasa Indonesia).
39. López-Olmedo, N.; Hernández-Cordero, S.; Neufeld, L.M.; García-Guerra, A.; Mejía-Rodríguez, F.; Méndez Gómez-Humarán, I. The associations of maternal weight change with breastfeeding, diet and physical activity during the postpartum period. *Matern. Child Health J.* **2016**, *20*, 270–280. [CrossRef] [PubMed]

nutrients

MDPI

Article

Daily Dietary Intake Patterns Improve after Visiting a Food Pantry among Food-Insecure Rural Midwestern Adults

Breanne N. Wright [1], Regan L. Bailey [1], Bruce A. Craig [2], Richard D. Mattes [1], Lacey McCormack [3], Suzanne Stluka [4], Lisa Franzen-Castle [5], Becky Henne [6], Donna Mehrle [7], Dan Remley [8] and Heather A. Eicher-Miller [1,*]

1 Department of Nutrition Science, Purdue University, West Lafayette, IN 47907, USA; wrigh197@purdue.edu (B.N.W.); reganbailey@purdue.edu (R.L.B.); mattes@purdue.edu (R.D.M.)
2 Department of Statistics, Purdue University, West Lafayette, IN 47907, USA; bacraig@purdue.edu
3 Health and Nutritional Sciences, South Dakota State University, Brookings, SD 57007, USA; lacey.mccormack@sdstate.edu
4 Extension, South Dakota State University, Brookings, SD 57007, USA; suzanne.stluka@sdstate.edu
5 Nutrition and Health Sciences, University of Nebraska-Lincoln, Lincoln, NE 68583, USA; lfranzen2@unl.edu
6 Extension, Michigan State University, Charlotte, MI 48813, USA; henner@msu.edu
7 Extension, University of Missouri, Columbia, MO 65212, USA; mehrled@missouri.edu
8 Extension, Ohio State University, Piketon, OH 45661, USA; remley.4@osu.edu
* Correspondence: heicherm@purdue.edu; Tel.: +1-765-494-6815

Received: 19 April 2018; Accepted: 7 May 2018; Published: 9 May 2018

Abstract: Emergency food pantries provide food at no cost to low-resource populations. The purpose of this study was to evaluate single-day dietary intake patterns before and after visiting a food pantry among food-secure and food-insecure pantry clients. This observational cohort study comprised a paired, before-and-after design with a pantry visit as the intervention. Participants (n = 455) completed a demographic and food security assessment, and two 24-h dietary recalls. Adult food security was measured using the U.S. Household Food Security Survey Module. Dietary intake patterns were assessed using Automated Self-Administered 24-h Recall data and classified by Healthy Eating Index (HEI-2010) scores, dietary variety, number of eating occasions, and energy intake. Paired t-tests and Wilcoxon signed-rank tests compared outcomes before and after a pantry visit. Mean dietary variety increased after the pantry visit among both food-secure (p = 0.02) and food-insecure ($p < 0.0001$) pantry clients. Mean energy intake (p = 0.0003), number of eating occasions (p = 0.004), and HEI-2010 component scores for total fruit ($p < 0.001$) and whole fruit ($p < 0.0003$) increased among food-insecure pantry clients only. A pantry visit may improve dietary intake patterns, especially among food-insecure pantry clients.

Keywords: emergency food assistance; food pantry; food insecurity; dietary patterns; dietary quality

1. Introduction

Approximately 16 million Americans utilize emergency food pantries, most of whom (67%) are classified as food-insecure [1]. Food insecurity is characterized by reports of reduced dietary quality and variety, disrupted eating patterns, and reduced food intake [2]. Food insecurity in adults is associated with lower intake of vegetables, fruits, dairy products, vitamins A and B6, calcium, magnesium, and zinc compared to food-secure adults [3]. Food insecurity is also associated with indicators of diet-related chronic diseases, including increased rates of diabetes, hypertension and hyperlipidemia, as well as poorer physical and mental health, and quality of life [4]. These health limitations may, in turn, increase the burden of food insecurity and perpetuate this cycle. Emergency food pantries provide food resources to food-insecure individuals at no cost and with minimal requirements. Use of emergency food pantries by clients was originally regarded as a response to a temporary situation, but may be increasingly used on a consistent basis as a dependable food source [5].

The nutritional contributions of food pantries to client diets is largely unknown [6]. Yet, it has been estimated that food pantries could be responsible for up to 25% of the household food supply among pantry users [6]. The impact of pantry foods on client diets may also vary based on food security status. There may be two distinct groups of emergency food pantry users; one group who relies on pantries because of a short-term or "emergency" change in their economic situation (indicating food insecurity), and another group who uses pantry resources for an extended period of time as one component of their ongoing food supply (as a buffer to retain food security) [7]. Consequently, the relationship between food insecurity and dietary intake patterns among food pantry clients should be evaluated to determine the differential potential of food pantries as an intervention to improve dietary intake patterns for households that may be using food pantries in different capacities.

The objectives of this study were to quantify and compare the short-term dietary intake patterns before and after a pantry visit among rural, Midwestern adult food pantry clients overall and then stratified by food security status. We hypothesized that dietary intake patterns, including the Healthy Eating Index-2010 (HEI-2010) score as a measure of dietary quality, the number of eating occasions, energy intake, and dietary variety, would increase significantly from before compared with after receipt of pantry foods, particularly for food-insecure pantry clients.

2. Materials and Methods

2.1. Study Design

This observational cohort study comprised a before-and-after design with a pantry visit as the intervention. This study was part of a larger multi-state intervention, "Voices for Food", which was administered through the Extension programs of universities in each of six states: Indiana, Michigan, Missouri, Nebraska, Ohio and South Dakota, and aimed to improve food security among rural, Midwestern food pantry clients. Four food pantries from counties defined as non-metro with poverty rates higher than 16% in 2011 [8], with Cooperative Extension presence, and without well-established food policy councils in each state were selected (totaling four food pantries per state). In each state, two of the food pantries were designated as "intervention" pantries and matched with "comparison" pantries based on several criteria, including: level of client choice, number of households served, pounds of food distributed per month, receipt of government commodity program assistance, food bank partnership, infrastructure and capacity (storage, shelving, etc.), and predominant racial/ethnic group served at the pantry.

2.2. Recruitment

From August to November 2014, a convenience sample of participants was recruited through flyers that advertised the study during pantry operation hours, and by approaching clients while they waited in line to receive food at selected pantries. Participants were screened by a trained interviewer. Only clients who were English speaking, adults $\geq$18 years (or $\geq$19 years in Nebraska where the legal age criteria classifying adult status is 19 years), who visited this food pantry at least one time prior to recruitment, and who were receiving foods from the pantry on the day of recruitment were invited to participate. The South Dakota State University and Ohio State University Institutional Review Boards approved research activities prior to beginning the study and participants gave consent before completing study materials. A sample size goal of 78 pantry clients in each food security subgroup was sought based on a meaningful change in HEI total score from a previous study [9], and estimates of correlation and standard deviation of the paired sample using pilot study data.

2.3. *Participants*

A total of 613 pantry clients were confirmed eligible and recruited. Four hundred and seventy-four (77%) participants completed two single-day 24-h dietary recalls. However, because of incomplete dietary and food security data, only 455 (74%) participants were included in the final analysis. Significant differences were found between pantry clients who completed multiple recalls compared to pantry clients who completed the initial recall only; significant differences were noted only for state ($p < 0.0001$) and soup kitchen use ($p = 0.005$; data not shown).

2.4. *Instruments*

The initial interview was conducted at the pantry by trained research staff in a semi-private area. Participants completed an electronic or paper version of a questionnaire that elicited information on demographic and pantry use characteristics, and included the validated 18-item U.S. Household Food Security Survey Module (US HHFSSM) [2]. Following this questionnaire, participants completed the Automated Self-Administered 24-h Dietary Recall (ASA24™-2014), an internet-based 24-h recall [10], with optional staff assistance. An additional dietary recall was self-completed, or completed through an assisted phone interview, within two weeks of the pantry visit. Participants received $10 as compensation in the form of a grocery store gift card upon completion of the initial interview (including the questionnaire and first dietary recall), and an additional gift card for completing the second dietary recall. Sixteen percent of initial recalls and 45% of 2nd recalls captured a weekend day.

2.5. *Data Analysis*

Food security status over the past 12 months was measured using the US HFSSM. Ten of the items were used to classify food security among household adults as per previous direction [11]. A raw score (number of affirmative responses on the food security scale) of zero was categorized as high food-secure, a score of 1–2 was categorized as marginal food-secure, a score of 3–5 was categorized as low food-secure and a score of 6–10 was categorized as very low food-secure. Food security status was dichotomized into two groups: "food-secure" (included high and marginal food-secure groups) and "food-insecure" (included low and very low food-secure groups).

Dietary information from ASA24™-2014 was used to determine the single-day dietary intake patterns (including before-pantry and after-pantry single-day energy intake, HEI-2010 scores, number of eating occasions, and number of unique USDA food codes). The total number of eating occasions was determined from the self-reported intake of meals, snacks, and beverages. The number of unique food items consumed for each participant was determined using the USDA food code, a unique, eight-digit number that is assigned to identify each food and beverage item included in nutrient composition databases. The HEI-2010 is an overall measure of diet quality that indicates conformance to the Dietary Guidelines for Americans and is comprised of 12 component scores: Total Fruit, Whole Fruit, Total Vegetables, Greens and Beans, Whole Grains, Total Dairy, Total Protein, Seafood and Plant Proteins, Fatty Acids, Refined Grains, Sodium, and Empty Calories (i.e., solid fat, alcohol, and added sugars) [12]. Each of the 12 components are weighted to yield a HEI-2010 total score that has a maximum value of 100, indicating full adherence to the Dietary Guidelines for Americans (DGA), and a minimum value of 0, indicating no adherence to the DGA [12]. Because the data were collected prior to the release of the 2015 DGA and HEI-2015, the HEI-2010 was the appropriate metric to use for this study.

2.6. *Statistical Analysis*

Prevalence of participant characteristics was compared across food security status using chi-square analysis (significance $p < 0.05$). The mean number of unique USDA food codes, mean number of eating occasions, mean HEI-2010 total and component scores, and mean energy intake were estimated for the pre-pantry and post-pantry recall and compared for all clients as well as food-secure and food-insecure subgroups. Wilcoxon signed rank tests determined differences in before-pantry and after-pantry intakes for the number of unique food codes (statistically significant when $p < 0.05$) and number of eating occasions (statistically significant when $p < 0.05/2$ sub-categories of eating occasions as 'Meals and Snacks' and 'Meals,' using Bonferroni-type adjustment for multiple comparisons of sub-groups). Paired *t*-tests determined differences in before-pantry and after-pantry intakes for mean energy intake (statistically significant when $p < 0.05$) and total and component HEI-2010 scores (statistically significant when $p < 0.05/13$ HEI total and component scores, using Bonferroni-type adjustment for multiple comparisons of sub-groups). A post-hoc analysis was performed to infer whether or not improvement in dietary outcomes was a direct result of the pantry visit. The mean, median and mode of lag time were determined. Linear regression models with the response being the change in HEI total and component scores (recall 2-recall 1) and the predictors being lag time and household size were performed (statistical significance $p < 0.05$). All analyses were completed using SAS version 9.4. (SAS Institute, Hong Kong, China) and R version 2.11.1.

3. Results

Pantry clients in the sample were predominately white (81%), female (72%), aged 45–65 (45%), and classified as food-insecure (78%) (Table 1). When characteristics were stratified by food security status, significant differences were observed for state, age, and the number of times the pantry was visited in the last 12 months. A greater proportion of food-secure pantry clients (35%) reported being >65 years old compared to food-insecure pantry clients (16%). A greater proportion of food-secure (63%) pantry clients reported visiting the pantry six or more times compared to food-insecure pantry clients (47%).

Table 1. Characteristics of a multistate sample of rural, Midwestern, adult emergency food pantry clients by food security status (n = 455).

	All Pantry Clients		**Food-Secure**		**Food-Insecure**		χ^2
	n	%	*n*	%	*n*	%	***p*-Value** [1]
Total [2]	455		100	22	355	78	
State							0.04
Indiana	117	26	23	23	94	26	
Michigan	87	19	13	13	74	21	
Missouri	102	22	21	21	81	23	
Nebraska	49	11	10	10	39	11	
Ohio	50	11	14	14	36	10	
South Dakota	50	11	19	19	31	9	
Age							0.0004
18–44 years	136	35	28	32	108	35	
45–64 years	176	45	29	33	147	48	
>65 years	81	20	31	35	50	16	
Sex							0.3
Male	107	28	28	32	79	26	
Female	280	72	59	68	221	74	
Race							0.3
White	305	81	67	78	238	82	
Black	32	8	10	12	22	8	
American Indian	28	7	8	9	20	7	
Other	12	3	1	1	11	4	
Ethnicity							0.1
Hispanic	15	4	1	1	14	5	
Not Hispanic	362	96	82	99	280	95	
Income							0.2
<$10,000	221	52	42	46	179	54	
$10,001–$15,000	91	22	26	28	65	20	
>$15,000	110	26	24	26	86	26	

Table 1. *Cont.*

	All Pantry Clients		Food-Secure		Food-Insecure		χ^2
	n	%	*n*	%	*n*	%	*p*-Value [1]
Number of Pantries Visited (past 12 months)							0.1
1 pantry	203	46	50	53	153	44	
≥2 pantries	239	54	44	47	195	56	
Household Food From Food Pantry							0.2
A few days' worth	191	45	34	40	157	46	
One to two weeks' worth	147	35	29	34	118	35	
More than half of the food for the month	86	20	23	26	63	19	
Times Visited This Pantry (past 12 months)							0.03
0–1 times	73	16	14	12	59	17	
2–5 times	153	34	24	24	129	36	
≥6 times	229	50	62	63	167	47	

[1] Statistical significance is p <0.05 for chi-square comparisons between food-secure and food-insecure adult food pantry clients. [2] Total numbers do not always add to sample size due to missing values; Percentages do not always add to 100 due to rounding.

A significant increase in mean energy intakes (before: 1400 ± 870, after: 1600 ± 880, $p < 0.0001$), mean number of eating occasions (before: 3.2 ± 1.1, after: 3.3 ± 1.1, $p = 0.002$) and mean number of unique food codes (before: 9 ± 5, after: 11 ± 5, $p < 0.0001$) was observed among all adult emergency food pantry clients from before to after the pantry visit (Table 2). However, when separated by food security status, a significant increase in the mean energy intake (before: 1400 ± 890, after: 1600 ± 890, $p = 0.0003$) and number of eating occasions (before: 3.1 ± 1.1, after: 3.3 ± 1.1, $p = 0.004$) was only noted among food-insecure food pantry clients, while a significant increase in the mean number of unique food codes was noted among both the food-secure (before: 11 ± 4, after: 12 ± 6, $p = 0.02$) and food-insecure (before: 9 ± 5, after: 11 ± 5, $p < 0.0001$) groups (Table 2).

Table 2. Comparison of before and after pantry dietary intake patterns (number of eating occasions, number of unique food codes reported consumed, energy intake and total HEI-2010 score) for all, food-secure, and food-insecure pantry clients in a multistate sample of rural, Midwestern, adult emergency food pantry clients (n = 455).

	All Pantry Clients				
	Before-Pantry		After-Pantry		
n = 455	Mean	SD	Mean	SD	*p*-value [1]
Number of Eating Occasions [2]	3.2	1.1	3.3	1.1	0.002 [3]
Meals and Snacks	2.7	1.0	2.8	1.0	0.02 [3]
Meals	2.2	0.8	2.3	0.8	0.03 [3]
Number of Unique Food Codes [2]	9	5	11	5	<0.0001 [3]
Energy Intake (kcal) [2]	1400	870	1600	880	<0.0001 [4]
Total HEI Score [2]	41	13	42	13	0.47 [4]
	Food-secure				
	Before-Pantry		After-Pantry		
n = 100	Mean	SD	Mean	SD	*p*-value
Number of Eating Occasions [2]	3.4	1.0	3.5	1.0	0.2 [3]
Meals and Snacks	3.0	0.9	3.0	0.9	0.3 [3]
Meals	2.4	0.7	2.5	0.8	0.7 [3]
Number of Unique Food Codes [2]	11	4	12	6	0.02 [3]
Energy Intake (kcal) [2]	1500	770	1600	840	0.1 [4]
Total HEI Score [2]	46	13	45	14	0.4 [4]

Table 2. *Cont.*

	Food-insecure				
	Before-Pantry		After-Pantry		
n = 355	Mean	SD	Mean	SD	p-value
Number of Eating Occasions [2]	3.1	1.1	3.3	1.1	0.004 [3]
Meals and Snacks	2.6	1.0	2.7	1.0	0.04 [3]
Meals	2.1	0.8	2.2	0.8	0.1 [3]
Number of Unique Food Codes [2]	9	5	11	5	<0.0001 [3]
Energy Intake (kcal) [2]	1400	890	1600	890	0.0003 [4]
Total HEI Score [2]	40	13	41	13	0.2 [4]

[1] Statistical significance is $p < 0.05$ for paired t-test and Wilcoxon signed rank test comparisons between before- and after-pantry energy intake and number of unique food codes; Statistical significance is $p < 0.025$ for paired t-test comparisons between before- and after-pantry number of eating occasions ($p < 0.05/2$ subcategories of 'Meals and Snacks' and 'Meals', Bonferroni-type adjustment for multiple comparisons of sub-groups); Statistical significance is $p < 0.004$ for paired t-test comparisons between before- and after-pantry HEI Scores ($p < 0.05/13$ HEI total and component groups, Bonferroni-type adjustment for multiple comparisons of sub-groups). [2] Indicates inclusion of all eating/drinking occasions: meals, snacks, and just a drink. [3] Indicates p-value was determined using the Wilcoxon signed rank test. [4] Indicates p-value was determined using the paired t-test.

Despite this increased in dietary intake patterns after a pantry visit, overall dietary quality, quantified using the mean total HEI score, was poor (mean HEI-2010 total score of 41), and a statistically significant difference in HEI-2010 total score before and after a pantry visit was not observed, regardless of food security status (Table 3). A significant increase in the mean HEI-2010 total fruit (before: 1.2 ± 1.9, after: 1.7 ± 2.2, $p < 0.0001$) and whole fruit (before: 0.9 ± 1.8, after: 1.4 ± 2.1, $p < 0.0001$) scores was observed among all pantry clients. After stratifying by food security status, there was a significant increase observed only among food-insecure pantry clients for the mean total fruit (before: 1.1 ± 1.9, after: 1.7 ± 2.1, $p < 0.001$) and whole fruit (before: 0.8 ± 1.7, after: 1.3 ± 2.0, $p = 0.0003$) HEI-2010 component scores.

Table 3. Comparison of before and after pantry HEI-2010 total and component scores in a multistate sample of rural, Midwestern, adult emergency food pantry clients for all pantry clients and for food-insecure pantry clients (n = 455).

		All Pantry Clients				
		Before-Pantry Score		After-Pantry Score		
n = 455	Max Score	Mean	SD	Mean	SD	p-Value [1]
Total Vegetables	5	2.9	2.0	2.9	1.9	0.9
Green Beans	5	0.8	1.7	0.6	1.5	0.1
Total Fruit	5	1.2	1.9	1.7	2.2	<0.0001
Whole Fruit	5	0.9	1.8	1.4	2.1	<0.0001
Whole Grain	10	2.1	3.3	1.9	3.0	0.4
Total Dairy	10	4.8	3.9	5.0	3.8	0.3
Total Protein	5	3.9	1.7	4.0	1.5	0.1
Seafood and Plant Protein	5	0.9	1.7	1.0	1.8	0.3
Fatty Acid	10	4.0	3.7	4.0	3.7	0.9
Sodium	10	3.3	3.6	3.2	3.5	0.5
Refined Grain	10	6.1	3.9	6.0	3.7	0.8
Empty Calories	20	10.3	7.0	9.9	6.7	0.4
Total HEI	100	41	13.0	42	13.0	0.5

Table 3. *Cont.*

		Food-insecure Pantry Clients [2]				
		Before-Pantry Score		After-Pantry Score		
$n = 355$	Max Score	Mean	SD	Mean	SD	p-Value [1]
Whole Fruit	5	0.8	1.7	1.3	2.0	0.0003
Total Fruit	5	1.1	1.9	1.7	2.1	<0.001
Total HEI	100	40	13	41	13	0.21

[1] p-value was determined using the paired t-test; Statistical significance is $p < 0.004$ for paired t-test comparisons between before- and after-pantry HEI Scores ($p < 0.05/13$ HEI total and components, Bonferroni-type adjustment for multiple comparisons of sub-groups). [2] Only HEI-2010 component scores that significantly changed from before to after a pantry visit among food-insecure pantry clients are shown.

Post-hoc analysis showed that the average lag time was 3.7 days with both a median and mode of two days (results not shown), and lag time was inversely associated with change in Whole Fruit score (data not shown).

4. Discussion

Research regarding the relationship between food insecurity and dietary intake among food pantry clients is limited [13–17]. This study represents the first investigation of single-day dietary intake patterns before and after food pantry use for food-secure and food-insecure pantry clients. Dietary variety increased for both food-insecure and food-secure pantry clients from before compared to after visiting a pantry, while an indicator of the fruit intake component to dietary quality, energy intake, and the number of eating occasions improved only for food-insecure pantry clients.

Overall dietary quality among food pantry clients was poor, a finding that is consistent with other studies evaluating dietary quality among food pantry clients [15]. The estimated HEI-2010 total score and component scores, indicating adherence to the Dietary Guidelines for Americans, for pantry clients observed in this study were low compared to the most recent estimate among the U.S. population (59.0 ± 1.0) [18]. Component scores for total fruit, whole fruit, greens and beans, and seafood and plant protein were especially low in this group, and indicate a critical need for improvement. These results are perhaps expected considering the high prevalence of food insecurity in the sample. Seventy-eight percent of participants were classified as food-insecure. Although much higher than the U.S. population, as expected [19], the prevalence of food insecurity in this rural Midwestern food pantry-user participant sample was consistent with other studies that have evaluated food security among emergency food system clients [9,15,17,20].

Dietary quality, dietary variety, number of eating occasions, and energy intake were expected to increase significantly after receipt of pantry foods based on the premise that pantry users visit the pantry to obtain more foods. Results revealed no significant increase in overall dietary quality from before compared with after pantry use, but did reveal a significant increase in the quality of the fruit dietary component. Providing enough food (quantity) may be more of a concern to emergency food pantry providers compared with the quality of foods provided. In support of this, studies have found that food packages provided to clients by food pantries do not meet recommended nutritional requirements and may be low in fruits, dairy, whole grains and fish [21–23], all of which are key components of the HEI-2010 index. This may explain why the quantity of food may increase after using a pantry, while the overall quality measured by the HEI-2010 total score may remain unchanged. While lower than U.S. averages [18], component scores for total fruit and whole fruit (total fruit excluding juice) significantly increased after receipt of pantry foods. The increase in whole fruit score suggest that the increase in the total fruit component score may not be entirely due to an increase in juice intake. Although many pantries may not offer the recommended amount of fruit [21–23], results from this study suggest that the fruit offered by pantries is an improvement upon what clients are otherwise able to obtain, or that foods offered by pantries allow clients to use other funds to purchase fruits and represents potential for the food pantry to enhance dietary quality.

Only food-insecure pantry clients experienced a significant increase in the number of eating occasions and energy intake after visiting the pantry. Food insecurity is characterized by reports of reduced dietary quality, dietary variety, disrupted eating patterns, and reduced food intake [2], suggesting greater need for resources to restore dietary patterns. This supports the hypothesis that food-secure and food-insecure groups may use pantries differently; food-insecure pantry clients may rely on pantries in response to a dire situation, while food-secure pantry clients may use pantries continually to serve as a buffer to maintain food security. In support of this idea, the results revealed a greater prevalence of pantry use ($\geq$6 times in the past 12 months) among food-secure pantry clients (63%) compared to food-insecure pantry clients. Therefore, food-insecure pantry clients may exhibit a higher degree of dietary restriction due to circumstance before visiting the pantry and consequently have a higher potential for improving their dietary intake patterns upon receipt of pantry foods. Both food security subgroups experienced an increase in dietary variety. Food-insecure pantry clients may receive foods from pantries that they cannot receive otherwise using non-pantry resources and therefore pantry use increases their food choices and improves dietary variety. On the other hand, food-secure pantry clients may rely on pantries consistently to acquire staple foods which they are able to supplement using other non-pantry resources, thereby improving dietary variety.

4.1. Strengths

Most prior studies evaluating the dietary intake of food pantry clients used only a single 24-h recall [14,15,24–26] with assessment completed on the day the client presented at the food pantry [15,24,25]. This study characterized the dietary patterns of pantry clients before and after visiting the pantry among a large multi-state sample of rural, Midwestern U.S. adults by assessing the dietary intake from two 24-h recalls.

4.2. Limitations

The observed changes in dietary intake patterns before and after pantry use may not be a direct effect of pantry use since food pantries are not the only source of foods for clients. Participants received a \$10 grocery store gift card upon completion of the initial recall, which may have been used to purchase foods that clients otherwise would not have been able to afford and thus impacted dietary patterns in their second recall; however, it was unethical to withhold compensation or provide it only to participants who completed two recalls. Additionally, the research team did not assess whether or not clients visited additional pantries between the initial dietary recall and the follow-up recall, and the present study and others have reported that clients may use multiple pantries [7,27,28]. A large proportion of the secondary recalls were collected on a weekend day; previous research has indicated that diet quality is lower and energy intake is higher on weekends compared to weekdays [29], which may have biased the results. The lag time between the first and second 24-h recall could range from two days to two weeks, and it was noted that the amount of food provided by pantries is typically small. This study population had an average lag time of 3.7 days with both a median and mode of two days. Thus, in a study population where most participants reported foods lasting a few days to two weeks, application of the results is appropriate. In support of this conclusion, lag time was inversely associated with change in Whole Fruit score, suggesting that improvement in whole fruit intake decreases as time passes after visiting the pantry. Finally, because of the nature of the emergency food system, the study sample was disproportionately food-insecure and therefore there was a discrepancy in the sample sizes of the food security groups after stratification. This may have resulted in increased power for statistically significant changes in dietary intake patterns in the food-insecure group compared to the food-secure group, and thus underestimated the impact of pantry foods on diet for food-secure clients. The sample size of the present study was based on a meaningful change in HEI total score; thus, the study may not have had statistical power to detect differences in HEI component scores before and after a pantry visit, and may explain the several non-significant results. This could be improved in future studies by increasing sample size, and ultimately statistical power.

5. Conclusions

Food pantries may be utilized to increase dietary variety for all patrons as well as energy intake, number of meals consumed, and fruit intake specifically among food-insecure pantry clients. Food pantries may be an ideal environment for a dietary intervention to improve food security and dietary intake patterns by improving the quality, quantity, and variety of foods offered. Future research should focus on determining the usual nutrient and food group intake of food pantry clients and comparing the intake by food security status while adjusting for potential confounders in efforts to examine how pantry foods may mediate dietary intake differently among and between food-secure and food-insecure pantry clients.

Author Contributions: H.A.E.-M. conceived the research question, supervised and directed analysis of the data; B.N.W. and H.A.E.-M. interpreted the data; B.N.W., L.M., S.S., L.F.-C., B.H., D.M., D.R. and H.A.E.-M. acquired the data; B.N.W. drafted the manuscript; B.N.W., R.L.B., B.A.C., R.D.M., L.M., S.S., L.F.-C., B.H., D.M., D.R. and H.A.E.-M. critically reviewed for important intellectual content and approved the final version.

Acknowledgments: This project was supported by U.S. Department of Agriculture, National Institute of Food and Agriculture, Voices for Food Grant 2013-69004-20401. The authors would like to thank Ashley G. Jacobs for her contributions to the research question, data analysis, data acquisition and early manuscript draft.

Conflicts of Interest: The authors declare no conflict of interest.

References

1. Coleman-Jensen, A.; Rabbitt, M.; Gregory, C.; Singh, A. *Statistical Supplement to Household Food Security in the United States in 2016*; Economic Research Service, AP-077; U.S. Department of Agriculture: Washington, DC, USA, 2017. Available online: https://www.ers.usda.gov/webdocs/publications/84981/ap-077.pdf?v=42979 (accessed on 17 April 2018).
2. Bickel, G.; Nord, M.; Price, C.; Hamilton, W.; Cook, J. *Guide to Measuring Household Food Security, Revised 2000*; Food and Nutrition Service; U.S. Department of Agriculture: Washington, DC, USA, 2000.
3. Hanson, K.L.; Connor, L.M. Food insecurity and dietary quality in US adults and children: A systematic review. *Am. J. Clin. Nutr.* **2014**, *100*, 684–692. [CrossRef] [PubMed]
4. Gundersen, C.; Ziliak, J.P. Food Insecurity and Health Outcomes. *Health Aff.* **2015**, *34*, 1830–1839. [CrossRef] [PubMed]
5. Kaiser, M.; Cafer, A. Understanding high incidence of severe obesity and very low food security in food pantry clients: Implications for social work. *Soc. Work Public Health* **2018**, *33*, 125–139. [CrossRef] [PubMed]
6. Verpy, H.; Smith, C.; Reicks, M. Attitudes and behaviors of food donors and perceived needs and wants of food shelf clients. *J. Nutr. Educ. Behav.* **2003**, *35*, 6–15. [CrossRef]
7. Kicinski, L. Characteristics of Short and Long-Term Food Pantry Users. *Mich. Sociol. Rev.* **2012**, *26*, 58–74.
8. U.S. Department of Agriculture Economic Research Service. County-Level Data Sets. 2011. Available online: https://data.ers.usda.gov/reports.aspx?ID=14843 (accessed on 1 August 2013).
9. Petrogianni, M.; Kanellakis, S.; Kallianioti, K.; Argyropoulou, D.; Pitsavos, C.; Manios, Y. A multicomponent lifestyle intervention produces favourable changes in diet quality and cardiometabolic risk indices in hypercholesterolaemic adults. *J. Hum. Nutr. Diet.* **2013**, *26*, 596–605. [CrossRef] [PubMed]
10. Subar, A.; Kirkpatrick, S.; Mittl, B.; Zimmerman, T.P.; Thompson, F.E.; Bingley, C.; Willis, G.; Islam, N.G.; Baranowski, T.; McNutt, S.; et al. The Automated Self-Administered 24-hour dietary recall (ASA24): A resource for researchers, clinicians, and educators from the National Cancer Institute. *J. Acad. Nutr. Diet.* **2012**, *112*, 1134–1137. [CrossRef] [PubMed]
11. U.S. Department of Agriculture Economic Research Service. U.S. Household Food Security Survey Module: Three-Stage Design, with Screeners. Available online: https://www.ers.usda.gov/media/8271/hh2012.pdf (accessed on 1 August 2014).

12. Guenther, P.; Casavale, K.; Reedy, J.; Kirkpatrick, S.I.; Hiza, H.A.; Kuczynski, K.J.; Kahle, L.L.; Krebs-Smith, S.M. Update of the Healthy Eating Index: HEI-2010. *J. Acad. Nutr. Diet.* **2013**, *113*, 569–580. [CrossRef] [PubMed]
13. Tarasuk, V.; Beaton, G. Household food insecurity and hunger among families using food banks. *Can. J. Public Health* **1999**, *90*, 109–113. [CrossRef] [PubMed]
14. Starkey, L.; Kuhnlein, H.; Gray-Donald, K. Food bank users: Sociodemographic and nutritional characteristics. *CMAJ* **1998**, *158*, 1143–1149. [PubMed]
15. Duffy, P.; Zizza, C.; Jacoby, J.; Tayie, F. Diet quality is low among female food pantry clients in Eastern Alabama. *J. Nutr. Educ. Behav.* **2009**, *41*, 414–419. [CrossRef] [PubMed]
16. Castetbon, K.; Mejean, C.; Deschamps, V.; Bellin-Lestienne, C.; Oleko, A.; Darmon, N.; Hercberg, S. Dietary behaviour and nutritional status in underprivileged people using food aid (ABENA study, 2004-2005). *J. Hum. Nutr. Diet.* **2011**, *24*, 560–571. [CrossRef] [PubMed]
17. Robaina, K.; Martin, K. Food insecurity, poor diet quality, and obesity among food pantry participants in Hartford, CT. *J. Nutr. Educ. Behav.* **2013**, *45*, 159–164. [CrossRef] [PubMed]
18. U.S. Department of Agriculture Center for Nutrition Policy and Promotion. Health Eating Index. Available online: http://www.cnpp.usda.gov/sites/default/files/healthy_eating_index/HEI-2010-Table.pdf (accessed on 1 August 2016).
19. Coleman-Jensen, A.; Rabbitt, M.; Gregory, C.; Singh, A. *Household Food Security in the United States in 2015*; Economic Research Service, ERR-215; U.S. Department of Agriculture: Washington, DC, USA, 2016. Available online: http://www.ers.usda.gov/media/2137663/err215.pdf (accessed on 24 March 2017).
20. Martin, K.S.; Wu, R.; Wolff, M.; Colantonio, A.G.; Grady, J. A novel food pantry program: Food security, self-sufficiency, and diet-quality outcomes. *Am. J. Prev. Med.* **2013**, *45*, 569–575. [CrossRef] [PubMed]
21. Neter, J.; Dijkstra, S.; Visser, M.; Brouwer, I. Dutch food bank parcels do not meet nutritional guidelines for a healthy diet. *Br. J. Nutr.* **2016**, *116*, 526–533. [CrossRef] [PubMed]
22. Nanney, M.; Grannon, K.; Cureton, C.; Hoolihan, C.; Janowiec, M.; Wang, Q.; Warren, C.; King, R. Application of the Healthy Eating Index-2010 to the hunger relief system. *Public Health Nutr.* **2016**, *19*, 1–9. [CrossRef] [PubMed]
23. Akobundu, U.; Cohen, N.; Laus, M.; Schulte, M.; Sousslof, M. Vitamins A and C, calcium, fruit, and dairy products are limited in food pantries. *J. Am. Diet. Assoc.* **2004**, *104*, 811–813. [CrossRef] [PubMed]
24. Lenhart, N.; Read, M. Demographic profile and nutrient intake assessment of individuals using emergency food programs. *J. Am. Diet. Assoc.* **1989**, *89*, 1269–1272. [CrossRef] [PubMed]
25. Bell, M.; Wilbur, L.; Smith, C. Nutritional status of persons using a local emergency food system program in middle America. *J. Am. Diet. Assoc.* **1998**, *98*, 1031–1033. [CrossRef]
26. Jacobs Starkey, L.; Gray-Donald, K.; Kuhnlein, H. Nutrient intake of food bank users is related to frequency of food bank use, household size, smoking, education and country of birth. *J. Nutr.* **1999**, *129*, 883–889. [CrossRef] [PubMed]
27. Campbell, E.; Hudson, H.; Webb, K.; Crawford, P. Food Preferences of Users of the Emergency Food System. *J. Hunger Environ. Nutr.* **2011**, *6*, 179–187. [CrossRef]
28. Greger, J.L.; Maly, A.; Jensen, N.; Kuhn, J.; Monson, K.; Stocks, A. Food pantries can provide nutritionally adequate food packets but need help to become effective referral units for public assistance programs. *J. Am. Diet. Assoc.* **2002**, *102*, 1126–1128. [CrossRef]
29. Jahns, L.; Conrad, Z.; Johnson, L.K.; Scheett, A.J.; Stote, K.S.; Raatz, S.K. Diet Quality Is Lower and Energy Intake Is Higher on Weekends Compared with Weekdays in Midlife Women: A 1-Year Cohort Study. *J. Acad. Nutr. Diet.* **2017**, *177*, 1080–1086. [CrossRef] [PubMed]

nutrients

MDPI

Article

Impact of a Pilot School-Based Nutrition Intervention on Dietary Knowledge, Attitudes, Behavior and Nutritional Status of Syrian Refugee Children in the Bekaa, Lebanon

Marwa Diab El Harake [1], Samer Kharroubi [1], Shadi K. Hamadeh [2] and Lamis Jomaa [1,3,*]

1 Department of Nutrition and Food Sciences, Faculty of Agriculture and Food Sciences, American University of Beirut, P.O. Box 11-0.236, Riad El Solh, Beirut 11072020, Lebanon; md106@aub.edu.lb (M.D.E.H.); sk157@aub.edu.lb (S.K.)
2 Environment and Sustainable Development Unit, Faculty of Agriculture and Food Sciences, American University of Beirut, P.O. Box 11-0.236, Riad El Solh, Beirut 11072020, Lebanon; shamadeh@aub.edu.lb
3 Refugee Health Program, Global Health Institute, American University of Beirut, Beirut 11072020, Lebanon
* Correspondence: lj18@aub.edu.lb; Tel.: +961-1-350000 (ext. 4544)

Received: 24 May 2018; Accepted: 13 July 2018; Published: 17 July 2018

Abstract: This study evaluated the impact of a 6-month school nutrition intervention on changes in dietary knowledge, attitude, behavior (KAB) and nutritional status of Syrian refugee children. A quasi-experimental design was followed; Syrian refuge children in grades 4 to 6 were recruited from three informal primary schools (two intervention and one control) located in the rural Bekaa region of Lebanon. The intervention consisted of two main components: classroom-based education sessions and provision of locally-prepared healthy snacks. Data on household socio-demographic characteristics, KAB, anthropometric measures and dietary intake of children were collected by trained field workers at baseline and post-intervention. Of the 296 school children enrolled, 203 (68.6%) completed post-intervention measures. Significant increases in dietary knowledge ($\beta = 1.22$, 95% CI: 0.54, 1.89), attitude ($\beta = 0.69$, 95% CI: 0.08, 1.30), and body mass index-for-age-z-scores ($\beta = 0.25$, 95% CI = 0.10, 0.41) were observed among intervention vs. control groups, adjusting for covariates ($p < 0.05$). Compared to the control, the intervention group had, on average, significantly larger increases in daily intakes of total energy, dietary fiber, protein, saturated fat, and several key micronutrients, $p < 0.05$. Findings suggest a positive impact of this school-based nutrition intervention on dietary knowledge, attitude, and nutritional status of Syrian refugee children. Further studies are needed to test the feasibility and long-term impact of scaling-up such interventions.

Keywords: nutrition; knowledge; refugees; children; school intervention; Lebanon

1. Introduction

Conflicts and forced displacement are among the main challenges facing our world today, with more people being displaced by conflicts than any other time since World War II. According to the United Nations High Commission for Refugees (UNHCR), a record number of 65.6 million people were uprooted from their homes by conflict and persecution at the end of 2016, 22.5 million of whom were refugees [1]. A refugee is defined as an individual who "owing to a well-founded fear of being persecuted for reasons of race, religion, nationality, membership of a particular social group or political opinion, is outside the country of his nationality, and is unable or unwilling to avail himself of the protection of that country" [2].

Refugees face tremendous challenges that affect their safety, health, livelihoods, and survival with food and nutrition insecurity being considered as one of their basic challenges. Yet, refugee children represent a particularly vulnerable population group that can suffer from the adverse consequences of conflicts, poverty and food insecurity. Studies have shown that the lack of consistent access to safe and nutritious food can have serious detrimental and long-lasting effects on the physical, cognitive, and psycho-social development of children [3–6]. Children in food insecure households and with poor dietary intakes may suffer from nutrient deficiencies, increased illnesses, poor general health, and increased cognitive and behavioral problems that can affect not only their educational attainment, but also their economic productivity later in life [7].

Despite the high vulnerability of refugee children to the adverse consequences of food insecurity and poverty, few studies to date were conducted to explore the health and nutritional status of refugee children in complex emergencies and protracted crises [8–10]. In fact, the limited research conducted within crisis-settings focuses primarily on assessing the prevalence of malnutrition among young children (<5 years), such as stunting, wasting, and anemia [11], with less emphasis being placed on the nutritional status of school-aged children. Recent evidence highlights the importance of considering older children, who may be equally, if not more, vulnerable to the adverse consequences of poverty and food insecurity compared to their younger siblings [7,12,13]. In addition, school children are at increased risk of poor dietary behaviors, including skipping breakfast, consuming low amounts of fruits and vegetables, and adopting unhealthy snacking behaviors that can affect their nutritional status and expose children to higher risk of weight gain and associated co-morbidities [14,15]. Although the first 1000 days of the child's life remain a critical period to ensure adequate growth and development [16–18], recent studies have shown that school-aged children and adolescents have the potential for catch-up growth, which makes them a suitable age group to target through well-designed nutrition interventions [19,20].

Schools can offer an optimal setting to reach out to a large number of children and to promote healthy eating habits and lifestyle behaviors through classroom-based nutrition education, role modeling of heathy behaviors and offering of nutritious snacks and meals [21,22]. Scientific evidence supports the effectiveness of multi-component, school-based interventions in improving the dietary and health-related knowledge and attitude of primary school-aged children [23–25]; however, evidence is less consistent in terms of the impact of such interventions on children's dietary behaviors [26,27]. A previous review on the effectiveness of school feeding programs in developing countries emphasized the importance of integrating interventions that include nutrition and health educational components to complement the provision of nutritious food and snacks within feeding programs to help alleviate hunger and improve the children's micronutrient status [28]. Despite the strong evidence supporting the positive impact of school-based interventions, the effectiveness of such interventions in improving the nutritional status of vulnerable children within conflict and displacement settings has not been adequately explored [9].

Today, the Syrian refugee crisis represents one of the largest humanitarian disasters worldwide with 5.5 million Syrian individuals fleeing the country since 2011 and seeking refuge in neighboring countries, including Turkey, Jordan, and Lebanon [29]. Lebanon is a small middle income country in the Middle East and North Africa region (MENA) region that has the highest per capita concentration of refugees worldwide [30–32]. As of April 2018, slightly less than a million Syrian individuals were registered with the UNHCR in Lebanon as refugees, of which, 36% (354,326 individuals) reside in the Bekaa, a rural and underdeveloped region that is geographically close to the Syrian–Lebanese border [33]. The high influx of Syrian refugees to the impoverished host communities in the Bekaa have added further strain to the limited resources and basic services available, including access to adequate food, water, shelter, education, and health services [34,35].

This study aimed to evaluate the impact of a 6-month pilot school-based nutrition intervention on changes in dietary knowledge, attitude, and behavior of Syrian refugee children enrolled in informal primary schools located in the rural region of the Bekaa in Lebanon. A secondary objective of the study was to explore the effect of the intervention on the dietary intake and nutritional status of children. Findings from this pilot project can provide the evidence for conducting multi-component interventions that aim at alleviating food insecurity and improving the nutritional status and health outcomes of children residing in low-income, conflict-affected settings.

2. Materials and Methods

2.1. Study Design and Population

This was a quasi-experimental study conducted as part of a larger two year-project called 'GHATA: Bringing Education to Informal Tented Settlements'. The GHATA project aimed to design three modular schools that provide Syrian refugee children aged 6 to 14 years with a credentialed education and adequate nutrition through offering healthy snacks and nutrition education. These informal schools served as spaces for provision of education and child protection programs targeting Syrian refugees living in some of the most underserved communities in the Bekaa. As of 2016, it has been estimated that more than 250,000 children, approximately half of school-aged Syrian children registered in Lebanon, are out of school [36], and only 15% of refugee children in the Bekaa valley are enrolled in schools [37].

The informal modular schools built within the GHATA project welcomed refugee children who dropped out of school due to the war in Syria and assisted in overcoming some of the main reported barriers limiting Syrian refugee children from enrolling within the Lebanese public school system. These barriers included the cost of education, the need for child labor, limited capacities for registration in schools, language and social integration difficulties [36]. Schools were structurally designed by the Center for Civic Engagement at the American University of Beirut (AUB) and were managed by the Kayany Foundation, a local non-governmental organization that provides education to disadvantaged Syrian refugee children.

For the purpose of this study, two of the three informal schools were randomly selected to serve as intervention schools and the third served as a control school. Schools had similar school enrollment capacities and community characteristics (such as the number of public schools in the area and number of hospitals). Each school had on average a total of 640 students enrolled in grades one to six. Each grade level had three sections with an average classroom size of 27 students. The three schools were located approximately 10–14 km away from each other and were situated in the three areas of Majdal Anjar, Saadneyil, and Bar Elias within the Bekaa valley, Lebanon. The intervention conducted in this study focused on school children enrolled in grades 4 to 6 within the three informal schools.

2.2. Sample Size and Recruitment

A power calculation was performed prior to the start of the study indicating that at least 64 students (32 students from intervention and 32 students from control) were required to detect a significant difference in dietary knowledge scores (effect size = 2.8) between intervention and control groups with 80% power and 95% confidence interval. The expected effect size was based on results from another school-based nutrition intervention conducted among children enrolled in grades 4 and 5 within public schools in Lebanon [14]. An additional 25% was added to the sample size to account for potential dropouts and incomplete data. The intended sample size was 80 school children, and the final sample enrolled at baseline consisted of 296 children (195 from intervention schools and 101 from control school), please see supportive material Figure S1 (flow diagram for study participants).

The present study was conducted over two academic years (2015–2016 and 2016–2017). Recruitment of the study population took place in September at the beginning of each of the consecutive school years during the registration period. After receiving approval from schools' administration, the research team approached parents of children enrolled in grades 4 to 6 during the school registration period explaining the purpose of the study. Parents who agreed to participate in the study were contacted to schedule interviews for data collection with children and their mothers at a date of their preference within a private classroom in their respective schools. Schools were considered a convenient site to conduct the interviews as they were located only a walking distance (5–10 min) from the informal tented settlements (refugee camps) where school children and their families reside. All study participants gave their informed consent for inclusion before participating in the study. The study was conducted in accordance with the Declaration of Helsinki, and the protocol was approved by the Ethics Committee of American University of Beirut (NUT.LJ.07).

2.3. Description of Intervention

The school-based nutrition intervention implemented in the present study was composed of two main components: (1) delivering health and nutrition education modules on a bi-weekly basis; and (2) providing children with locally-prepared nutritious snacks. Children in grades 4 to 6 within the intervention schools received the combination of both components, whereas children in the control school received their usual curriculum and a standard snack. Children in the control group received all the intervention material at the end of the second year of the project. The research team conducted field trip observations, meetings with school supervisors, and short evaluation surveys with children to assess fidelity to the project. Results from this process evaluation showed good adherence to the intervention components and any challenges were addressed throughout the study duration.

2.3.1. Classroom-Based Educational Sessions

The classroom-based health and nutrition education modules developed in this study were tailored for children in the upper elementary school levels and were based on the social cognitive theory, focusing primarily on observational learning, behavioral capability and self-efficacy. Prior school-based interventions showed modest effectiveness of this theory and its constructs to help increase the cognitive and behavioral skills of children and improve their dietary behaviors both at home and at school [21,38,39]. A total of 12 interactive classroom-based health and nutrition sessions were delivered by classroom teachers on a bi-weekly basis over a period of 6 months. Each of the educational sessions lasted approximately 45 min. Topics covered within these educational sessions included basic hygienic practices, importance of consuming breakfast daily, role of fruits and vegetables in a healthy diet, benefits of consuming water versus sugar-sweetened beverages, healthy snacking behaviors, and importance of physical activity. Hands-on activities and games were incorporated as part of these educational sessions to reinforce the main messages within each module. In addition, school teachers within the intervention schools were given a resource box that included visually-appealing and culturally-sensitive posters and printed material, such as the Lebanese food guide pyramid, the World Health Organization (WHO) poster for an adequate hand washing technique, to be mounted on the walls within the classrooms and throughout the school facilities. These visual aids were intended to reinforce and promote healthy eating behaviors, handwashing, among other basic hygiene practices among children. Intervention schools were also provided with physical activity resources that can be used as part of the physical education and activity sessions, such as skipping ropes, hula hoops, and balls.

To assist teachers with implementing the health and nutrition sessions, two-day training-of-trainers workshops were conducted at the beginning of the school year and a refresher training was conducted mid-year to ensure fidelity to the intervention. During the training workshops, intervention toolkits that included educational lesson plans, games, activities, and other supportive material were provided to all trained school teachers. Teachers were also provided with knowledge, skills, and relevant resources required for effective delivery of the intervention. The toolkit and all educational lesson plans were developed by a team of nutrition experts at the Department of Nutrition and Food Sciences at AUB using a variety of resources including the United States Department of Agriculture (USDA) online resources, age-appropriate science textbooks adopted by the Lebanese public schools, and published material and evidence available from similar low-to-middle-income country (LMIC) settings [12,14,40].

All educational materials were pilot tested with the school teachers at the beginning of the intervention to ensure cultural-sensitivity and appropriateness.

2.3.2. Locally-Prepared Nutritious Snacks

One of the main components of the GHATA project was to establish small kitchens or cooking units within the three newly established schools and to provide training to kitchen employees hired from the local Syrian refugee community to prepare nutritious and safe snacks to children during the school year. Children in the intervention group were provided with one snack item on a daily basis during the school break according to a pre-planned weekly menu. Food availability and children acceptability were taken into consideration by the research team when planning for the weekly snack menus. Snacks consisted of cheese or 'labneh' sandwiches, spinach pies, or thyme pastries (known as 'manakeesh'). In addition, children were offered fruits (oranges, apples, or bananas) twice a week, depending on seasonality, availability, and cost. The snack offered to children in the intervention schools supplied on average 357 kcal per day, 11 g protein, 58 g carbohydrates, and 9 g of fat. Dietary needs of children for calcium, iron, vitamins A and C were also considered as part of the snack planning and composition using the Dietary Reference Intakes (DRI) as a reference. Children in the control group also received standard daily snacks that consisted of thyme pastries, a locally-acceptable and affordable choice offered in public schools in the country. The standard snack supplied children on average with 294 kcal per day, 4.9 g protein, 31 g carbohydrates, and 17 g of fat. Children in the intervention and control schools found the offered snacks to be favorable and consumed them regularly. Only few children in the intervention schools expressed a preference to spread cheeses rather than locally-produced white cheese varieties at the beginning of the study, and were thus offered alternative sandwich options. It is worth noting that shortly afterwards, children expressed content with the offered white cheese options after noticing their peers in the school consuming and enjoying these varieties. All children in the intervention and control groups received daily snacks, regardless of their involvement in the study.

2.4. Data Collection (Instruments and Outcomes)

Face-to-face interviews with children and their mothers, who served as proxy respondents, were conducted by a team of trained field workers at the beginning of each of the academic years (September–October; 2015–2016 and 2016–2017) to collect baseline data. Measurements included sociodemographic characteristics of households, dietary knowledge, attitude and behavior (KAB) of children, as well as children's anthropometric measurements and dietary intake. Measurements of KAB, anthropometrics, and dietary intake were repeated at the end of each of the school years (May–June). Interviews lasted on average 45 min.

2.4.1. Socio-Demographic Characteristics

Information on child's gender and age, maternal age, educational level, employment, income, access to food assistance, and living conditions of household were obtained during interviews with the mother of the child. The crowding index (CI) is a proxy measure of household socio-economic status that has been previously used in Lebanon and other LMIC settings providing reliable results [41–43]. CI was calculated as the total number of household members divided by the total number of rooms in a household (excluding kitchens, bathrooms and balconies) [41]. Household food security status was also assessed using an Arabic-translated, locally validated version of the Household Food Insecurity Access Scale (HFIAS) [43]. The HFIAS consisted of nine questions that ask about modifications households made in their diet or food consumption patterns due to limited resources to acquire food, each of which can be answered as 'No', 'Rarely', 'Sometimes', and 'Often' with an individual score of "0", "1", "2", and "3", respectively. This 9-question scale produces a total score between 0 and 27 with higher scores indicating higher food insecurity [44].

2.4.2. Knowledge, Attitude and Behavior (KAB)

The dietary knowledge, attitude and behavior (KAB) of children were assessed at baseline and at 6 months follow-up using a 32-item questionnaire. The questionnaire included three sections: (1) nutrition knowledge section (15 questions); related to the importance of breakfast, fruits, vegetables and water consumption, healthy snacking, benefits of being physically active; (2) nutrition attitude section (10 questions); it included statements about healthy eating and making healthy food choices; and (3) dietary and lifestyle behaviors' section (7 questions), such as frequency of fruits, vegetables, dairy consumption, snacking, skipping meals and watching TV. The KAB-related questions were either formulated or adapted from published questionnaires and school-based studies conducted in Lebanon [14] and other middle-income country settings [12,40,45]. All questions were reviewed by one academic coordinator and 3 school teachers from the participating schools and were also pre-tested with 20 school children (aged 11–14 years) from the local Syrian refugee community to ensure accuracy, clarity and cultural-adequacy. Minor modifications were made to the questions according to feedback from children and teachers.

The questions on dietary knowledge, attitude and behaviors were separately analyzed. For the nutrition knowledge questions, each correct response was allocated a score of 1 point and an incorrect or no response was allocated 0 point. The total knowledge score ranged between 0 and 15 points with higher scores indicating the child displayed better nutritional knowledge. For the attitude statements, each question was measured on a 3-point Likert scale (1 = I agree, 2 = I am not sure, 3 = disagree) using faces that expressed these scales to make it easier for children to report their answers. The 10 attitude statements were also summed into a single score (range 0–10); whereby the favorable options (I agree) were given 1 point each and unfavorable options (I am not sure or disagree) were given 0 point. A higher attitude score reflected more positive attitude towards healthy eating. For questions related to dietary and lifestyle behaviors, favorable options were also given a score of 1 and unfavorable options were given a score of 0. The total behavior score ranged between 0 and 22 points with a higher score reflecting good dietary and lifestyle behaviors of children. Details related to the number of options for each of the KAB questions and the coding of correct answers are presented as supporting material (Table S1).

2.4.3. Dietary Intake

The dietary intake of children was assessed at baseline and at follow up by trained nutritionists using the 24-h dietary recall approach. Mothers were present at the time of the interview and served as proxy respondents. Interviewers followed the 5-steps USDA multiple pass method when collecting data on the food, beverage, and snack intake of children during the previous 24-h period or any other typical day during that week. Only few children reported dietary intake from a day different to that of the previous day. An atypical day included limited food availability at home for the child or the child was fasting for religious purposes during a month different than the fasting month of 'Ramadan', typically observed by Muslims. The steps included (1) the quick list; (2) the forgotten foods list; (3) time and occasion at which foods were consumed; (4) the detail cycle; and (5) the final probe [46]. To assist children and their mothers in assessing the portion sizes and amounts of food consumed at home and at school by the child, two-dimensional portion size posters, household measures and graduated food models were used (Millen and Morgan, Nutrition Consulting Enterprises, Framingham, MA, USA). Daily energy, macronutrient and micronutrient intake of children were computed from the 24-h recalls using the food composition database of the Nutritionist Pro software (Nutritionist Pro, Axxya Systems, San Bruno, CA, USA, version 5.1.0, 2018). The software food database was expanded by adding analyses of locally consumed foods and recipes [47]. Given that there are no gender- or age-specific DRIs for Middle Eastern populations, values arising from the analyzed data were compared to the US-based DRIs for children, as recommended by the Institute of Medicine [48].

2.4.4. Anthropometric Measures

Anthropometric measurements of children (weight, height, waist circumference) and their mothers (weight and height) were obtained by the trained nutritionists. Measurements were carried out only at baseline for mothers and at baseline and follow up for children using standard protocols and equipment. Weight was measured to the nearest 0.1 kg in light indoor clothing and with bare feet or stockings, using a portable standard calibrated balance (Seca model 877, Germany) and height was measured, without shoes, to the nearest 0.1 cm using a portable stadiometer (Seca, model 213, Hamburg, Germany). A non-stretchable measuring tape (Seca model 201, Germany) was used to measure waist circumference of children at the level of the umbilicus to the nearest 0.1 cm, with the subject standing and after normal expiration. All measurements were taken twice and the average of the 2 values was reported. Body mass index (BMI) (kg/m^2) was calculated by dividing the weight (kg) over the height squared (m^2). Mothers were categorized as normal, overweight or obese based on the WHO classifications [49]. Age and gender-specific BMI z-scores (BAZ), height for age z-scores (HAZ) and weight for age z-scores (WAZ) were calculated for children using the WHO Anthro Plus software (1.0.4) [50]. Children were classified as thin, normal weight, overweight, and obese based on the WHO age and gender-specific cut-offs [51]. Stunting and underweight were defined as HAZ < −2 SD and WAZ < −2 SD of the WHO child growth standards median, respectively [51]. In addition, the Waist to height ratio (WHtR) was calculated by dividing waist circumference (WC) by height, both measured in centimetres [52]. The cut-off point of ≥0.5 was used to identify children with elevated WHtR, an indicator of abdominal obesity among children [52,53].

2.5. Data Analysis

Data were entered and analyzed using Stata/SE version 12 (StataCorp., College Station, TX, USA). Descriptive statistics were performed and presented as means and standard error (SE) for continuous variables or as frequencies and proportions for categorical variables. At baseline, comparisons of sociodemographic and anthropometric characteristics of participants between intervention and control groups were assessed using clustered independent *t*-tests and chi-square analyses (stata command clttest and clchi). Paired *t*-tests were used to compare independently the differences in KAB scores, energy and nutrient intakes between baseline and 6-months follow up within each of the intervention and control groups (within-group differences). In addition, between-group differences (intervention versus (vs.) control groups) in mean changes of scores (i.e., follow-up minus baseline scores) were evaluated using clustered independent *t*-tests. Additionally, two-way analysis of variance was conducted to test differences in mean changes of KAB scores and anthropometric measurements between intervention/control and school year. No significant interactions were found between group status and school year with mean change in dietary knowledge, attitude or behavior scores and with anthropometric measurements ($p > 0.05$). Multiple linear regression analyses were conducted to test the effect of the nutrition intervention on mean changes in dietary KAB and anthropometric measures (BMI for age *z*-score (BAZ), waist to height ratio (WHtR), HAZ, and WAZ) among children, adjusting for covariates found significantly different at baseline between intervention and control groups. In case two variables were highly correlated (*p*-value < 0.001), then one of the variables was excluded from the model to avoid multicollinearity. Linear regressions were performed using the wild cluster bootstrap-t procedure (stata command cgmwildboot) [54,55]. This procedure provides adequate power and desirable false rejection rates for performing statistical inference, even for data with small numbers of clusters [55]. Sensitivity analyses were conducted to determine whether our conclusions were biased by incomplete data. We accounted for missing values, which were assumed to be missing at random, using a simulation-based statistical technique (namely, multiple imputations). Imputed models showed that the majority of results were similar to the complete case analyses; see Tables S2 and S3 in supportive material. A *p*-value of <0.05 was considered statistically significant.

3. Results

Survey data were collected at baseline from 296 school children out of 318 that were contacted to take part in the study (93% response rate). Data at baseline and at follow up was available for 203 children (completion rate = 68.6%). The sample size was reduced to $n = 183$ due to clustering effect. At baseline, the mean age of children was 11.04 ± 0.23 years with an approximately equal gender distribution among the study sample (50.7% females and 49.3% males). Almost a third of their mothers had intermediate level education or more, whereas 42% of fathers had similar educational levels. The majority of mothers (94.4%) and 43% of fathers were unemployed. Approximately 63% of households reported an average monthly income less than 200 USD and the majority received some form of assistance in the past three months, either in the form of food baskets, e-card, or as conditional cash. Significant socio-demographic and anthropometric differences were observed between the intervention and control groups at baseline ($p < 0.05$) and are presented in Table 1. No significant differences were noted between intervention and control groups at baseline with respect to dietary knowledge (range 0–15) and behavior scores (range 0–22). However, dietary attitude scores (range 0–10) were found to be on average significantly higher at baseline among children in the intervention compared to the control group (8.18 ± 0.18 vs. 7.47 ± 0.23, $p = 0.047$).

Table 1. Baseline socio-demographic and anthropometric characteristics of school-aged children enrolled in intervention and control elementary schools in the Bekaa region, Lebanon ($n = 203$).

	Total Sample ($n = 203$)	Intervention ($n = 114$)	Control ($n = 89$)	p-Value [1]
Socio-demographic characteristics				
Child's age (years), Mean ± Standard Error (SE)	11.04 ± 0.23	11.16 ± 0.31	10.89 ± 0.47	0.651
Child's gender, n (%)				
Males	100 (49.3)	58 (50.9)	42 (47.2)	0.458
Females	103 (50.7)	56 (49.1)	47 (52.8)	
Mother's age (years), Mean ± SE	35.75 ± 0.41	36.16 ± 0.67	35.25 ± 0.75	0.395
Mother's education, n (%)				0.0001
No school	51 (25.9)	18 (16.2)	33 (38.4)	
Primary school	76 (38.6)	37 (33.3)	39 (45.3)	
≥Intermediate school	70 (35.5)	56 (50.5)	14 (16.3)	
Mother's employment, n (%)				0.910
Unemployed	186 (94.4)	105 (94.6)	81 (94.2)	
Employed	11 (5.6)	6 (5.4)	5 (5.8)	
Father's education, n (%)				0.003
No school	35 (17.9)	11 (10.0)	24 (27.9)	
Primary school	78 (39.8)	45 (40.9)	33 (38.4)	
≥Intermediate school	83 (42.3)	54 (49.1)	29 (33.7)	
Father's employment, n (%)				0.715
Unemployed	84 (43.1)	47 (42.7)	37 (43.5)	
Employed	111(56.9)	63 (57.3)	48 (56.5)	
Monthly income (USD dollars), n (%)				0.754
<200	121 (62.7)	70 (64.8)	51 (60.0)	
200–399	61 (31.6)	31 (28.7)	30 (35.3)	
≥400	11 (5.7)	7 (6.5)	4 (4.7)	
Crowding index [2], Mean ± SE	5.83 ± 0.53	4.72 ± 0.26	7.14 ±0.28	0.0004
Household Food insecurity score, Mean ± SE	15.37 ± 0.71	14.31 ± 0.83	16.64 ± 1.09	0.132
Household Food Insecurity status [3], n (%)				0.021
Non-severely food insecure	41 (20.9)	30 (27.3)	11 (12.8)	
Severely food insecure	155 (79.1)	80 (72.7)	75 (87.2)	
Receive assistance (Yes), n (%)	161 (82.6)	88 (80.0)	73 (85.9)	0.250
Food assistance: food basket [4] (Yes), n (%)	43 (22.1)	17 (15.5)	26 (30.6)	0.010
Food assistance: e-card [5] (Yes), n (%)	152 (77.9)	80 (72.7)	72 (84.7)	0.069
Conditional cash [6] (Yes), n (%)	12 (6.2)	6 (5.5)	6 (7.1)	0.670

Table 1. *Cont.*

	Total Sample (n = 203)	Intervention (n = 114)	Control (n = 89)	p-Value [1]
Anthropometric characteristics [7]				
Mothers (n = 171)				
Body Mass Index (BMI) (kg/m^2), Mean ± SE	29.66 ± 0.35	29.09 ± 0.59	30.33 ± 0.64	0.197
BMI status [8], n (%)				0.189
Normal (≤24.9 kg/m^2)	35 (18.5)	22 (21.4)	13 (15.1)	
Overweight (25.0–29.9 kg/m^2)	67 (35.4)	39 (37.9)	28 (32.6)	
Obese (≥30 kg/m^2)	87 (46.0)	42 (40.8)	45 (52.3)	
Children				
Weight (kg), Mean ± SE	35.62 ± 1.37	37.24 ± 1.62	33.58 ± 2.34	0.239
Height (cm), Mean ± SE	141.63 ± 1.70	143.86 ± 1.98	138.82 ± 2.89	0.193
Waist Circumference (cm), Mean ± SE	67.27 ± 1.03	68.22 ± 1.43	66.10 ± 2.02	0.412
BMI for Age Z-score (BAZ), Mean ± SE	0.03 ± 0.06	0.11 ± 0.10	−0.06 ± 0.12	0.297
BAZ, n (%)				0.524
Thin (BAZ ≤ −2)	5 (2.5)	2 (1.8)	3 (3.4)	
Normal (−2 < BAZ ≤ +1)	162 (80.6)	87 (77.7)	75 (84.3)	
Overweight (+1 < BAZ ≤ +2)	22 (10.9)	14 (12.5)	8 (9.0)	
Obese (BAZ > +2)	12 (6.0)	9 (8.0)	3 (3.4)	
Waist to Height ratio (WHtR), Mean ± SE	0.48 ± 0.003	0.48 ± 0.006	0.48 ± 0.007	0.926
WHtR, n (%)				
WHtR < 0.5	142 (75.1)	76 (71.0)	66 (80.5)	
WHtR ≥ 0.5 (elevated)	47 (24.9)	31 (29.0)	16 (19.5)	
Height for age Z-score (HAZ), Mean ± SE	−0.40 ± 0.11	−0.16 ± 0.11	−0.71 ± 0.12	0.011
HAZ, n (%)				0.438
HAZ ≥ −2	178 (88.6)	100 (89.3)	78 (87.6)	
HAZ < −2 (stunted)	23 (11.4)	12 (10.7)	11 (12.4)	
Weight for age Z-score (WAZ) [9], Mean ± SE	−0.003 ± 0.21	0.31 ± 0.39	−0.34 ± 0.58	0.418
WAZ, n (%)				0.538
WAZ ≥ −2	74 (96.1)	37 (97.4)	37(94.9)	
WAZ < −2 (underweight)	3 (3.9)	1 (2.6)	2 (5.1)	
Knowledge Attitude Behavior (KAB) scores [10]				
Knowledge scores, Mean ± SE	9.85 ± 0.14	10.06 ± 0.20	9.69 ± 0.22	0.260
Attitude scores, Mean ± SE	7.88 ± 0.20	8.18 ± 0.18	7.47 ± 0.23	0.047
Behavior scores, Mean ± SE	9.07 ± 0.46	9.82 ± 0.53	8.31 ± 0.71	0.133

[1] Comparison of baseline characteristics between intervention and control groups was conducted for continuous and for categorical variables using clustered independent and chi-squared tests. Statistical significance was determined at p-value <0.05. [2] Crowding index: the average number of people per room, excluding the kitchen and bathroom. [3] Households were grouped into four levels of food insecurity: food secure (2.6%); mildly food insecure (2.5%); moderately food insecure (15.8%); and severely food insecure (79.1%). [4] World Food Programme (WFP) distributes a food basket tailored to beneficiaries' nutrition needs, preferences, activity levels and other factors (climate condition, demographic profile, and existing levels of malnutrition and disease [56]. [5] WFP provides electronic vouchers that allow beneficiaries to purchase food at local shops [57]. [6] Cash transfers given to stimulate beneficiaries to invest in their health, nutrition and education [58]. [7] Anthropometric measurements of mothers and children were categorized based on World Health Organization (WHO) classification [49,51]. [8] Mothers with underweight BMI (n = 3) were added to the normal BMI group. [9] Weight for age z-scores were assessed only for children ≤10 years old (n = 68) as per the WHO growth charts [51]. [10] The total knowledge, behavior and attitude scores ranged: 0–15 points, 0–10 points and 0–22 points, respectively.

Table 2 presents between-group differences (intervention versus control) with respect to mean change from baseline to 6-months follow up in dietary knowledge, attitude and behavior scores as well as anthropometric measures of children in the study sample. Compared to the control group, a greater change in knowledge scores was observed among the intervention group (2.25 ± 0.22 vs. 0.89 ± 0.24, p = 0.002). Similarly, greater changes in BAZ and HAZ scores were noted among children in the intervention compared to control groups, (0.10 ± 0.06 vs. −0.10 ± 0.08, p = 0.039 and 0.39 ± 0.04 vs. 0.24 ± 0.05, p = 0.024). No other significant differences in mean changes of attitude, behavior, WAZ scores and WHtR were noted between intervention and control groups. Within-group differences in KAB and anthropometric measures were presented in Table S4, as supplementary material.

Using linear regression models, the mean change in dietary knowledge scores increased on average by 1.22 units (95% CI = 0.54, 1.89; $p < 0.001$) among children in the intervention compared to the control group, even after adjusting for other covariates (Table 3). Similarly, the mean change in dietary attitude scores increased by 0.69 units (95% CI = 0.08, 1.30, $p = 0.026$) in the intervention group within the regression model, while the mean change in behavior scores was not found to be significantly different by group status (intervention vs. control) (see Table 3).

Table 2. Between-group differences (intervention versus control) in mean change of nutrition knowledge, attitude, behavior scores and anthropometric measures of school-aged children ($n = 183$).

	Intervention ($n = 102$)	Control ($n = 81$)	p-Value [1]
	Mean Change ± SE		
Knowledge Attitude Behavior (KAB) scores [2]			
Knowledge scores	2.25 ± 0.22	0.89 ± 0.24	0.002
Attitude scores	0.97 ± 0.17	0.82 ± 0.19	0.294
Behavior scores	0.36 ± 0.72	0.43 ± 0.96	0.521
Anthropometric measurements			
BMI for Age Z-score (BAZ)	0.10 ± 0.06	−0.10 ± 0.08	0.039
Waist to Height ratio (WHtR)	−0.01 ± 0.008	−0.02 ± 0.008	0.260
Height for age Z-score (HAZ)	0.39 ± 0.04	0.24 ± 0.05	0.024
Weight for age Z-score (WAZ) [3]	0.32 ± 0.12	0.08 ± 0.18	0.177

[1] Differences in mean changes (follow up minus baseline) of KAB scores and anthropometric measures between intervention and control groups were conducted using clustered independent tests. Statistical significance was determined at p-value < 0.05. [2] The total knowledge, behavior and attitude scores ranged: 0–15 points, 0–10 points and 0–22 points, respectively. [3] Weight for age z-scores were assessed only for children ≤10 years old ($n = 68$) as per the WHO growth charts [51].

Table 3. General linear regression models for mean change in nutrition knowledge, attitude and behavior scores among school-aged children in the study sample † ($n = 183$).

	Mean Change in Knowledge Scores Adjusted β (95% CI)	Mean Change in Attitude Scores Adjusted β (95% CI)	Mean Change in Behavior Scores Adjusted β (95% CI)
Group status (Intervention)	1.22 (0.54, 1.89), $p < 0.001$	0.69 (0.08, 1.30), $p = 0.026$	−0.20 (−2.53, 2.14)
School year (Year 2)	0.26 (−0.63, 1.15)	−0.63 (−1.07, −0.19), $p = 0.005$	0.37 (−0.99, 1.73)
Child's age	−0.18 (−0.49, 0.13)	0.02 (−0.24, 0.28)	1.56 (0.45, 2.68), $p = 0.006$
Gender (Females)	0.04 (−0.60, 0.68)	0.33 (−0.26, 0.93)	0.80 (−1.06, 2.65)
Mother's education			
No school (Ref.)	—	—	—
Primary	−0.19 (−1.04, 0.65)	0.02 (−0.80, 0.84)	−1.54 (−3.82, 0.75)
Intermediate to higher	0.02 (−0.89, 0.93)	−0.17 (−0.97, 0.62)	−1.73 (−4.28, 0.83)
Father's education			
No school (Ref.)	—	—	—
Primary	−0.54 (−1.14, 0.06)	−0.29 (−0.98, 0.40)	−1.23 (−3.50, 1.03)
Intermediate to higher	−1.59(−2.14, −1.05), $p < 0.001$	−0.54 (−1.32, 0.23)	−0.07 (−2.39, 2.25)
Crowding Index	−0.01 (−0.17, 0.15)	0.12 (0.01, 0.24), $p = 0.040$	0.05 (−0.25, 0.35)
Food basket (Yes)	−0.84 (−1.38, −0.30), $p = 0.002$	0.67 (−0.01, 1.36)	1.50 (−0.68, 3.69)
Household food insecurity status			
Non-severely food insecure (Ref.)	—	—	—
Severely food insecure	−0.40 (−1.13, 0.32)	0.19 (−0.35, 0.74)	2.20 (0.93, 3.48), $p = 0.001$
Height for age Z-score (HAZ)	0.23 (−0.01, 0.46)	−0.12 (−0.36, 0.13)	0.53 (−0.02, 1.08)

† Variables adjusted for in the three models testing the impact of group status were variables found significantly different at baseline between intervention group (IG) and control group (CG). These variables include school year, child's age, mother's and father's educational levels, crowding index, receiving assistance (food basket), household food insecurity status, and children's anthropometric measures (HAZ).

As for the anthropometric measures, there was a significant increase in mean BAZ scores among children in the intervention compared to the control group (β = 0.25, 95% CI =0.10, 0.41; p = 0.001). No other significant differences were noted between intervention and control groups in the regression models with respect to WAZ, HAZ, or WHtR (see Table 4).

Table 4. General linear regression models for mean change in anthropometric measurements (BAZ, WHtR, HAZ, and WAZ) among school-aged children in the study sample [1] (n = 183).

	Mean Change in BAZ Adjusted β (95% CI)	Mean Change in WHtR Adjusted β (95% CI)	Mean Change in HAZ Adjusted β (95% CI)	Mean Change in WAZ [2] Adjusted β (95% CI)
Group status (Intervention)	0.25 (0.10, 0.41), p = 0.001	0.02 (−0.01, 0.05)	0.19 (−0.07, 0.45)	0.25 (−0.04, 0.54)
School year (Year 2)	−0.05 (−0.14, 0.04)	0.01 (−0.03, 0.05)	−0.11 (−0.24, 0.02)	−0.05 (−0.11, −0.003), p = 0.039
Mother's education				
No school (Ref.)	—	—	—	—
Primary	0.01 (−20, 0.22)	0.02 (−0.06, 0.11)	0.10 (−0.80, 0.28)	0.02 (−0.13, 0.17)
Intermediate to higher	−0.04 (−0.22, 0.13)	−0.002 (−0.07, 0.06)	0.06 (−0.30, 0.42)	0.04 (0.02, 0.06), p < 0.001
Father's education				
No school (Ref.)	—	—	—	—
Primary	−0.17 (−0.35, −0.001), p = 0.048	−0.02 (−0.07, 0.03)	−0.04 (−0.34, 0.26)	−0.15 (−0.22, −0.07), p < 0.001
Intermediate to higher	−0.17 (−0.39, 0.06), p < 0.001	−0.002 (−0.06, 0.05)	0.01 (−43, 0.44)	−0.16 (−0.23, −0.10), p < 0.001
Crowding Index	−0.01 (−0.03, 0.01)	0.002 (−0.05, 0.01)	0.01 (−0.02, 0.05)	−0.002 (−0.02, 0.01)
Food basket (Yes)	0.05 (−0.21, 0.30)	0.02 (−0.02, 0.06)	0.07 (−0.02, 0.16)	−0.004 (−0.17, 0.16)
Household food insecurity status				
Non-severely food insecure (Ref.)	—	—	—	—
Severely food insecure	0.02 (−0.10, 0.15)	0.008 (−0.01, 0.03)	0.06 (−0.14, 0.26)	0.01 (−0.07, 0.09)

[1] Variables adjusted for in the three models testing the impact of group status were variables found significantly different at baseline between IG and CG. These variables include school year, mother's and father's educational levels, crowding index, receiving assistance (food basket), and household food insecurity status. [2] Weight for age z-scores were assessed only for children ≤10 years old (n = 68) as per the WHO growth charts [51].

Between-group differences (intervention vs. control) with respect to mean change of energy intake and macro-and micro-nutrients are presented in Table 5. Compared to the control group, children in the intervention group had on average significantly higher mean changes in daily intakes of total energy (kcal), dietary fiber, protein, and saturated fat (p < 0.05). In addition, children in the intervention group had significantly higher mean changes in intakes of key micronutrients, including vitamin K (p < 0.001), zinc (p = 0.037), calcium (p = 0.017), and magnesium (p = 0.007). It was also noted that between-group differences for vitamin E and phosphorus approached statistical significance (p = 0.05). Within-group differences were also noted in the study sample and were presented in supportive material (Table S5).

Table 5. Between-group differences (intervention versus control) in mean change of total energy (kcal/day) and macro-and micronutrient intakes (g/day) among school-aged children (n = 183).

	Intervention (n = 102)	Control (n = 81)	
	Mean Change Mean ± SE		p-Value †
Energy intake (Kcal)	94.71 ± 68.80	−110.00 ± 77.02	0.0469
Macronutrients			
Carbohydrates (g)	9.76 ± 9.89	−8.31 ± 11.07	0.132
Sugar (g)	−1.36 ± 3.63	0.99 ± 4.07	0.661
Dietary fiber (g)	1.03 ± 1.01	−2.60 ± 1.19	0.027
Protein (g)	5.95 ± 1.94	−0.38 ± 2.17	0.033
Total fat (g)	3.25 ± 4.60	−8.35 ± 5.17	0.064
MUFA (g)	1.76 ± 3.49	−5.45 ± 4.76	0.130
PUFA (g)	−6.45 ± 1.07	−2.04 ± 1.25	0.212
Saturated fat (g)	1.48 ± 0.82	−1.76 ± 0.92	0.017
Trans fat (g)	−0.05 ± 0.04	0.03 ± 0.05	0.893

Table 5. *Cont.*

	Intervention (n = 102)	Control (n = 81)	
	Mean Change Mean ± SE		p-Value †
Micronutrients			
Vitamin C (mg)	10.41 ± 5.27	0.08 ± 5.90	0.116
Vitamin A (μg)	90.31 ± 53.18	−0.05 ± 69.22	0.167
Vitamin D (μg)	0.34 ± 0.20	0.12 ± 0.22	0.242
Vitamin E (mg)	0.12 ± 0.65	−1.70 ± 0.75	0.055
Vitamin K (μg)	124.08 ± 20.49	−36.90 ± 24.87	0.0001
Vitamin B1 (mg)	0.10 ± 0.08	−0.0001 ± 0.08	0.196
Vitamin B2 (mg)	0.08 ± 0.18	−0.01 ± 0.22	0.375
Vitamin B3 (mg)	1.36 ± 0.79	−0.03 ± 0.88	0.140
Vitamin B6 (mg)	0.11 ± 0.05	−0.01 ± 0.06	0.094
Vitamin B12 (μg)	0.06 ± 0.24	0.24 ± 0.30	0.676
Folate (μg)	12.41 ± 24.10	−19.97 ± 32.24	0.224
Iron (mg)	0.94 ± 1.21	−2.40 ± 1.65	0.073
Zinc (mg)	0.30 ± 0.55	−1.58 ± 0.70	0.037
Calcium (mg)	141.19 ± 40.61	−28.75 ± 50.59	0.017
Phosphorus (mg)	73.11 ± 34.11	−23.73 ± 38.20	0.050
Magnesium (mg)	26.76 ± 9.32	−18.29 ± 10.43	0.007
Sodium (g)	0.25 ± 0.13	0.03 ± 0.14	0.143
Potassium (g)	0.18 ± 0.10	−0.03 ± 0.12	0.109

† Differences in mean changes of nutrient intakes between intervention and control groups were conducted using clustered independent tests. Statistical significance was determined at p-value < 0.05.

4. Discussion

The present study evaluated the impact of a pilot school-based nutrition intervention on the dietary knowledge, attitude, behaviors and nutritional status of refugee children enrolled in primary-level informal schools. To the best of our knowledge, this is the first school-based nutrition intervention that combines nutrition education with provision of healthy snacks among primary-level school children residing in refugee camp settings.

Findings from this pilot nutrition intervention suggest significant improvements in the dietary knowledge and attitude of children post-intervention, even after adjusting for other covariates. These results are consistent with findings from previous school-based interventions conducted among primary-school children in LMIC settings [12,14,38,59]. The positive results in the present study could be explained by the adoption of a theory-driven approach in our intervention, mainly the social cognitive theory, when developing the nutrition and health educational curriculum. Examples are the use of evidence-base constructs suggested to be effective in changing dietary knowledge and behaviors [60,61], such as observational learning through the role modeling of healthful behaviors by school teachers and promoting behavioral capability and self-efficacy among children through games and activities that build the confidence of children to identify what are healthy meal and snack choices, and how to not skip breakfast and engage in fun and culturally-acceptable physical activities within their context. In addition, the use of a multi-component approach that included classroom-based health and nutrition education combined with provision of healthy snacks could have contributed to the positive increases in children's knowledge scores and to improvement in their attitude scores.

On the other hand, mean change in behavior scores was not found to be significantly different between children from the intervention and control groups in the regression models. This finding was not surprising as other school-based studies conducted in LMIC settings have shown mixed results with respect to behavioral changes and outcomes. The HEALTH-E-PALS, a multi-component school-based pilot intervention conducted in Lebanon among primary-level school children (9–11 years), showed significant improvements in the nutritional knowledge, self-efficacy, and children's dietary behaviors, such as daily breakfast intake and lower consumption of chips and sweetened drinks, yet limited to no significant increases in fruits and vegetables intake or in the children's physical activity-related behaviors. Similarly, Francis et al., 2010 reported reductions in intakes of sugar, fat and salt-dense snacks and sodas, but no significant impact on the physical activity level of primary-school children enrolled in a short-term school-based nutrition and physical activity intervention in Trinidad and Tobago [38]. On the other hand, the HealthKick, a primary school nutrition intervention conducted in low-income schools in Western Cape Province (South Africa), showed no significant improvements in the snacking behaviors or the overall diet quality of grade 4 children [27].

Differences in results between our study and others may be attributed to a number of factors, such as variations in intervention components, duration, or mode of delivery of intervention (by school teachers vs. dedicated research team members or expert dietitians). Evidence in this field also shows that nutrition education may improve the knowledge of children towards healthy eating and active lifestyles; however, changing behaviors is a much more complex process that may be influenced by a multitude of economic, environmental, cultural and social factors [39,62,63]. In the case of the present study, it is worth considering the unique study population and the harsh context where the school intervention was conducted within informal tented settlements (refugee camps). In fact, baseline results show that the majority of children's households in the study sample were experiencing severe forms of food insecurity, had low socioeconomic status, and were dependent on some form of humanitarian assistance. The poor living conditions of Syrian refugee children in parallel with the limited resources available for their families within a refugee camp setting [64,65] can make it reasonably challenging for children to access adequate food resources or make healthy dietary and lifestyle choices, despite the significant improvements in their dietary knowledge. Other factors that may hinder the ability of children to make significant behavioral changes may be related to their psychological and mental health status. Most school-based interventions conducted within similar refugee settings report the high levels of anxiety, fear, and depression experienced by children after fleeing a war [26,27,66], in addition to the daily environmental stressors that they are exposed to in the host country making healthier dietary choices more challenging and less attainable [67,68].

Our pilot intervention showed improvements in the dietary intake of refugee children as assessed using the 24-h recall data. Compared to the control group, children in the intervention group had on average significantly larger increases in intakes of total energy (kcal), dietary fiber, protein, and saturated fats, as well as larger increases in intakes of vitamin K, zinc calcium, and magnesium. These dietary changes may be attributed to the healthy snacks provided to children during the school days. In fact, the snacks contributed on average to a 357 kcal per day, representing 16% of daily dietary needs of children in this age group, while also meeting their daily needs for several micronutrients, including calcium, iron, vitamins A and C (11–77% of dietary reference intakes). Although the mean change in intake of saturated fats was significantly higher among children in the intervention compared to the control group, this increase may be explained by the consumption of full-fat dairy products, which are rich in saturated fats. Nevertheless, dairy products represent a rich source of protein and micronutrients including calcium, phosphorus and B-vitamins, and these products were not frequently consumed among refugee children in the study sample. In addition, when examining the intake of saturated fats as percent of total daily energy intake at follow up among children in the intervention group, it was found to contribute to 7.2% of energy intake, which is still below the WHO upper limits for saturated fat in this age group [69].

Findings from the present study showed a significant increase in mean BAZ scores among children in the intervention group compared to control, even after adjusting for other covariates. Nevertheless, the mean changes in WHtR (an indicator of abdominal obesity) [52,53] was not found to be statistically significant between the intervention and control groups. In fact, when considering within-group analyses, results showed that the proportion of overweight children did not differ significantly between baseline and follow up within the intervention (20.5% vs. 21.4%) or control groups (12.5% vs. 9.1%), rather the proportion of thin children decreased slightly in the intervention group (1.8% to 0.8%) while it increased in the control group (3.4% to 4.5%), see supportive material Table S6. Although, HAZ and WAZ scores were not found to be statistically significant between the intervention and control groups in the complete case analysis, a larger increase in these scores could have been detected with a larger sample size, as observed in the imputed models (Tables S2 and S3). These results suggest that the intervention did not contribute to an increase in overweight and obesity levels among children in the study sample, but rather to a potential improvement in their overall growth. This increase could be explained by increases in energy intake among children receiving the healthy snacks as part of the school intervention or it can be attributed to improvements in some of the dietary behaviors of children post-intervention, even though the overall behavior scores did not reach statistical significance. A previously published Cochrane review that examined the effectiveness of obesity-prevention interventions supported the beneficial impact that programs conducted in schools can have on BMI of children, particularly targeting those aged 6–12 years [70]. Interventions that were found to be promising in that review were those that included a school curriculum addressing healthy eating and physical activity, improving the nutritional quality of foods offered at schools and teacher involvement, many of which were covered in the present study.

The present study has a number of strengths. This is the first study, to the best of our knowledge, evaluating the impact of a multi-component school-based nutrition intervention on dietary knowledge, behaviors and nutritional status of primary-level school children residing in refugee camp settings. The sustainability of the intervention beyond the study duration was considered through training school teachers on the educational curriculum and the establishment of cooking units within schools and training kitchen employees to plan and prepare safe and nutritious snacks for children during the school year. Another strength of the study is the overall acceptability and satisfaction of children with the health and nutrition educational sessions and daily snack choices as assessed through field observations, student evaluations, and meetings with teachers and school administration.

Although the findings of this pilot intervention were promising, the study has a number of limitations that need to be considered. First, the study was conducted in one area of the country with a small number of schools that may not be representative of the entire refugee population. Differences between intervention and control groups were also noted at baseline and may have biased the results. However, adjustments for all covariates found to be statistically significant between both groups were done in the regression models. Lessons learned from this pilot intervention can provide insights for future studies to be conducted in similar vulnerable population groups in order to reduce potential selection bias between intervention and control groups. For example, the duration of the refugees' stay in the host country and their place of residence (rural or urban context) prior to migration are important to consider when setting the inclusion and exclusion criteria, as these factors may contribute to their socioeconomic, cultural background and potential differences. Another limitation of the study is the use of a single 24-h recall to estimate dietary intake, which may have been subject to recall bias. Nevertheless, every attempt was exerted to minimize recall bias through collecting dietary data from children in the presence of their mothers (as proxy respondents). In addition, interviewers were trained nutritionists who received extensive training to reduce judgmental verbal and non-verbal communication and underwent a 2-day training workshop to ensure the standardization of data collection protocol. The research team also faced several challenges when conducting this intervention, such as the high turnover of teachers in schools due to their refugee status and their relocation into other areas in Lebanon or immigration to other countries. Nevertheless, training of new teachers was conducted throughout the school year, in addition to the pre-scheduled training and refresher workshops at the beginning and middle of the academic year to ensure fidelity to the intervention protocol. Another limitation was the high attrition rate (31.4%) noted in the study and that can be attributed to the low attendance of children at the end of the school year when post-intervention visits were scheduled, as children were skipping school days to assist their families in agriculture-related activities during the harvest season. Nevertheless, sensitivity analyses showed that the majority of results were still similar between the complete case and imputed model analyses.

In conclusion, findings from the present study suggest a promising impact of a combined nutrition education and healthy snack intervention on the dietary knowledge and nutritional status of refugee primary-school children. Future studies are needed to test the feasibility of scaling up such nutrition interventions within low-income and conflict-affected settings and to evaluate their long-term impact on children's overall health and nutritional status.

Supplementary Materials: The following are available online at http://www.mdpi.com/2072-6643/10/7/913/s1, Figure S1: Flow diagram for study Participants; Table S1: Dietary and lifestyle-related knowledge attitude and behavior (KAB) questionnaire and coding criteria; Tables S2 and S3: Imputed general linear regression models for mean change in nutrition knowledge, attitude and behavior scores among school-aged children in the study sample ($n = 296$); Table S4: Within-group differences (baseline versus follow up) in mean change of nutrition knowledge, attitude, behavior scores and anthropometric measures of school-aged children ($n = 183$); Table S5: Within-group differences (baseline versus follow up) in mean change of total energy (kcal/day) and macro- and micronutrient intakes (g/day) among school-aged children ($n = 178$); Table S6: Post-intervention nutritional status of school-aged children enrolled in intervention and control elementary schools in the Bekaa region, Lebanon ($n = 183$).

Author Contributions: L.J. conceptualized the research design and objectives and coordinated data collection, entry and analysis. M.D.E.H. collected and analyzed data and contributed to the writing of the manuscript. S.K. provided substantial statistical advice and contributed to data interpretation. S.K.H. contributed to the overall design and implementation of the intervention. All authors read and approved the final manuscript.

Funding: This study was funded by the Reach Out to Asia (ROTA): Education Above All Foundation in Qatar, as part of the GHATA project.

Acknowledgments: The authors would like to first express their sincere gratitude to all study participants and to school teachers and staff who contributed to the delivery of this project. We also would like to thank the Center for Civic Engagement and Community Services, Kayany Foundation, and the Environment and Sustainable Development Unit at the American University of Beirut for the field support provided. We would like to extend our appreciation to all the field workers and to the following people for their relentless support and dedication during the study period: Romy Abi Fadel, Rabih Shibli, Hala Fleihan Lamia Masri, Dominique Anid, and Marwa Soubra.

Conflicts of Interest: The authors declare no conflict of interest. The founding sponsors had no role in the design of the study; in the collection, analyses, or interpretation of data; in the writing of the manuscript, and in the decision to publish the results.

References

1. Figures at a Glance. Available online: http://www.unhcr.org/afr/figures-at-a-glance.html (accessed on 24 April 2018).
2. Refugees: Risks and Challenges Worldwide. Available online: https://www.migrationpolicy.org/article/refugees-risks-and-challenges-worldwide (accessed on 17 April 2018).
3. Food Insecurity in Households with Children: Prevalence, Severity, and Household Characteristics, 2010–11. Available online: https://www.ers.usda.gov/webdocs/publications/43763/37672_eib-113.pdf?v=41424 (accessed on 5 March 2018).

4. Nord, M. What have we learned from two decades of research on household food security? *Public Health Nutr.* **2014**, *17*, 2–4. [CrossRef]
5. Bronte-Tinkew, J.; Zaslow, M.; Capps, R.; Horowitz, A.; McNamara, M. Food insecurity works through depression, parenting, and infant feeding to influence overweight and health in toddlers. *J. Nutr.* **2007**, *137*, 2160–2165. [CrossRef] [PubMed]
6. Gundersen, C.G.; Garasky, S.B. Financial Management Skills Are Associated with Food Insecurity in a Sample of Households with Children in the United States. *J. Nutr.* **2012**, *142*, 1865–1870. [CrossRef] [PubMed]
7. Schmeer, K.K.; Piperata, B.A. Household food insecurity and child health. *Matern. Child Nutr.* **2017**, *13*. [CrossRef] [PubMed]
8. Collier, E.; Grant, M.J. A literature review on the experience of long-term mental illness. *Issues Ment. Health Nurs.* **2017**, 1–8. [CrossRef] [PubMed]
9. Abuhaloob, L.; Carson, S.; Richards, D.; Freeman, R. Community-based nutrition intervention to promote oral health and restore healthy body weight in refugee children: A scoping review. *Community Dent. Health* **2018**, *35*, 81–88. [CrossRef] [PubMed]
10. Carroll, G.J.; Lama, S.D.; Martinez-Brockman, J.L.; Pérez-Escamilla, R. Evaluation of Nutrition Interventions in Children in Conflict Zones: A Narrative Review. *Adv. Nutr.* **2017**, *8*, 770–779. [CrossRef] [PubMed]
11. Hossain, S.M.; Leidman, E.; Kingori, J.; Al Harun, A.; Bilukha, O.O. Nutritional situation among Syrian refugees hosted in Iraq, Jordan, and Lebanon: Cross sectional surveys. *Confl. Health* **2016**, *10*, 26. [CrossRef] [PubMed]
12. Zalilah, M.; Siti, S.; Norlijah, O.; Normah, H.; Maznah, I.; Zubaidah, J. Nutrition education intervention improves nutrition knowledge, attitude and practices of primary school children: a pilot study. *Int. Electron. J. Health Educ.* **2008**, *11*, 119–132.
13. Piperata, B.A.; Schmeer, K.K.; Hadley, C.; Ritchie-Ewing, G. Dietary inequalities of mother–child pairs in the rural Amazon: Evidence of maternal-child buffering? *Soc. Sci. Med.* **2013**, *96*, 183–191. [CrossRef] [PubMed]
14. Habib-Mourad, C.; Ghandour, L.A.; Moore, H.J.; Nabhani-Zeidan, M.; Adetayo, K.; Hwalla, N.; Summerbell, C. Promoting healthy eating and physical activity among school children: findings from Health-E-PALS, the first pilot intervention from Lebanon. *BMC Public Health* **2014**, *14*, 940. [CrossRef] [PubMed]
15. Global School-Based Student Health Survey. 2011. Available online: http://www.who.int/ncds/surveillance/gshs/2011_Lebanon_GSHS_Questionnaire.pdf (accessed on 17 April 2018).
16. Assessing the Nutritional Status of Primary School Children in Wakiso District Uganda. 2013. Available online: http://d-scholarship.pitt.edu/17928/ (accessed on 21 June 2018).
17. School Age Children their Health and Nutrition. 2002. Available online: https://www.unscn.org/web/archives_resources/files/scnnews25.pdf (accessed on June 21 2018).
18. Prentice, A.M.; Ward, K.A.; Goldberg, G.R.; Jarjou, L.M.; Moore, S.E.; Fulford, A.J.; Prentice, A. Critical windows for nutritional interventions against stunting. *Am. J. Clin. Nutr.* **2013**, *97*, 911–918. [CrossRef] [PubMed]
19. Black, R.E.; Victora, C.G.; Walker, S.P.; Bhutta, Z.A.; Christian, P.; De Onis, M.; Ezzati, M.; Grantham-McGregor, S.; Katz, J.; Martorell, R.; et al. Maternal and child undernutrition and overweight in low-income and middle-income countries. *Lancet* **2013**, *382*, 427–451. [CrossRef]
20. The Nutritional Health of Young Refugee Children Resettling in Washington State. 2016. Available online: https://www.migrationpolicy.org/.../FCD-Dawson-Hahn-FINAL.pdf (accessed on 14 May 2018).
21. Gortmaker, S.L.; Cheung, L.W.; Peterson, K.E.; Chomitz, G.; Cradle, J.H.; Dart, H.; Fox, M.K.; Bullock, R.B.; Sobol, A.M.; Colditz, G.; et al. Impact of a school-based interdisciplinary intervention on diet and physical activity among urban primary school children: eat well and keep moving. *Arch. Pediatr. Adolesc. Med.* **1999**, *153*, 975–983. [CrossRef] [PubMed]
22. Rao, D.R.; Vijayapushpam, T.; Rao, G.S.; Antony, G.; Sarma, K. Dietary habits and effect of two different educational tools on nutrition knowledge of school going adolescent girls in Hyderabad, India. *Eur. J. Clin. Nutr.* **2007**, *61*, 1081–1085. [CrossRef] [PubMed]
23. Verstraeten, R.; Roberfroid, D.; Lachat, C.; Leroy, J.L.; Holdsworth, M.; Maes, L.; Kolsteren, P.W. Effectiveness of preventive school-based obesity interventions in low-and middle-income countries: A systematic review. *Am. J. Clin. Nutr.* **2012**, *96*, 415–438. [CrossRef] [PubMed]

24. Prelip, M.; Slusser, W.; Thai, C.L.; Kinsler, J.; Erausquin, J.T. Effects of a School-Based Nutrition Program Diffused Throughout a Large Urban Community on Attitudes, Beliefs, and Behaviors Related to Fruit and Vegetable Consumption. *J. School Health* **2011**, *81*, 520–529. [CrossRef] [PubMed]
25. Schultz, B.K.; Evans, S.W. *A Practical Guide to Implementing School-Based Interventions for Adolescents with ADHD*; Springer: New York, NY, USA, 2015.
26. Oosthuizen, D.; Oldewage-Theron, W.; Napier, C. The impact of a nutrition programme on the dietary intake patterns of primary school children. *S. Afr. J. Clin. Nutr.* **2011**, *24*, 75–81. [CrossRef]
27. Steyn, N.P.; de Villiers, A.; Gwebushe, N.; Draper, C.E.; Hill, J.; de Waal, M.; Dalais, L.; Abrahams, Z.; Lombard, C.; Lambert, E.V. Did HealthKick, a randomised controlled trial primary school nutrition intervention improve dietary quality of children in low-income settings in South Africa? *BMC Public Health* **2015**, *15*, 948. [CrossRef] [PubMed]
28. Jomaa, L.H.; McDonnell, E.; Probart, C. School feeding programs in developing countries: Impacts on children's health and educational outcomes. *Nutr. Rev.* **2011**, *69*, 83–98. [CrossRef] [PubMed]
29. Syria Conflict at 5 Years: The Biggest Refugee and Displacement Crisis of Our Time Demands a Huge Surge in Solidarity. 2016. Available online: http://www.unhcr.org/news/press/2016/3/56e6e3249/syria-conflict-5-years-biggest-refugee-displacement-crisis-time-demands.html (accessed on 17 May 2018).
30. Lebanon Plan of Action for Resilient Livelihoods: Food Security Response and Stabilization of Rural Livelihoods Addressing The Impacts of The Syria Crisis (2014–2018). 2014. Available online: http://www.fao.org/3/a-i4379e.pdf (accessed on 7 April 2018).
31. Lebanon: Syria Crisis. 2017. Available online: https://ec.europa.eu/echo/files/aid/countries/factsheets/lebanon_syrian_crisis_en.pdf (accessed on 27 April 2018).
32. Vulnerability Assessment of Syrian Refugees (VASyR) in Lebanon. 2017. Available online: https://reliefweb.int/sites/reliefweb.int/files/resources/VASyR%202017.compressed.pdf (accessed on 20 May 2018).
33. Lebanon-Situation Syria Regional Refugee Response. 2018. Available online: http://data2.unhcr.org/en/situations/syria/location/71 (accessed on 20 May 2018).
34. Cherri, Z.; González, P.A.; Delgado, R.C. The Lebanese–Syrian crisis: impact of influx of Syrian refugees to an already weak state. *Risk Manag. Healthc. Policy* **2016**, *9*, 165. [CrossRef] [PubMed]
35. Lebanon Facts & Figures. Available online: https://ec.europa.eu/echo/files/aid/countries/factsheets/lebanon_syrian_crisis_en.pdf (accessed on 20 May 2018).
36. Barriers to Education for Syrian Refugee Children in Lebanon Education for Children from Syria Who Live in Lebanon. 2013. Available online: https://www.hrw.org/report/2016/07/19/growing-without-education/barriers-education-syrian-refugee-children-lebanon (accessed on 20 May 2018).
37. Reaching all Children with Education in Lebanon: Opportunities for Action. 2015. Available online: https://www.alnap.org/system/files/content/resource/files/main/269-425e9dbef2c7ca9980-tom6bga7x.pdf (accessed on 20 May 2018).
38. Francis, M.; Nichols, S.S.; Dalrymple, N. The effects of a school-based intervention programme on dietary intakes and physical activity among primary-school children in Trinidad and Tobago. *Public Health Nutr.* **2010**, *13*, 738–747. [CrossRef] [PubMed]
39. Keshani, P.; Mousavi, S.M.; Mirzaei, Z.; Hematdar, Z.; Maayeshi, N.; Mirshekari, M.; Ranjbaran, H.; Faghih, S. Effect of a School-based Nutrition Education Program on the Nutritional Status of Primary School Children. *Nutr. Food Sci. Res.* **2016**, *3*, 27–34. [CrossRef]
40. Townsend, M.S.; Johns, M.; Shilts, M.K.; Farfan-Ramirez, L. Evaluation of a USDA nutrition education program for low-income youth. *J. Nutr. Educ. Behav.* **2006**, *38*, 30–41. [CrossRef] [PubMed]
41. Melki, I.; Beydoun, H.; Khogali, M.; Tamim, H.; Yunis, K. Household crowding index: A correlate of socioeconomic status and inter-pregnancy spacing in an urban setting. *J. Epidemiol. Community Health* **2004**, *58*, 476–480. [CrossRef] [PubMed]
42. Nasreddine, L.; Naja, F.; Akl, C.; Chamieh, M.C.; Karam, S.; Sibai, A.-M.; Hwalla, N. Dietary, lifestyle and socio-economic correlates of overweight, obesity and central adiposity in Lebanese children and adolescents. *Nutrients* **2014**, *6*, 1038–1062. [CrossRef] [PubMed]
43. Naja, F.; Hwalla, N.; Fossian, T.; Zebian, D.; Nasreddine, L. Validity and reliability of the Arabic version of the Household Food Insecurity Access Scale in rural Lebanon. *Public Health Nutr.* **2015**, *18*, 251–258. [CrossRef] [PubMed]

44. Household Food Insecurity Access Scale (HFIAS) for Measurement of Food Access: Indicator Guide. 2007. Available online: https://www.fantaproject.org/monitoring-and-evaluation/household-food-insecurity-access-scale-hfias (accessed on 19 April 2018).
45. Kemirembe, O.M.; Radhakrishna, R.B.; Gurgevich, E.; Yoder, E.P.; Ingram, P.D. An evaluation of nutrition education program for low-income youth. *J. Ext.* **2011**, *49*, 1–7. [CrossRef]
46. Conway, J.M.; Ingwersen, L.A.; Moshfegh, A.J. Accuracy of dietary recall using the USDA five-step multiple-pass method in men: An observational validation study. *J. Am. Diet. Assoc.* **2004**, *104*, 595–603. [CrossRef] [PubMed]
47. Pellet, P.; Shadarevian, S. *Food Composition Tables for Use in the Middle East*, 2nd ed.; American University of Beirut: Beirut, Lebanon, 1970; p. 126.
48. Dietary Reference Intakes Tables and Application. Available online: http://nationalacademies.org/HMD/Activities/Nutrition/SummaryDRIs/DRI-Tables.aspx (accessed on 17 February 2018).
49. Obesity: Preventing and Managing the Global Epidemic-Report of a WHO Consultation (WHO Technical Report Series 894). Available online: http://www.who.int/nutrition/publications/obesity/WHO_TRS_894/en/ (accessed on 18 June 2018).
50. Global Database on Child Growth and Malnutrition. Available online: http://www.who.int/nutgrowthdb/software/en/ (accessed on 23 May 2018).
51. Training Course on Child Growth Assessment: WHO Child Growth Standards. Available online: http://www.who.int/childgrowth/training/module_c_interpreting_indicators.pdf (accessed on 16 February 2015).
52. Maffeis, C.; Banzato, C.; Talamini, G. Waist-to-height ratio, a useful index to identify high metabolic risk in overweight children. *J. Pediatr.* **2008**, *152*, 207–213. [CrossRef] [PubMed]
53. McCarthy, H.D.; Ashwell, M. A study of central fatness using waist-to-height ratios in UK children and adolescents over two decades supports the simple message–'keep your waist circumference to less than half your height'. *Int. J. Obes.* **2006**, *30*, 988. [CrossRef] [PubMed]
54. Cameron, A.C.; Gelbach, J.B.; Miller, D.L. Bootstrap-based improvements for inference with clustered errors. *Rev. Econ. Stat.* **2008**, *90*, 414–427. [CrossRef]
55. Menger, A. *CLUSTSE: Stata Module to Estimate the Statistical Significance of Parameters When the Data is Clustered with a Small Number of Clusters*; Boston College: Chestnut Hill, MA, USA, 2017.
56. The WFP Food Basket. Available online: https://www.wfp.org/food-assistance/kind-food-assistance/wfp-food-basket (accessed on 18 April 2018).
57. WFP. Syrian Refugees Get E-Cards to Buy Food in Lebanon. 2013. Available online: https://www.wfp.org/stories/syrian-refugees-get-e-cards-buy-food-lebanon (accessed on 14 April 2018).
58. Cash Transfers. Available online: http://www1.wfp.org/cash-transfers (accessed on 15 April 2018).
59. Shah, P.; Misra, A.; Gupta, N.; Hazra, D.K.; Gupta, R.; Seth, P.; Agarwal, A.; Gupta, A.K.; Jain, A.; Kulshreshta, A.; et al. Improvement in nutrition-related knowledge and behaviour of urban Asian Indian school children: Findings from the 'Medical education for children/Adolescents for Realistic prevention of obesity and diabetes and for healthy aGeing' (MARG) intervention study. *Br. J. Nutr.* **2010**, *104*, 427–436. [CrossRef] [PubMed]
60. Perez-Rodrigo, C.; Aranceta, J. Nutrition education in schools: experiences and challenges. *Eur. J. Clin. Nutr.* **2003**, *57*, S82. [CrossRef] [PubMed]
61. Nixon, C.; Moore, H.; Douthwaite, W.; Gibson, E.; Vogele, C.; Kreichauf, S.; Wildgruber, A.; Manios, Y.; Summerbell, C.D.; ToyBox-Study Group. Identifying effective behavioural models and behaviour change strategies underpinning preschool-and school-based obesity prevention interventions aimed at 4–6-year-olds: A systematic review. *Obes. Rev.* **2012**, *13*, 106–117. [CrossRef] [PubMed]
62. Kaiser, L.L.; Townsend, M.S. Food insecurity among US children: Implications for nutrition and health. *Top. Clin. Nutr.* **2005**, *20*, 313–320. [CrossRef]
63. Sherman, J.; Muehlhoff, E. Developing a nutrition and health education program for primary schools in Zambia. *J. Nutr. Educ. Behav.* **2007**, *39*, 335–342. [CrossRef] [PubMed]
64. Survey Finds Syrian Refugees in Lebanon Became Poorer, More Vulnerable in 2017. 2018. Available online: http://www.unhcr.org/news/briefing/2018/1/5a548d174/survey-finds-syrian-refugees-lebanon-poorer-vulnerable-2017.html (accessed on 24 January 2018).
65. Vulnerability Assessment of Syrian Refugees in Lebanon—VASYR 2017. 2017. Available online: https://data2.unhcr.org/en/documents/details/61312#_ga=2.171737248.1402681600.1526641303-1754322128.1511439035 (accessed on 13 June 2018).

66. Tyrer, R.A.; Fazel, M. School and community-based interventions for refugee and asylum seeking children: A systematic review. *PLoS ONE* **2014**, *9*, e89359. [CrossRef] [PubMed]
67. Holmboe-Ottesen, G.; Wandel, M. Changes in dietary habits after migration and consequences for health: a focus on South Asians in Europe. *Food Nutr. Res.* **2012**, *56*, 18891. [CrossRef] [PubMed]
68. Curtis, P.; Thompson, J.; Fairbrother, H. Migrant children within Europe: A systematic review of children's perspectives on their health experiences. *Public Health* **2018**, *158*, 71–85. [CrossRef] [PubMed]
69. Healthy Diet—World Health Organization. 2015. Available online: http://www.who.int/news-room/fact-sheets/detail/healthy-diet (accessed on 29 June 2018).
70. Waters, E.; de Silva-Sanigorski, A.; Burford, B.J.; Brown, T.; Campbell, K.J.; Gao, Y.; Armstrong, R.; Prosser, L.; Summerbell, C.D. Interventions for preventing obesity in children. *Cochrane Libr.* **2011**. [CrossRef] [PubMed]

nutrients MDPI

Article

Best Practices and Innovative Solutions to Overcome Barriers to Delivering Policy, Systems and Environmental Changes in Rural Communities

Lindsey Haynes-Maslow [1,*], Isabel Osborne [2] and Stephanie B. Jilcott Pitts [3]

[1] Department of Agricultural and Human Sciences, North Carolina State University, Raleigh, NC 27695, USA
[2] Department of Global Studies, University of North Carolina, Chapel Hill, NC 27514, USA; iosborne@live.unc.edu
[3] Department of Public Health, East Carolina University, Greenville, NC 27834, USA; jilcotts@ecu.edu
* Correspondence: lhmaslow@ncsu.edu; Tel.: +919-515-9125

Received: 6 July 2018; Accepted: 30 July 2018; Published: 3 August 2018

Abstract: To better understand the barriers to implementing policy; systems; and environmental (PSE) change initiatives within Supplemental Nutrition Assistance Program-Education (SNAP-Ed) programming in U.S. rural communities; as well as strategies to overcome these barriers, this study identifies: (1) the types of nutrition-related PSE SNAP-Ed programming currently being implemented in rural communities; (2) barriers to implementing PSE in rural communities; and (3) common best practices and innovative solutions to overcoming SNAP-Ed PSE implementation barriers. This mixed-methods study included online surveys and interviews across fifteen states. Participants were eligible if they: (1) were SNAP-Ed staff that were intimately aware of facilitators and barriers to implementing programs, (2) implemented at least 50% of their programming in rural communities, and (3) worked in their role for at least 12 months. Sixty-five staff completed the online survey and 27 participated in interviews. Barriers to PSE included obtaining community buy-in, the need for relationship building, and PSE education. Facilitators included finding community champions; identifying early "wins" so that community members could easily see PSE benefits. Partnerships between SNAP-Ed programs and non-SNAP-Ed organizations are essential to implementing PSE. SNAP-Ed staff should get buy-in from local leaders before implementing PSE. Technical assistance for rural SNAP-Ed programs would be helpful in promoting PSE.

Keywords: rural populations; food assistance; low-income

---

1. Introduction

The prevalence of obesity in the United States (U.S.) creates a significant public health problem for both children and adults. In 2016, nearly 30% of children were overweight or obese and 30% of adults were obese [1]. Low-income individuals have the greatest risk of obesity, with 18% of children living below the federal poverty line being obese versus 10% of those living above the poverty level [2–4]. Geographically, nearly 16% of individuals in rural areas live below the poverty line, in contrast to 12% of individuals in urban areas [5]. Due to these income disparities, 16% of households in rural counties participate in the Supplemental Nutrition Assistance Program (SNAP) compared to 13% of household in urban counties [5]. Additionally, both children and adults living in rural areas are more likely to be obese than those living in urban areas [1,6,7]. These disparities in obesity prevalence may be partially due to disparities in access to healthy eating and physical activity opportunities. Compared to residents living in urban areas, residents in rural community have less access to healthy food and safe places to be active [8–10].

To help address food insecurity among low-income individuals in the U.S., the federal government created the SNAP in the 1960s [11]. Since its creation, SNAP has shifted its focus to also include improving dietary quality with the creation of federal nutrition education programs such as SNAP-Education (SNAP-Ed) [11]. The SNAP-Ed program was created in the 1980s as an optional cost-sharing federal program, to increase the likelihood that SNAP recipients make healthy food choices within a limited budget [11]. Individuals are eligible for SNAP-Ed if their incomes are at or below 185% of the Federal Poverty Level. SNAP-Ed reaches approximately 95 million low-income Americans in all 50 states, the District of Columbia, and three territories. Nationally, there are seven SNAP-Ed geographic regions. These regions include a range of states, and each state has at least one state SNAP-Ed implementing agency. Currently, there are 138 SNAP-Ed implementing agencies across the U.S. [11].

Prior to 2010, the majority of SNAP-Ed programming was traditional, direct- nutrition education (i.e., series-based classes or single session classes). Under traditional, direct-nutrition education, SNAP-Ed implementing agencies in rural areas faced barriers with recruiting families to attend sessions due to transportation, time, and lack of Internet access (for those living in mountainous regions) [12]. A 2004 national report concluded that more research was needed to determine whether SNAP-Ed behavior changes among low-income audiences was due to SNAP-Ed programs or other factors [13]. In 2010, the Healthy, Hunger-Free Kids Act added an additional component to SNAP-Ed encompassing broader policy, systems, and environmental (PSE) changes [11]. The Interpretive Guide to the SNAP-Ed Evaluation Framework defines a policy change as involving "a written plan or course of action designed to influence and determine decisions (includes the passing of laws, ordinances, resolutions, mandates, regulations or rules)." A system change "involves changes made to the rules or procedures within an organization—this can be a worksite, faith setting, school, non-profits, for-profit organizations." An environmental change includes "changes made to the physical, social, or economic environment. SNAP-Ed interventions can be customized for different geographic regions, ages, and cultural settings" [14].

Utilizing PSE approaches to encourage healthy dietary changes can help overcome recruitment and attendance barriers, since PSE changes are typically meant to "make the healthy choice the easy choice" for a variety of populations. When PSE changes are implemented, a large segment of the SNAP-Ed population can be affected compared to a smaller segment of those who choose to enroll in traditional direction-education classes. However, SNAP-Ed implementing agencies vary widely in their ability and capacity to implement PSE interventions in their programs [15]. Two years after SNAP-Ed implementing agencies were encouraged to deliver PSE, nationally, approximately 98% were still focusing on direct education [16]. Furthermore, there have been prior studies that broadly covered rural PSE change implementation barriers, identifying barriers such as cultural differences, population size, and resulting limited human capital [17]. Strategies to overcome such barriers include building partnerships, and utilizing existing infrastructure [18,19]. There is also a great need to rigorously evaluate PSE in rural areas to determine effectiveness for future implementation [19,20]. Thus, more work is needed to learn how SNAP-Ed staff in rural areas view PSE, how they implement PSE, and how implementation and evaluation of PSE could be improved within the SNAP-Ed program, especially in rural areas.

Therefore, the purpose of this study was to better understand the barriers to implementing PSE approaches within SNAP-Ed programming in rural communities, as well as the strategies to overcome these barriers to SNAP-Ed programming in rural communities. In this study, we identified: (1) the types of nutrition-related PSE SNAP-Ed programming currently being implemented in rural communities, (2) barriers to implementing PSE in rural communities, and (3) common best practices and innovative solutions to overcoming SNAP-Ed PSE implementation barriers in rural communities.

2. Materials and Methods

To gain a better understand of the barriers to implementing SNAP-Ed PSE changes in rural communities, as well as the strategies to overcoming these barriers, we employed a mixed-method approach. We triangulated data obtained from an online survey administered to SNAP-Ed Staff across the United States, and subsequently conducted qualitative in-depth interviews among a sub-set of those SNAP-Ed staff who completed the online survey. Below, we outline additional details regarding methods of each data collection method.

2.1. Online Survey: Participant Recruitment and Analysis

We recruited staff at SNAP-Ed programs across the country to complete an online survey by using the Association for SNAP Education Nutrition Administration (ASNNA) and the CDC-funded Nutrition and Obesity Policy Research and Evaluation Network Rural Food Access Working Group (RFAWG) email listservs. The RFAWG includes academic researchers, public health and cooperative extension practitioners, and other experts focused on rural food access. Several RFAWG members connected us with SNAP-Ed implementing agency contacts in their respective states. The following were eligibility criteria to complete the survey and subsequent qualitative interview: (1) a SNAP-Ed staff member that was intimately aware of facilitators and barriers to implementing programs in the community; (2) individuals who have worked for a SNAP-Ed program that provides at least 50% of programming in rural communities; and worked in their role for at least 12 months.

This study was approved by North Carolina State University's Institutional Review Board and all participants signified consent after being read an information sheet and agreeing to take part in the online survey and/or interview.

We used Qualtrics, an online survey program, to obtain information about PSE knowledge and experience, PSE activities, and partners engaged in PSE activities. Participants were asked to rate their level of knowledge with PSE approaches to behavior change using a 4-point Likert scale, ranging from "not knowledgeable at all" (=1) to "very knowledgeable" (=4). Participants were also asked to rate their level of experience with PSE using a 4-point Likert scale, ranging from "not experienced at all" to "very experienced". Among those with experience implementing PSE, we asked in what types of community settings PSE initiatives were being implemented, with response options including community gardens, schools, farmers' markets, healthy food retail and food pantries. We also asked what types of partners they were working with to implement those PSE initiatives, with response options including managers, principals, teachers, staff, food policy councils. SNAP-Ed staff could choose as many settings and partners that were applicable. Participants were asked about relevant outcome or evaluation data collected on PSE initiatives as an optional question. Data from the Qualtrics survey were exported from the program as a report, and simple descriptive statistics were calculated to determine frequencies of various responses.

2.2. In-Depth Interview Recruitment, Administration and Analysis

The last survey question asked study participants if they were interested in participating in an in-depth interview about barriers and facilitators to implementing SNAP-Ed within rural communities. Participants were asked to include their name and email and a member of the research team contacted them to schedule an interview. SNAP-Ed staff participated in telephone-administered interviews lasting 45–60 min using NoNotes, a professional telephone recording and audio sharing platform. Each interview was conducted by either Dr. Lindsey Haynes-Malsow (LHM) or Dr. Stephanie B. Jilcott Pitts (SJP) or using a semi-structured interview guide.

Participants were asked about their general experience with the SNAP-Ed program, such as how long they had worked with SNAP-Ed and in what capacity; what types of PSE initiatives in which their agency was currently engaged; what their favorite PSE initiative was and which initiative they felt was most effective; specific barriers to implementing PSE initiatives in rural communities; strategies that they used to overcome these barriers; future PSE initiatives that they were planning to implement in the following year, and how or if they were evaluating PSE initiatives.

Interviews were transcribed verbatim and analyzed using Atlas.ti version 7.0 (Scientific Software Development Gmbh, Berlin, Germany). LHM and SJP created a codebook based on independently coding a subset of three interviews. LHM and Isabel Osborne (IO) then independently applied these codes to all interview transcripts. Codes were reconciled and code memos, a 1–2 page summary based on each code, were written based on the all the codes. Final themes were compiled based on questions included on the interview guide. While participants were not asked specifically about "innovative" or "best" practices, LHM and SJP created an "innovative practice" code based on reviewing all PSE initiatives in accordance with SNAP-Ed guidelines, a description of how well the PSE initiative worked, and whether other participants had mentioned this practice. If the practice was mentioned only once, it was deemed "innovative". If it was mentioned by more than one respondent, it was coded as a "best practice".

3. Results

3.1. Online Survey

A total of 65 SNAP-Ed staff in rural implementing agencies completed online surveys. Sixteen (24.6%) responded they were somewhat knowledgeable, 26 (40.0%) knowledgeable, and 23 (35.4%) were very knowledgeable about PSE approaches to behavior change. However, when asked to rate their level of experience with PSE, 5 (7.8%) responded that they were not experienced at all, 25 (39.1%) were somewhat experienced, 23 (35.9%) were experienced, and 11 (17%) were very experienced. Table 1 shows that the top three settings in which respondents worked were schools (96%), food pantries (89%), and farmer's markets (83%). The least frequently reported setting was supermarkets/supercenters, in which only 24% of respondents said they were implementing PSE initiatives. Among the "other" settings, 5 out of 11 respondents reported working in gardens. The type of partner varied by setting. For example, in schools, most SNAP-Ed staff partnered with the school staff such as principals or teachers. Surprisingly, those working in healthy food retail settings, such as corner stores and grocery stores, only reported working with the retail setting owner or manager as a partner approximately 25% of the time. Other partners they worked with in retail settings were health departments, food policy councils, and worksite staff (not owners or managers).

Table 1. PSE Settings and Partners.

Where SNAP-Ed PSE Programming is Located		Partner				
Settting	I Work in This Setting	Health Departments	Retail Food Store Owner	Food Policy Councils	Worksite Staff	Other
Childcare center	61%	11%	0%	4%	30%	18%
School	96%	7%	5%	11%	50%	23%
Workplace	64%	12%	2%	9%	19%	22%
Senior Center	68%	15%	0%	7%	22%	25%
Faith-based locations	66%	5%	2%	12%	20%	27%
Corner store	54%	11%	22%	3%	6%	12%
Grocery store	53%	7%	26%	2%	4%	14%
Supermarket/supercenter	24%	2%	10%	2%	4%	6%
Food Pantry	89%	15%	4%	17%	27%	27%
Farmer's Market	83%	13%	3%	13%	22%	32%
Other Setting	44%	2%	0%	2%	12%	18%

In terms of outcome or evaluation data collected on PSE initiatives (an optional question), responses varied greatly; however, some of the common responses were pounds of produce donated or sold; national SNAP-Ed indicators such as reach (the number of people that were in contact with the PSE initiative) and impact (behavior change such as fruit and vegetable intake). Among those that answered the optional question of whether they would be interested in participating in an interview 27 (41.5%) responded "yes" and 38 (58.5%) responded "no".

3.2. In-Depth Interviews

A total of 27 interviews were conducted with SNAP-Ed staff in 15 states across all 7 SNAP-Ed regions (see Figure 1). The majority of interviewees had been working for SNAP-Ed for approximately 0–2 years (40.7%); were an average age of 39 years, female (81.5%), white/Caucasian (70.0%); conducted more than 75% of their work in rural communities (94.1%); contributed more than 75% of their time to PSE activities (37.0%); and less than 25% to direct-education (51.9%). See Table 2 for more information.

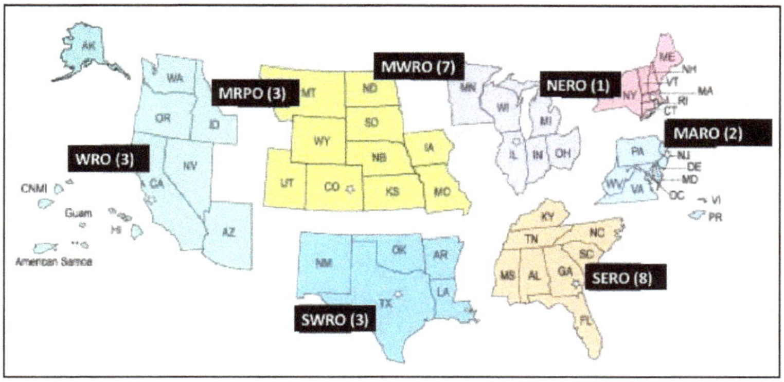

Figure 1. Interview Respondent Locations. Note: SERO (Southeast Regional Office); SWRO (Southwest Regional Office); MARO (Mid-Atlantic Regional Office); NERO (Northeast Regional Office); MWRO (Midwest Regional Office); MRPO (Mountain Regional Plains Office); WRO (West Regional Office)

Table 2. Interview Participant Demographics (n = 27).

Characteristic	Number	Percent
Number of years working for SNAP-Ed		
0–2	11	40.7%
3–5	6	22.2%
6–10	3	11.1%
>10	5	18.5%
Mean Age (years)		39
Gender		
Male	2	7.4%
Female	22	81.5%
Race/Ethnicity		
White	19	70.0%
Native American/American Indian	1	3.7%
Hispanic or Latino	2	7.4%
African American or Black	2	7.4%
Work Conducted in Rural Communities		
25–50%	5	18.5%
51–75%	4	14.8%
>75%	16	94.1%
PSE Work		
<25%	6	22.2%
25–50%	5	18.5%
51–75%	4	14.8%
>75%	10	37.0%
Direct-Ed Work		
<25%	14	51.9%
25–50%	4	14.8%
51–75%	4	14.8%
>75%	3	11.1%

A total of 10 codes were created based on interviewees' responses (see Table 3). These codes focused on PSE initiatives, barriers to implementing PSE, and facilitators to implementing PSE.

Table 3. Codebook for Interviews.

Code	Definition	Illustrative Quote	Frequency
PSE Initiative: Garden-based	Mention of garden-based PSE strategies	"The biggest thing is that I have worked with a sort of small coalition of people in the community to start a new community garden park, we found a big three-acre parcel of land and then got a garden park sort of design put together that includes garden plots and a playground and a walking trail and a pavilion and a hoop house and all kinds of things that make it both a place where people can exercise and come and gather as a community, and then also grow food for themselves in these plots that are free."	27
PSE Initiative: School Wellness-Based	Mention of school-wellness PSE strategies	"We've worked on developing a training module for the staff and teachers to learn more about the school wellness policy. The school system has had a wellness policy for a number of years and it is a pretty good wellness policy, but we did a survey last year and found out most of the staff don't really know anything about it, so the idea is that they have to complete these online little video modules every year before the start of the school year."	21
PSE Initiative: Healthy Food Retail	Mention of healthy food retail PSE strategies, such as corner stores, grocery stores, supermarkets	"There is a PSE in the region that's a corner store makeover, which it's super popular around the country, so I'm sure you've heard of that one."	21
PSE Initiative: Farmers' Market	Mention of farmers' market PSE strategies	"We work in farmers markets doing food demonstrations and recipe kind of hand outs and other direct education, kind of very brief handouts."	13
PSE Initiative: Food Pantries	Mention of food pantry PSE strategies	"I've partnered our regional food bank, and we are working on a nudging pilot. SNAP-Ed has partnered with them to provide signage. We're offering volunteer education. I've done food demos and recipe cards for produce items that they know they'll have excess of."	12
Lack of healthy food and physical activity Infrastructure	There is lack of infrastructure in rural communities that make access to healthy food and physical activity difficult for the population.	"Somebody in a rural area might have to drive like a half hour or an hour to go get groceries that doesn't have anything fresh."	59
Partnerships	Partnering with other community initiatives or organizations, building relationships with partners, coalitions, wellness committees, advisory groups, ect.	"One of my favorite PSE strategies, is really having SNAP-Ed partners who are connecting with existing opportunities in their communities and regions to bring the SNAP-Ed lens to these coalitions that have some kind of health focus and then identifying strategies that allows those multi-sector partners around the table to leverage resources and work to advance PSE work that some of that's SNAP-Ed, but it also goes beyond SNAP-Ed."	65
Short-term PSE wins	Recognizing the importance of having short term wins to prove that PSE can be an effective strategy for behavior change, this includes being intentional where you work choosing locations where you think your programming will be successful.	"Over the past couple of years, we have been required to look at that environmental level and think about the short-term piece, so your partnerships, needs and readiness, that kind of stuff."	11
Level of understanding of PSEs	Mentions the lack of understanding of PSE as a barrier to implementation	"We're definitely going to start with a statewide training so that everybody understands the importance of PSE, and when I say everybody, we're talking about not just people who are health educators. We're trying to be pretty strategic in who we invite to the training and who we invite as a coach. We're talking about our parks department, our state, and city, and town planners, our faith-based leaders, trying to really be all-inclusive of everybody who impacts health to really help folks understand that everybody has an impact on health."	33
Funding	Lack of funding for the amount of work that needs to be done; also includes SNAP-Ed's lack of ability to cover incentives for participants	"I would like to have the time or staffing to go out and really spend time with our educators and their partners developing relationships where our partners understood the importance of PSE work. I need them to do direct education and PSE work and get their reporting done on time;, I just don't have a lot of time left for them. And so I would say I would just need a bigger chunk of money so I could have more people to really dive in."	52

3.3. Types of Nutrition-Related SNAP-Ed PSE Initiatives Being implemented in Rural Communities

The most common PSE initiatives mentioned were gardens, school wellness-based initiatives, healthy food retail, farmers' markets, and food pantries. In terms of implementing PSE initiatives in rural communities, the main challenges were funding, and level of PSE understanding among SNAP-Ed staff and stakeholders. However, strategies to overcome these challenges included working through partnerships and finding short-term PSE wins to demonstrate the importance of this approach to behavioral change. Below, we discuss the setting-based themes in more detail.

3.3.1. Gardens

In the in-depth interviews, the most commonly mentioned PSE initiative was gardens. Many interviewees mentioned PSE initiatives related to gardening such as community gardens, school gardens, and personal gardens. These initiatives included activities such as teaching adults basic gardening skills, ways to increase garden viability such as bee keeping and composting, as well gardening education for students by showing them how and where fruits and vegetables grow, and generating general community interest in the value of gardening. A participant from SNAP-Ed Southeast Region commented: "I started a garden program at one of the schools, so we're introducing the fourth grade students how to garden and where their food comes from because a lot of students, believe it or not, don't know where their food comes from. They think it comes from Food Loin or Walmart. I'm tell them, 'Well, technically yes, but it's grown. It's a process. Right now, I'm just at one school doing the garden program, but my goal is to eventually spread out and work with multiple grade levels, not just at the fourth grade levels, with that particular program."

Setting-specific barriers—Gardens: Some SNAP-Ed staff mentioned barriers to implementing garden-based initiatives related to weather (late freezes, extreme heat, and droughts) or when working in schools, having to compete for time with schools' teaching requirements and curriculum standards.

Setting-specific best practices—Gardens: Several interviewees mentioned potential facilitators to increase school gardening PSE programs, such as encouraging all schools to have a garden (making it the cultural norm) and full support from the community.

Setting-specific innovative solutions—Gardens: One innovative solution mentioned was having work meetings in gardens. As a participant from SNAP-Ed Mountains Plains Region said, "Our educator partnered with Extension and they helped tell her (worksite owner) what kind of plants grow well there and taught her about companion plants and that kind of thing. And she partnered with other agencies so they could have working meetings and actually work in the garden while they were discussing business." This increased both awareness of the garden and helped build a better partnership between the SNAP-Ed staff and worksite.

3.3.2. School Wellness Initiatives

Many of the interviewees described effective PSE strategies within schools in their rural communities. These strategies included smarter lunchrooms, farm-to-school projects, school gardens, and taste tastings. In addition, many SNAP-Ed staff encouraged schools to connect direct-education to PSE initiatives so could reinforce lessons learned in class and maximize exposure to healthy living initiatives. As a participant from SNAP-Ed Western Region said, "I would have to say that for all our counties, our PSE work is primarily in the school setting. We do edible school gardens, local school wellness policy participation, school stenciling projects and mural projects, physical activity integration, technical and training assistance for teachers, and, Smarter Lunchroom Movement activities."

Setting Specific Barriers—School-Wellness: Several SNAP-Ed staff discussed competing for class time as a barrier to implementing PSE-based programs. Since some regional elementary schools have end-of-year grade exams, schools are fairly focused on ensuring that students are well prepared for these exams; time that is taken away from teaching for this test is seen as a competing interest.

Additionally, not having buy-in from school principals or teachers was also a barrier for newer SNAP-Ed staff.

Setting-specific best practices—School Wellness: To increase school interest in SNAP-Ed programming, some SNAP-Ed staff explained how they created programs that did not require teacher participation. Some staff explained that if teachers were required to help with programming, they would find it burdensome on an already heavy teaching load. Other SNAP-Ed staff let school leadership choose which PSE initiative(s) they wanted to implement. Generally, schools with PSE initiatives were more likely to have community partners helping them sustain their activities, such as donating school garden produce to food pantries.

Setting-specific innovative solution—School-Wellness Based: One innovative practice used at a school involved converting an old and outdated pool into a garden and converting the pool house for produce processing, and tool and lumber storage. As a participant from SNAP-Ed Northeast Region stated about the initiative, "It's been very successful ... and after all this time finally getting produce into the cafeteria."

3.3.3. Healthy Food Retail

Many SNAP-Ed staff discussed healthy food retail in the context of working with grocery stores and corner stores. These initiatives included posting new signage to direct people towards healthier food items, graphically designing advertisements for healthy food specials, deals, and sales, and creating healthy food check-out lines where produce and other healthy "grab and go" snacks were easily accessible. Some healthy food retail projects were well-received in the community, as one participant in the SNAP-Ed Northeast Region said their "corner store makeover" was extremely popular among community members.

Setting Specific Barriers—Healthy Food Retail: When working on healthy food retail, some SNAP-Ed staff experienced lack of buy-in from store owners—as they did not want to change their food inventory and what they sold to customers. Additionally, several SNAP-Ed staff had difficulty measuring the impact of their healthy food retail initiatives to determine how effective they were, as well as ensuring that store owners and managers continued to post signage and stock fresh produce.

Setting-specific best practices—Healthy Food Retail: To help overcome lack of buy-in, many SNAP-Ed staff described ensuring that they communicated regularly with the store owners and discussing with stores the benefits of how these small, no or low cost changes could improve the community's diet and health. One SNAP-Ed staff member from Southeast Region summarized their experience as, "Just getting my foot in the door with the corner store was very difficult because the owner wasn't on-board at first, which I can understand because of the community and the dynamics of it. His store was known for hot dogs and ice cream—and getting him to implement change in the store did not come easy for his customers. He was trying to think on that aspect, but then as I continued to work and talk with him, he was open to the idea of stocking fruits. He started to put the fruits out and just to see what would happen, and on the first day he did it, he said he had to stock up twice."

Setting-specific innovative solutions—Healthy Food Retail: One SNAP-Ed staff member encouraged bundling (combining multiple food products and selling them together) healthy foods with other high demand foods. Essentially, making the bundled price (the high demand food item plus healthy snacks) cheaper than the price of a high demand food item plus an unhealthy snack. Additionally, another SNAP-Ed staff member was working with an independent grocery store owner to develop a mobile grocery store to increase access to healthy food in areas with limited access. As the SNAP-Ed interviewee from the Southeast Region stated, "We're really trying to work on every level to help with this opportunity, help with the funding, and help our educators. We've got just a stellar independent grocer here locally. And thank goodness for me he's local so I can work directly with him and we can work out models and look at the economics around the model and things of that nature. And he actually is—they're about to pilot starting in the first quarter of 2018 online SNAP acceptance."

3.3.4. Farmer's Markets

SNAP-Ed staff commented on working with their community farmer's markets using PSE approaches or how they had plans to improve it in the future. Many SNAP-Ed staff worked on encouraging farmer's markets to accept SNAP as part of their PSE initiative. SNAP-Ed staff would also provide food tastings and cooking demonstrations at farmer's markets, and provide hand-outs with recipes or health tips. Additionally, SNAP-Ed staff collaborated with other organizations to help work with farmer's markets.

Setting Specific Barriers—Farmer's Markets: Some communities did not have farmer's markets, so SNAP-Ed staff worked on trying to create one. However, this process is time consuming, expensive, and can be logistically challenging as many farmer's markets are usually not located in areas that low-income individuals frequent. Additionally, even if a rural community did have a farmer's market, they lacked SNAP, which was seen as a major barrier for low-income customers.

Setting-specific best practices—Farmer's Markets: Several SNAP-Ed staff talked about partnering with other organizations to implement incentive programs. As one SNAP-Ed staff from the Mountains Plains Region explained, "We worked to encourage them (the farmer's market) to do incentive programs, so if people do redeem SNAP benefits they may get 'double up bucks', they may get extra matching funds for whatever they redeem with their SNAP benefits, or they might get like an extra basket of fruits and vegetables in addition to what they would go buy."

Setting-specific innovative solution—Farmer's Markets: One farmer's market PSE initiative involved a policy practice. "One of the PSE changes that we did put in place at our farmer's market was demonstrating healthy recipes utilizing some of the fruits and vegetables that were being featured there that week, so anybody that came in and did a food demonstration had to serve fruits and vegetables. It had to be healthy. Water is served as the beverage of choice there, whereas before they may have been doing punch or something like that," said a participant from SNAP-Ed Southeast Region.

3.3.5. Food Pantries

Many interviewees commented on the prevalence of working with food pantries as part of their PSE programming. The majority of work with food pantries was in collaboration with others organizations or projects—building on behavioral economic movements such as nudging customers towards healthier foods [13]. Food pantries often offered direct food to pantry clients, and SNAP-Ed staff discussed coming into the pantry and using a client choice model, where food pantry customers could choose their food contents—but they were encouraged to choose healthy options. One SNAP-Ed agent from the Southeast Region described a specific example of this: "This particular pantry, there's a box that's pre-made—it has meat, some pasta, and canned goods. They get a box of these staple food items, but then they get to choose their produce items afterwards. It's a little bit of a client choice model, but not entirely. There are other pantries that allow you to choose every single food item that you want. That way, you don't end up with food that's unhealthy if you don't want it. The clients have a choice in that. This one is kind of a half client choice, but they still get a pre-made box."

Setting-specific barriers—Food Pantries: Several SNAP-Ed staff discussed the lack of buy-in from food pantry owners—as they did not want to change food distributions policy. Even when SNAP-Ed staff did get food pantry owners to try behavioral economics, they had to check-in frequently to ensure that the food pantry director or coordinator continued to use behavioral economics to encourage clients to choose healthy foods.

Setting-specific best practices—Food Pantries: SNAP-Ed staff discussed working with food pantry owners and managers and moving towards providing healthier food options within the pantries.

Setting-specific innovative solution—Food Pantries: One SNAP-Ed staff explained partnering with a medium-security prison on their produce-growing contest—prisons try to grow the most produce and after the contest, the produce is donated across the community. While SNAP-Ed funding does not allow funds to be spent within the prison population, SNAP-Ed staff members were initially invited by the warden to encourage volunteers to help find places to distribute the produce. As a

SNAP-Ed staff from the Midwest Region explained, "All of a sudden, we have this huge group of volunteers that wants to help distribute 12,000 pounds of produce, because one or two people can't distribute all of that. So all of a sudden, we have all of these volunteers who are on-board to help take all the produce to a central location, and then they'll take it to these food pantries or these programs that are low income. Our summer day camp that the YMCA runs is like 75% free and reduced lunch, so they'll get some, and distribute it to places that (A) don't have a budget to buy it, but (B) desperately need it for the clients that they're serving. I think that one of the biggest things with communities is just having the support of the people who live there, play there, work there."

3.4. *Barriers to Implementing SNAP-Ed PSE in Rural Communities*

There were three general barriers participants discussed when implementing SNAP-Ed PSE initiatives in rural communities: funding, lack of infrastructure, and lack of PSE understanding.

3.4.1. Funding

In terms of funding, most participants discussed the lack of funding available for PSE initiatives. As one SNAP-Ed Midwest Region participant said, "The biggest barrier is funding because lot of people like these (PSE) ideas, but there's very little extra money laying around". Additionally, due to SNAP-Ed allowable and unallowable costs, as defined by the U.S. Department of Agriculture (USDA), grantees cannot use SNAP-Ed funds for infrastructure (such as building sidewalks or playground) or to purchase food (such as funding "double up bucks" program).

3.4.2. Lack of PSE Understanding

Even though PSE has been a part of SNAP-Ed programming for several years now, there is still a lack of PSE understanding among some SNAP-Ed staff and stakeholders. Several interviewees discussed SNAP-Ed staff and stakeholders (community members, local leaders) as not having as high a regard for PSE as traditional direct-education. SNAP-Ed staff explained that some stakeholders wondered why PSE initiatives were important and questioned whether they would truly make an impact. Other SNAP-Ed staff and stakeholders misinterpreted the definition of policy, "Even though I'm comfortable with PSE, many of our SNAP-Ed assistants are not. 'Policy' is a scary word to them and I think a training to make them feel more comfortable about it, and realize that it's not always about talking to senators, would be helpful". (Participant from the SNAP-Ed Mid-Atlantic Region)

3.5. *Best Practices' to Overcoming SNAP-Ed PSE Implementation Barriers in Rural Communities*

While some barriers to SNAP-Ed programming cannot be overcome with SNAP-Ed grant funding, interviewees discussed strategies they have used to overcome challenges.

3.5.1. Overarching Best Practice: Partnerships

The most frequently cited facilitator to implementing SNAP-Ed programming was partnering with other community initiatives or organizations, building relationships with coalitions, wellness committees, advisory groups, or food policy councils. Partnerships were often useful with SNAP-Ed, as funds could not be used to cover the cost of a certain project, such as renovating a walking trail, but another organization could. Additionally, being in a rural community was seen as an advantage since, "everybody knows each other, so they have the ability to network and build or enhance partnerships"—(participant from the SNAP-Ed Midwest Region). Partnerships were also seen as a way to ensure sustainability of projects—especially beyond SNAP-Ed funding periods. Another interviewee from the SNAP-Ed Midwest Region stated, "SNAP-Ed is an important piece of what people are doing, but we don't want them to do it in a silo, and we want to have community buy-in to advance PSE strategies, right? So working at that broader level with multisector representatives really helps set those changes up not only for adoption but also for sustainability in the future".

3.5.2. Overarching Best Practice: Communicating Short-Term PSE Wins in the Community

Due to the fact that some SNAP-Ed staff and stakeholders did not understand the definition or value of PSE, many interviewees talked about the need for "short-term PSE wins" to demonstrate how impactful it could be in the community. Recognizing that SNAP-Ed funding is renewed every year and that PSE can take years to implement and achieve desired results, many SNAP-Ed staff talked about finding PSE work that was already underway in the community and assisting with those projects. One participant from the SNAP-Ed Midwest Region discussed helping with a complete street initiative and promoting connector trails to a major walking trail in the community: "I think a really helpful thing is to find a way to partner with and plug into things that are already sort of 'easy wins' that are already starting or initiated in some way and then trying to help shape them and direct them to the more healthy direction." Visually demonstrating to the staff, community, and other stakeholders that PSE can be an extremely influential and impactful strategy for behavior change is key to local buy-in and longer term success.

4. Discussion

The results of this study provide a deeper understanding of the types of nutrition-related SNAP-Ed PSE initiatives being implemented currently in rural communities, implementation barriers, and both "best practice" strategies and innovative solutions to overcoming SNAP-Ed PSE implementation barriers in rural communities.

Based on online surveys and interviews, we found that SNAP-Ed PSE initiatives in rural areas included working with schools, gardens, food pantries, farmers' markets, and food retail settings like corner stores and supermarkets. Nearly 96% of the participants reported working with schools. Another study conducted with 15 public health practitioners about environmental and policy changes to support healthy eating and physical activity in rural communities also identified schools as a main setting to implement initiatives [17].

Interviewees offered a variety of creative solutions to overcome barriers, including worksite meetings in gardens, repurposing an old pool, and working with an independent grocer on mobile markets. Such creativity and partnering with appropriate organizations and stakeholders are two vital components to overcome challenges to PSE in rural areas. Building partnerships and having buy-in from local leaders, such as the city council, was also seen as an important strategy in implementing environmental and policy interventions to support physical activity and healthy eating in rural communities, in another study [17].

One major barrier included funding restrictions due to SNAP-Ed allowable and unallowable costs. The barrier of funding restrictions was often overcome by partnering with other community groups, foundations, or grantees. Partnerships were noted in prior studies [18,19] as important solutions to PSE implementation barriers, and were a key best practice in the current study. Barnidge et al. found that the most important partners for implementing physical activity and healthy eating in rural communities were city councils or mayors, local businesses, schools, health promotion organizations, healthcare facilities or healthcare providers [17]. Similarly, partners mentioned in the current study included school staff, food policy council members, health department staff, and worksite staff.

The goal of PSE strategies is to make a healthy choice, an easy choice, or even the default choice. This quality of PSE makes it appealing, as it does not require attendance from SNAP-Ed participants, overcoming commonly cited transportation and time barriers [15]. In rural communities, PSE could have greater reach and impact due to transportation and infrastructure barriers that these communities face. In a recent study, researchers found that socioeconomic status, rather than geographic location, was a better predicator of transportation barriers. In a systematic literature review across 25 studies, between 10–51% of lower-income individuals reported transportation as a barrier [21]. In terms of infrastructure as barrier to health living, one study among eight southeastern rural communities in the U.S. found that rural communities lack policies and programs to support safe places to be active, especially sidewalks or policies related to schools, allowing the community to use their facilities outside of school hours (such as shared use policies) [22]. Additionally, access to healthy foods in rural communities is limited, as residents have greater exposure to retail food outlets that sell a limited selection of healthy food items [23–26]. Fortunately, research has suggested that healthy retail initiatives in small food stores, which can be supported by SNAP-Ed, can be a strategy to improve the quality of food in stores [27,28].

As mentioned in the interviews, some SNAP-Ed staff have varying levels of understanding PSE and some stakeholders do not fully comprehend PSE. A solution that others have recommended is to not use the words, "policy, systems, or environmental" change when talking with other community members, organizational leaders, and other stakeholders. Our study showed that these terms were perceived as very top-down, high-level, and abstract—all of which were not viewed as favorable among rural community members.

One way to demonstrate the impact of PSE on behavior change is through rigorous impact and outcome evaluation. Demonstrating that a policy, system, or environmental change can actually transform the environment and result in more positive and healthy behaviors is critical to indicating the utility of PSE for various stakeholder groups and can provide evidence of a "short term win". For example, a SNAP-Ed program assisted a local non-profit with renovation of a trail by providing signage and promoting the trail opening. However, the majority of SNAP-Ed interviewees expressed difficulties in evaluating PSE and evaluation methods as settings varied greatly across the different SNAP-Ed programs. Others have called for more rigorous evaluation of PSE in rural communities [18]. While the SNAP-Ed Evaluation Framework and Interpretive Guide offers many examples and suggestions on how to collect data, one barrier to evaluating programs is the lack of funding and time for SNAP-Ed programs to rigorously evaluate PSE initiatives [14]. SNAP-Ed implementers could have successful partnerships with evaluators of neighboring research institutes or universities to conduct rigorous evaluation of PSE initiatives.

5. Conclusions

The goal of SNAP-Ed is to help improve the chances of lower-income children and families making healthy food choices within a limited budget. Using a multi-level approach by combining direct education with PSE efforts gives SNAP-Ed the opportunity to facilitate positive behavior change. However, this requires that SNAP-Ed implementing agencies be knowledgeable and comfortable with delivering both types of programming [15]. The current study illustrates barriers, and creative solutions that other rural SNAP Ed staff can implement, to increase the success and sustainability of rural PSE initiatives.

This study has several strengths and limitations. First, it included SNAP-Ed staff from all seven SNAP-Ed regions. Additionally, this study is strengthened by having two trained qualitative researchers conduct all interviews, double-code transcripts, and reconcile all codes. Some of the limitations are the potential selection bias for those who chose to participate in the interviews. Since the online survey asked many questions about PSE, SNAP-Ed staff with more experience and interest in implementing PSE might have volunteered for an interview, rather than those with less experience or interest.

Few studies have investigated implementing SNAP-Ed PSE initiatives in rural communities [22]. This study revealed innovative strategies and best practices for implementing PSE in rural areas, which can assist similar SNAP-Ed implementing agencies working in rural communities to overcome barriers to PSE. The ultimate goal of implementing SNAP-Ed PSE initiatives is to empower low-income individuals to make healthy choices within their homes, schools, worksites, and communities. Future studies should focus on disseminating innovative strategies and best practices for implementing PSE in rural communities and evaluate whether these strategies are effective at positively changing health behaviors.

Author Contributions: Conceptualization, L.H.-M. and S.B.J.P.; Methodology, L.H.-M. and S.B.J.P.; Formal Analysis, L.H.-M., S.B.J.P., and I.O.; Writing—Original Draft Preparation, L.H.-M.; Writing—Review & Editing, L.H.-M. and S.B.J.P.; Supervision, L.H.-M.; Project Administration, L.H.-M.

Funding: This research was funded by Lindsey Haynes-Maslow and Stephanie Jilcott Pitts.

Acknowledgments: This research was supported by a grant from Healthy Eating Research, a national program of the Robert Wood Johnson Foundation. The views expressed here do not necessarily reflect the views of Healthy Eating Research or of the Foundation. The authors would like to thank SNAP-Ed staff for their time participating in this study.

Conflicts of Interest: The authors declare no conflict of interest. The founding sponsors had no role in the design of the study; in the collection, analyses, or interpretation of data; in the writing of the manuscript, and in the decision to publish the results.

References

1. Lundeen, E.A.; Park, S.; Pan, L.; O'Toole, T.; Matthews, K.; Blanck, H.M. Obesity Prevalence Among Adults Living in Metropolitan and Nonmetropolitan Counties—United States, 2016. *MMWR* **2018**, *67*, 653–658. [CrossRef] [PubMed]
2. Ogden, C.L.; Carroll, M.D.; Kit, B.K.; Flegal, K.M. Prevalence of childhood and adult obesity in the United States, 2011–2012. *JAMA* **2014**, *311*, 806–814. [CrossRef] [PubMed]
3. Singh, G.K.; Siahpush, M.; Kogan, M.D. Rising social inequalities in U.S. childhood obesity, 2003–2007. *Am. Educ. J.* **2010**, *20*, 40–52.
4. Skelton, J.A.; Cook, S.R.; Auinger, P.; Klein, J.D.; Barlow, S.E. Prevalence and trends of severe obesity among U.S. children and adolescents. *Acad. Peds.* **2009**, *9*, 322–329. [CrossRef] [PubMed]
5. Food Research Action Center. Participation in the Supplemental Nutrition Assistance Program (SNAP) Highest in Rural Areas and Small Towns, New Data Tool Reveals. Available online: http://frac.org/news/participation-supplemental-nutrition-assistance-program-snap-highest-rural-areas-small-towns-new-data-tool-reveals (accessed on 1 July 2018).
6. Davis, A.M.; Bennett, K.J.; Befort, C.; Nollen, N. Obesity and related health behaviors among urban and rural children in the United States: Data from the National Health and Nutrition Examination Survey 2003–2004 and 2005–2006. *J. Ped. Psychol.* **2011**, *36*, 669–676. [CrossRef] [PubMed]
7. Johnson, A.; Mohamdi, A. Urban-rural differences in childhood and adolescent obesity in the United States: A systematic revie and meta-analysis. *Child. Obes.* **2015**, *11*, 233–241. [CrossRef] [PubMed]
8. Murimi, M.W.; Harpel, T. Practicing preventive health: the underlying culture among low-income rural populations. *J. Rural Health* **2010**, *26*, 273–282. [CrossRef] [PubMed]
9. Hennessy, E.; Kraak, V.I.; Hyatt, R.R.; Bloom, J.; Fenton, M.; Wagoner, C.; Economos, C.D. Active living for rural children: Community perspectives using PhotoVOICE. *Am. J. Prev. Med.* **2010**, *39*, 537–545. [CrossRef] [PubMed]
10. Moore, J.B.; Jilcott, S.B.; Shores, K.A.; Evenson, K.R.; Brownson, R.C.; Novick, L.F. A qualitative examination of perceived barriers and facilitators of physical activity for urban and rural youth. *Health Educ. Res.* **2010**, *25*, 355–367. [CrossRef] [PubMed]
11. U.S. Department of Agriculture (USDA). Supplemental Nutrition Assistance Program Education (SNAP-Ed). Available online: www.fns.usda.gov/snap/supplemental-nutrition-education-assistance-program-education-snap-ed (accessed on 12 April 2018).
12. Leung, C.W.; Hoffnagle, E.E.; Lindsay, A.C.; Lofink, H.E.; Hoffman, V.A.; Turrell, S.; Willett, W.C.; Blumenthal, S.J. A Qualitative Study of Diverse Experts' Views about Barriers and Strategies to Improve the Diets and Health of Supplemental Nutrition Assistance Program (SNAP) Beneficiaries. *JAND* **2013**, *113*, 70–76. [CrossRef] [PubMed]
13. United States General Accounting Office. Nutrition Education: USDA Provides Services through Multiple Programs, but Stronger Linkage among Efforts Are Needed. 2004. Available online: http://www.gao.gov/new.items/d04528 (accessed on 8 February 2012).
14. U.S. Department of Agriculture (USDA). Interpretive Guide to the SNAP-Ed Evaluation Framework. Available online: https://snaped.fns.usda.gov/evaluation/evaluation-framework-and-interpretive-guide (accessed on 15 June 2016).

15. Frank, K. Delphi Study Summary: Barriers, Facilitators, and Training Needs for Successful PSE Implementation in SNAP-Ed and EFNEP. 2016. Available online: http://snapedpse.org/resources/RNECE-PSE%20Delphi%20summary%202016 (accessed on 1 June 2017).
16. United States Department of Agriculture (USDA). Food Stamp Nutrition Education Systems Review: Final Report. Available online: http://www.fns.usda.gov/ora/MENU/Published/NutritionEducation/Files/FSNESystemsReviewExecSummary (accessed on 8 February 2012).
17. Barnidge, E.K. Understanding and addressing barriers to implementation of environmental and policy interventions to support physical activity and healthy eating in rural communities. *J. Rural Health* **2013**, *29*, 97–105. [CrossRef] [PubMed]
18. Calancie, L.; Leeman, J.; Pitts, S.B.; Khan, L.K.; Fleischhacker, S.; Evenson, K.R.; Schreiner, M.; Byker, C.; Owens, C.; McGuirt, J.; et al. Nutrition-Related Policy and Environmental Strategies to Prevent Obesity in Rural Communities: A Systematic Review of the Literature, 2002–2013. *Prev. Chron. Dis.* **2015**, *12*, 140540. [CrossRef] [PubMed]
19. Wilson, N.L.; Just, D.R.; Swigert, J.; Wansink, B. Food pantry selection solutions: A randomized controlled trial in client-choice food pantries to nudge clients to targeted foods. *J. Public Health* **2016**, *39*, 366–372. [CrossRef] [PubMed]
20. Wyker, B.A.; Jordan, P.; Quigley, D.L. Evaluation of supplemental nutrition assistance program education: application of behavioral theory and survey validation. *JNEB* **2012**, *44*, 360–364. [CrossRef] [PubMed]
21. Syed, S.T.; Gerber, B.S.; Sharp, L.K. Traveling towards disease: Transportation barriers to health care access. *J. Community Health* **2013**, *38*, 976–993. [CrossRef] [PubMed]
22. Robinson, J.C.; Carson, T.L.; Johnson, E.R.; Hardy, C.M.; Shikany, J.M.; Green, E.; Willis, L.M.; Marron, J.V., Jr.; Li, Y.; Lee, C.H.; et al. Assessing environmental support for better health: Active living opportunity audits in rural communities in the southern United States. *Prev. Med.* **2014**, *66*, 28–33. [CrossRef] [PubMed]
23. Jilcott, S.B.; Liu, H.; Moore, J.B.; Bethel, J.; Wilson, J.; Ammerman, A.S. Commute times, food retail gaps, and weight status in rural and urban North Carolina counties. *Prev. Chron. Dis.* **2010**, *7*, A107.
24. D'Angelo, H.; Ammerman, A.; Gordon-Larsen, P.; Linnan, L.; Lytle, L.; Ribisl, K. Small food store retailers' willingness to implement healthy store strategies in rural North Carolina. *J. Community Health* **2016**, *42*, 109–115. [CrossRef] [PubMed]
25. McGuirt, J.T.; Pitts, S.B.J.; Ammerman, A.; Prelip, M.; Hillstrom, K.; Garcia, R.E.; McCarthy, W.J. A mixed methods comparison of urban and rural retail corner stores. *AIMS Public Health* **2015**, *2*, 554–582. [CrossRef] [PubMed]
26. Pinard, C.A.; Shanks, C.B.; Harden, S.M.; Yaroch, A.L. An integrative literature review of small food store research across urban and rural communities in the US. *Prev. Med. Rep.* **2016**, *3*, 324–332. [CrossRef] [PubMed]
27. Gittelsohn, J. Interventions in small food stores to change the food environment, improve diet, and reduce risk of chronic disease. *Prev. Chron. Dis.* **2012**, *9*, E59. [CrossRef]
28. Langellier, B.A.; Garza, J.R.; Prelip, M.L.; Glik, D.; Brookmeyer, R.; Ortega, A.N. Corner Store Inventories, Purchases, and Strategies for Intervention: A Review of the Literature. *Calif. J. Health. Promot.* **2013**, *11*, 1–13. [PubMed]

nutrients

MDPI

Article

What Drives Food Insecurity in Western Australia? How the Perceptions of People at Risk Differ to Those of Stakeholders

Lucy M. Butcher [1,2,*], Maria M. Ryan [3], Therese A. O'Sullivan [1], Johnny Lo [4] and Amanda Devine [1]

1 School of Medical and Health Sciences, Edith Cowan University, Joondalup, WA 6027, Australia; t.osullivan@ecu.edu.au (T.A.O.); a.devine@ecu.edu.au (A.D.)
2 Foodbank Western Australia, Perth Airport, WA 6105, Australia
3 School of Business and Law, Edith Cowan University, Joondalup, WA 6027, Australia; m.ryan@ecu.edu.au
4 School of Science, Edith Cowan University, Joondalup, WA 6027, Australia; j.lo@ecu.edu.au
* Correspondence: lucy.butcher@foodbankwa.org.au; Tel.: +61-08-9463-3215

Received: 13 July 2018; Accepted: 7 August 2018; Published: 9 August 2018

Abstract: Food insecurity is considered a "wicked" problem due to the highly complex and at times undefined casual factors. Although many stakeholders are working to address the problem, a possible divergence exists between their views on food insecurity and those of the people who are actually experiencing the problem. The purpose of this study was to investigate whether there was a difference between the opinions of those "at risk" and stakeholders. A total of seven focus groups (two stakeholder groups $n = 10$, five "at-risk" groups $n = 34$) and three interviews (stakeholders $n = 3$) were conducted to ascertain perceptions. Thematic analysis generated 329 (209 "at-risk" and 120 stakeholder) coded statements related to food insecurity drivers. Respondents were in agreement for the majority of factors, and limited income was considered the primary driver of food insecurity. However, there were notable deviations in the perceived importance of certain drivers, particularly around the price of food and the lack of food literacy. Differences in the perception of causes of food insecurity may in part be attributed to the varied role each group plays in working towards the resolution of the problem, either at the household or system level.

Keywords: vulnerable groups; food poverty; food insecurity; food literacy; public health; socioeconomics

1. Introduction

Food security is broadly defined as when all people, at all times, have sufficient food to meet their needs. It is underpinned by four pillars: food availability, access, utilisation and stability [1]. Availability refers to sufficient quantities of appropriate food, access refers to having economic and physical resources to obtain appropriate foods for a nutritious diet, utilisation is knowledge of basic nutrition and cooking skills, and stability refers to continued access that can withstand climatic or economic disasters or seasonal events [1]. Ultimately, the disruption of any of the abovementioned pillars may be the catalyst for food insecurity [2,3]. Often oversimplified as an issue of poverty, the problem remains largely hidden in developed countries such as Australia. The reported Australian prevalence of food insecurity varies considerably, depending on the definition and measurement used, between 4% [4] and 36% [5].

Food insecurity is considered a "wicked" problem due to the vast, highly complex and at times undefined casual factors [6]. Part of the challenge of making a tangible difference is the dynamic nature of the issue. Changes to the political, economic and social environments have a flow-on effect on the pillars of food security and thus affect a range of sectors within a population [7]. Although many stakeholders employed in the food relief sector are working to address the problem, a possible divergence exists between their views and those of food-insecure people [8]. Deviations in the perceived underlying casual factors between these two key groups may further complicate the process of resolving the issue of food insecurity. The purpose of this study was to compare and contrast opinions on household and systems level food insecurity drivers by those "at risk" and by stakeholders in Western Australia. To our knowledge, this study was the first to investigate the potential differences of opinions between these two key groups within an Australian context.

2. Materials and Methods

2.1. Sample Groups and Recruitment

Two groups were purposefully targeted for inclusion in either focus groups or in-depth interviews. The first group included stakeholders, who worked in the area of food insecurity (from government, academic and not for profit sectors) and acted as an expert source of information. The second group consisted of individuals who were determined to be at high risk of food insecurity, termed "at risk" (AR), in order to provide contextual information about the lived experience. Initially, stakeholders were recruited through an email sent to a professional interest group. Snowball sampling and word of mouth were utilised to increase recruitment, as recommended for studies of "hidden" issues [9].

A review of adult (≥18 years old) groups most at risk of food insecurity in Australia has identified tertiary students [10], individuals living in regional and remote areas [11], Aboriginal people [12], refugees [13], Culturally and Linguistically Diverse (CALD) people, low-income earners [14], single parents [15], the homeless [16] and those with chronic medical conditions [17]. The tertiary student groups were recruited via Facebook, posts on university message boards and personal invitations at lectures or conferences. Stakeholders were asked for recommendations or referral to other organisations that could provide access to groups whom they considered to be at a high risk of food insecurity. Individuals who met one or more of these criteria were targeted for inclusion in this study. Simplified definitions of food security and food insecurity were explained to all participants. The research topic was framed, during recruitment, as exploring the reasons why some people can't access enough or the right types of food in Australia. A $20 food voucher was offered to the AR respondents as compensation for their time and effort.

2.2. Data Collection

Data collection was conducted between December 2015 and November 2016. A semi-structured format, considered appropriate for open, in-depth discussion of sensitive topics with vulnerable groups [18], was utilised. Both respondent groups were offered inclusion via either focus group or interview. An interview guide with prompts was developed for the stakeholder and AR groups. The guide had the same underlying research aims, and questions, but was worded differently to ensure appropriateness for each group. All questions were open-ended and included the following topic areas: food insecurity prevalence, food affordability, barriers and personal experience. The content of the guide was informed by current literature and consultation from stakeholders and co-authors. The interview guide and research questions are available in the Supplementary Materials.

Individual interviews were also offered to both stakeholders and the AR individuals as an alternative to focus group participation. This interview format was intended to enable flexibility around attendance and to allow discussion of sensitive topics in a more private setting. All focus groups and interviews were conducted in Perth, Western Australia, but included participants who worked or had lived in regional or remote areas of the state.

2.3. Data Analysis

The Clarke and Braun [19] thematic analysis framework guided the identification of concepts and patterns. Conversations were recorded with permission and transcribed verbatim. Data was de-identified and transcripts were read twice to check for accuracy prior to being imported into NVivo qualitative data analysis software; (QSR International Pty Ltd., Version 11, 2015, Doncaster, VIC, Australia). NVivo was employed for the thematic analysis to increase the efficiency and trustworthiness of results in this qualitative research [20]. In addition to audio recording of the focus groups and interviews, notes were taken during both to assist the generation of themes and key concepts. Triangulation was employed to increase validity the data collection, quality of coding and rigour of the thematic analysis [20]. Investigator triangulation was achieved by co-authors (1) attendance one or more focus groups, review of the transcripts and audio recordings and (2) joint discussion of themes to ensure consistency. The use of this technique ensured that the multiple perspectives provided by the AR group and stakeholders were interpreted correctly and there was a consensus among multiple investigators [21].

The four pillars of food security and the research question formed the basis for the initial framework for coding. Twenty-one traditionally associated factors of food insecurity were identified in the literature and these were listed as potential nodes. New or emerging concepts relevant to the research questions were also coded into nodes. Themes and sub-themes, within these four pillars of food security, were created though the amalgamation and separation of the nodes. Data saturation point was ascertained when no additional themes were identified, and the generation of new nodes had ceased. Data saturation, when used in conjunction with investigator triangulation, is considered an appropriate and sufficient methodology for qualitative research [22]. Matrix coding queries, word clouds, text enquiries and frequencies were used for the data analysis.

Edith Cowan University's Human Research Ethics Committee approved the study (Project Number: 11118).

3. Results

Twenty stakeholders were invited to participate via email. Of those, 13 agreed to participate, five did not respond and two declined. Reasons given included a lack of time or an absence of expertise in food security. A total of seven organisations were emailed the study information letter and AR groups were invited to participate. Three organisations agreed to take part: a homeless refuge, a multi-cultural domestic violence group and a food relief agency, from which 34 AR individuals agreed to participate in the study. Of the four organisations that did not take part, three organisations did not feel their groups were suitable and one did not respond. In all, a total of 47 respondents participated in focus groups or interviews. A total of seven focus groups (two stakeholder groups $n = 10$, five AR groups $n = 34$) and three interviews (stakeholders $n = 3$) were conducted.

Of the three stakeholders who accepted the offer for an interview, two were face-to-face, and one interview was via telephone. All interested AR individuals opted to participate in a focus group. Two tertiary student focus groups were conducted, one with undergraduate students and one with post graduate students. Participant characteristics are outlined in Tables 1 and 2.

Table 1. Characteristics of stakeholders ($n = 13$).

Characteristic	*n*	%
Age (years)		
20–29	4	31
30–39	2	15
40–49	3	23
50+	4	31
Sex		
Female	11	85
Education		
<Tertiary	1	8
Tertiary	12	92
Employer		
Not for profit	9	69
Government	1	8
Academic institution	3	23

Tertiary = obtained a tertiary qualification (e.g., diploma, academic degree).

Table 2. Characteristics of 'at risk' (*n* = 34).

Characteristic	*n*	%
Age (years)		
20–29	15	44
30–39	6	17
40–49	5	15
50+	8	24
Gender		
Female	28	82
Education		
<Tertiary	25	74
Tertiary	9	26
Aboriginal and Torres Strait Islander	3	9
Culturally and Linguistically Diverse	10	29

Tertiary obtained a tertiary qualification (e.g., diploma, academic degree).

When asked, approximately two-thirds (68%) of the AR individuals and all stakeholders thought food insecurity was a problem in Australia. Thematic analysis generated 378 individually coded statements. Of these codes, 329 (209 AR and 120 stakeholder) were considered as drivers, either positively or negatively affecting an individual's healthy food acquisition, and were categorised into the four pillars of food security that formed the primary themes. The remaining 49 codes related to determinants of food security have not been included in this paper. Encompassed within these four primary themes were 15 drivers of food insecurity or sub-themes. Both groups noted similar drivers of food insecurity; however, the most apparent difference was the relative importance attributed to each of these factors. Figure 1 is a graphic comparison of the themes and sub-themes cited by both the stakeholders and AR group.

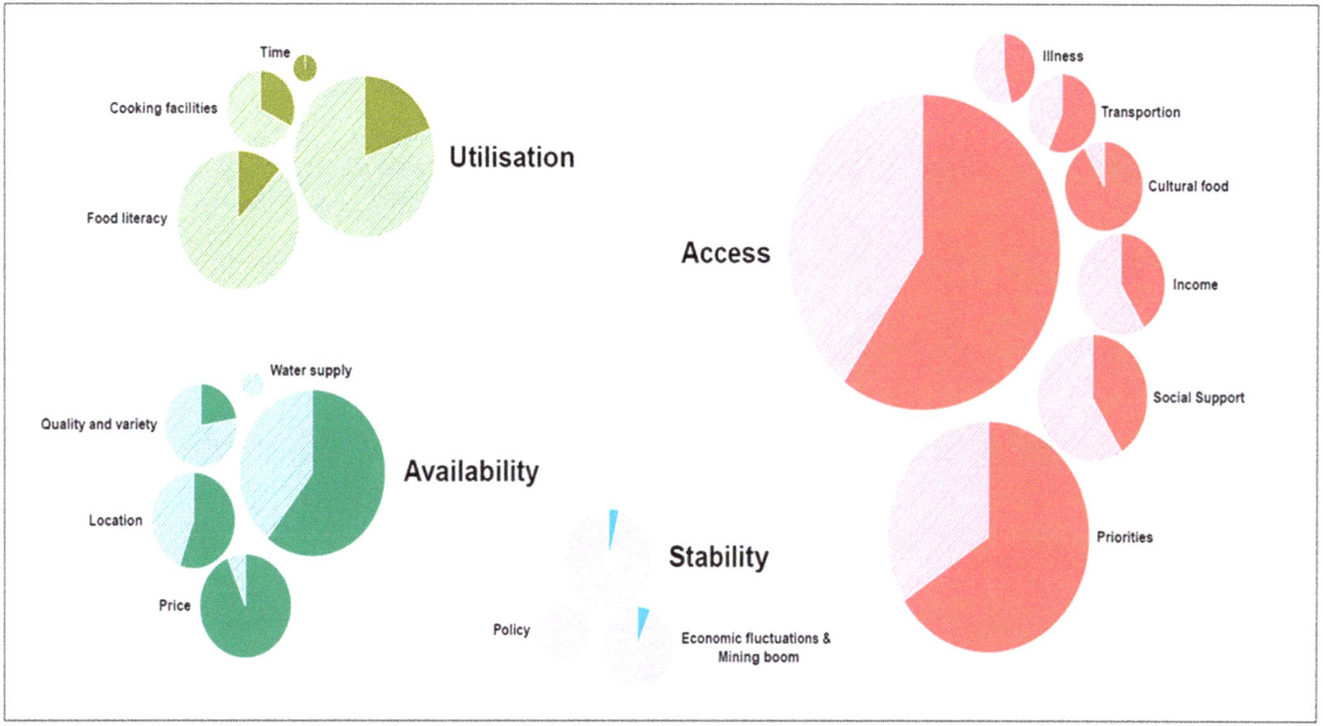

Figure 1. The proportions of the food insecurity drivers cited by stakeholders and at-risk group. The size of the circle indicates the frequency of the driver cited. An even distribution of solid and striped colours indicates that the driver was cited equally by stakeholders and at-risk individuals. A larger proportion of solid colour indicates that the driver was more frequently cited by at-risk individuals than stakeholders, and vice versa.

3.1. Food Access Pillar

Access was the most frequently referenced pillar (n = 211, 64%); 73% for the AR group (n = 152) and 49% for the stakeholder group (n = 59). From both groups, six subthemes were identified within the Access pillar: income, priorities, social, cultural foods, transport, and illness and mobility.

3.1.1. Income

Unexpected bills or costs added an extra burden on already strained finances. AR respondents felt there was no flexibility in the budget for luxuries and that food relief, theft and their social support networks were sometimes used as a means to access additional food. Both respondent groups discussed the concepts of household budget elasticity; competing costs and increasing daily compromises to ensure food supply.

"It relates back to money, but living week to week. If you don't have savings and you have used all your money for the week. You've got $10 left and your food is going to cost $30 dollars. Then there is that gap."

Stakeholder, Female, 40–49

"The self-serve juggle. If you put everything through fast enough they don't realise you're not paying everything. I mean you can just put through eleven milk cartons when you're only paying for three. You can do that kind of thing just to save money".

At-risk male, 20–29

3.1.2. Priorities

When income is limited, extensive prioritisation by food-insecure individuals was required to try to ensure perceived basic needs were met. Several compromises were reported by AR respondents and observed by stakeholders: including decreasing the variety of food or buying "cheap" unhealthy options to prevent hunger.

"It's about how can I make this last and in the home that there are still three meals being placed on the table. The quality of the meal they have also has to be in question as part of that food insecurity. Yes, it lacks any nutritional value, but there are three meals on the table . . . "

Stakeholder, Female, 50+

All of the AR respondents acknowledged that eating nutritious food and their health was important; however, avoiding hunger was their principal focus. One respondent conceded that they had stolen from supermarkets as means to feel full.

"All your health foods like fruit, veggies and nuts are quite expensive. A piece of bread and Vegemite might suffice on a particular day . . . You know it's not great over the long term, but in the short term it's cheap. It's not sustaining your health, but it is sustaining your need for food."

At-risk female, 50+

Housing and essential bills were items prioritised by the AR group; and for several AR individuals, so were vices such as alcohol, drugs or cigarettes.

"Well if I only have so much money, I would rather have cigarettes than food. I'll be honest with you."

At-risk female, 50+

3.1.3. Social Network

Both stakeholders and the AR group identified that a person's social network could have either a positive or negative affect on food security status. Families or group dwellings could share food, transport and resources, ultimately reducing financial burden and potentially increasing the enjoyment associated with food and meal preparation.

"If there were more people in the house the money would share as well. And I feel like if I did cook a big dish ... Then I would have to have left overs for the rest of the week and I would just get sick of it and I wouldn't want that dish anymore."

At-risk male, 20–29

Participants reported that living in shared housing or in emergency accommodation meant food could be stolen, or they felt obligated to feed other people who were not able or willing to share the expense. For Aboriginal communities, the transient nature of their society and strong extended family ties made meal planning and budgeting challenging, as it was difficult to predict the size of a household week to week.

"We have Aboriginal clients here ... There are lots of funerals in their families, but every time you have a funeral you have to feed everyone. Often you will get food insecurity if there have been a number of deaths in the family. Families stay after the funerals, so you have to feed all these people afterwards".

Stakeholder, Female, 40–49

More broadly, criminal behaviour of family members may burden households when grandparents or relatives are required to care for children while their parents are incarcerated. Instances of domestic violence may result in isolation, financial strain or a fear of going outside inhibiting access to food.

"If you're on a single pension then all of a sudden it puts your budget over or if your daughter or son goes to prison then you become the carer of their kids. Well, Centrelink doesn't know that. Often carer assistance isn't given or granted. They have five people in a family and they are living on a widow's pension."

Stakeholder, Female, 40–49

3.1.4. Cultural Food

AR respondents indicated cultural food, especially halal products, were often inaccessible, expensive or required extensive travel to obtain. Where halal products could not be sourced or were viewed as too expensive, some individuals would go without food on religious grounds.

"In Australia we have to find certain products like halal meats and it's difficult to find. We have to go 40 km to find the halal meats ... It's a big problem ... We have to travel a lot to get it. The Muslim people are struggling in most areas of Perth, because most of the shops don't sell halal meat."

At-risk female, 30–39

A stakeholder also indicated that their clients have difficulty obtaining cultural food (including halal foods).

3.1.5. Transport

Individuals without access to a car must walk or use public transport, and are limited by the amount of food they could carry in a single trip. The inability to buy in bulk and the need to undertake frequent shopping trips was seen by respondents as increasing the cost associated with healthy food and meal preparation. Alternatively, respondents relied on friends or family members for travel, but this often required payment for fuel and prior planning.

"I find it difficult to get to the shops when I don't have a car. Because you can't get everything you want in one shop. I don't have license so I have to walk everywhere."

At-risk female, 20–29

3.1.6. Illness and Mobility

Medications and doctors' visits represented unexpected costs and made budgeting challenging. Those with mental illness could have intense anxiety or fear about going to shops/supermarkets that are heavily populated, and this could hinder a person's ability to get nutritious food.

> *"I've got illness. Well I suffer from panic attacks, so I don't like to go to the shops. I like to be able to see the exit and go quick and get out. I don't want to go to the big shops."*
>
> At-risk female, 50+

Illness and older age can be related to taste changes, decreased appetite and fatigue, resulting in reduced motivation to purchase and prepare food. Stakeholders expressed concern about the elderly and those with disabilities for who reduced mobility could impact their ability to obtain food.

3.2. Food Availability Pillar

Availability was the second most noted theme overall (18%, n = 59); 21% for the AR group (n = 43) and 13% for the stakeholder group (n = 16). Four sub-themes of food availability that emerged included price, location, quality, variety and water supply. These are discussed below.

3.2.1. Price

The majority (56%) of AR respondents considered food to be expensive or unaffordable. Fruit, vegetables and seafood were the most frequently cited as the least affordable foods; rice, flour, bread and "junk" foods were perceived to be the cheapest options. Understandings of healthy food varied within the AR group. Some individuals felt food needed to be organic (frequently a more costly option) to be considered healthy. Healthy foods, such as avocados and mangoes, were considered luxury items for the AR group due to their prohibitive price.

> *"When I first got here, I took a picture and put it on Facebook, because an avocado cost $3..."*
>
> At-risk female, 40–49

However, stakeholders primarily mentioned the "subsidization" of processed foods and referenced supermarkets using marketing strategies, such as "loss leaders" as incentives. Promotional tactics were cited as taking advantage of vulnerable populations and encouraging an obesogenic environment where overconsumption of high-energy food was the social norm.

3.2.2. Location

Both stakeholders and the AR group agreed location affected variation in the price, quality and variety of food. An inconsistency in the price of food was noted across Australian states, but respondents largely spoke about the disparity between metropolitan, regional and remote areas within Western Australia. Respondents who worked or had lived in regional or remote areas spoke about the struggle to obtain healthy food due to climatic conditions, distance and community store processes.

> *" ... a local regional and remote community store ... wasn't providing any fresh fruit and vegetables because they thought it would be wasted, and there is a higher profit margin of white bread, sugar, coke and so on."*
>
> Stakeholder, Female, 20–29

Stakeholders commented that food outlets were strategically located to take advantage of vulnerable groups.

> *"It's the ease of fast food being available and they do it to prey on the weak (fast food company) put a (store) right at the corner of the park ... They absolutely knew there were some very vulnerable*

people and very low economic consumers that could buy their $1 or $2 or whatever it costs burger and they put themselves absolutely purposely in that spot ... We know that it's mostly plastic cheese and disgraceful meat, but people eat it because it's cheap..."

Stakeholder, Male, 40–49

AR respondents acknowledged that junk or fast food often provided a convenient and cost effective option. Opening hours and the distance to supermarkets were barriers to availability mentioned by the AR group. Shops and restaurants that closed by 9 p.m. limited the choice of those working late hours to expensive convenience stores or cheaper fast food options.

" ... especially when I was living far away from a shopping centre, I mean there were times when I was so hungry that I would just pop down to the servo to grab a pie or something."

At-risk male, 20–29

3.2.3. Quality and Variety (Including Water Supply)

Both stakeholders and the AR group considered the variety and quality of food within the metropolitan area was generally good. Stock was perceived as superior in quality and variety when compared to food sold in regional areas. Imported and exported foods were front of mind for both those AR and stakeholders. The AR respondents felt imported foods were inferior and at times not safe to consume.

Stakeholders were concerned about the net result of the export of healthy unprocessed foods and the subsequent import of processed non-nutritious foods.

"Because technically we have an abundant food supply, so it does come down to the individual, community and food policy side of things. There is such a great availability of non-nutritious foods."

Stakeholder, Female, 30–39

The concept that food security was inclusive of the availability of both adequate safe food and drinks.

"It encompasses the adequate availability of water. We don't have too much of an issue in metropolitan WA, but on the flip side how available the non-nutritious drinks are. Because that's an area of concern as well'."

Stakeholder, Female, 30–39

3.3. *Food Utilisation Pillar*

Overall, food utilisation was considered the third most significant driver of food insecurity (13%, $n = 44$); however, this pillar was perceived as more important for the stakeholder group (26%, $n = 31$) than for the AR group (6%, $n = 13$). Another notable point of difference was the primary sub-theme for each group; food literacy was the most referenced sub-theme for stakeholders while cooking facilities was paramount for the AR group.

3.3.1. Food Literacy

Stakeholders identified limited cooking skills or nutrition education as a food security barrier and current initiatives were often already preaching to the converted. Aggressive food marketing and advertising was viewed as affecting people's food choices, especially those with either lower education levels or poor food literacy. There was also a perception that their clients could not afford to experiment or try new recipes, in fear of their families not eating the food and increasing food waste.

"I think the low food literacy is a big part of it. Teaching people about food budgeting and that fresh healthy food per kg is cheaper and then teaching them the skills to cook it. Also having enough food

to meet their nutrient requirements. So if they are just getting the cheap take away or the sausages, white bread. They might have enough food, do they have enough nutrients."

Stakeholder, Female, 30–39

The AR group largely did not view their food literacy skills as impacting their ability to obtain enough healthy food. Only the six male student respondents commented that their lack of confidence in cooking and nutrition knowledge had been an issue in the past.

3.3.2. Cooking Facilities and Resources

Sharing cooking and storage facilities was highlighted by the AR group as a barrier to food security. For those at risk of food insecurity, a lack of, or unclean cooking facilities, made food preparation challenging and time consuming.

"I live in a communal place or area in a refuge. Everyone has to share the kitchen, so that makes it really hard. As opposed to having your own kitchen. I find it really frustrating, to be honest. I can't wait to be out of there. Especially when you have a little kid and when other people aren't clean. They just leave their stuff there and you have to work around it. It's not your job to clean up after them, but they don't do it as quickly as you do. I ended up saying something to someone yesterday and it ended up being a huge confrontation. It doesn't really make you want to cook."

At-risk female, 30–39

Stakeholders spoke about a general lack of very basic cooking facilities and how this ultimately impacted consumption of healthy food by people experiencing food insecurity.

"This affects Aboriginal people as well. Something like 40% of them doesn't have a kitchen. Or a stable address either. And those who have home the equipment still doesn't work. We see that a lot with our clients, a lot of them don't have fridge so they can't buy in bulk so they buy little bits and pieces. They basically have to use it all up within the day. Especially in the summer."

Stakeholder, Female, 20–29

Additionally, stakeholders and the AR group agreed that cooking could be a large financial investment. For example, a lack of pantry staples makes cooking from scratch expensive, as all ingredients need to be purchased. People who move frequently may not be able to take pantry ingredients with them.

The other thing is cooking a meal, when you have is a small amount of money. It's relatively large investment to go to get everything you need, because you won't use all of it in the meal and some of that doesn't last all that long. So unless you're cooking meals regularly it looks a lot worse on paper than the fast food options out there.

At-risk male, 20–29

3.3.3. Time

Time as barrier to food security was only mentioned by the AR group. Careful budgeting, strategic shopping and healthy meal preparation were all considered to be time consuming tasks, which presented a challenge when individuals were already overcommitted.

"It requires you to make a lot of trips and you've got to be checking it out really often and there are people that won't go to spend time for that."

At-risk male, 20–29

3.4. Stability Pillar

Stability (5%, $n = 15$) had the least number of themes emerged for stakeholders (12%, $n = 14$) and the AR group (<1%, $n = 1$). Policy and economic fluctuations were the sub-themes discussed.

3.4.1. Policy

Stakeholders conceded that the current public perception was that obtaining healthy food was a personal choice. Stakeholders expressed concern that governments shifted excessive responsibility for obtaining healthy food onto individuals, and that too little attention was given to the role played by policy and industry.

"It's like they have a choice, but they don't actually have a choice. They don't have access. It's unavailable. It's that sort of rhetoric of it's their choice to eat healthier or not to budget. It's kind of short changing all these other factors. It's really a right wing platitude. They are just the ignorant mass."

Stakeholder, Female, 50+

3.4.2. Economic Fluctuations

Stakeholders discussed the impact of the recent mining boom and bust in Western Australia on the gap between rich and poor. This gap increased as the prices went up with demand, but stakeholders also noted that when the mining boom stopped, the gap still existed as jobs were lost. The cost of living has continued to rise despite the reduction in wages and job losses.

"Look, there are many reasons, with the economic downturn there are redundancies. There could be people that are very highly geared, so that they were thinking that the mining boom or the gravy train was just going to continue. They might have just got the big house and lots of cars. You know completely geared themselves to have this lifestyle and possibly it fell unstuck that way".

Stakeholder, Female, 30–39

When prompted, all of the AR respondents agreed that the cost of living had remained high despite the resulting economic downturn.

4. Discussion

There was general agreement between people at risk of food insecurity and stakeholders working in the area on many of the factors considered to be driving food insecurity in Western Australia. Of interest was the most apparent deviation in regard to the relative importance attributed to each of the pillars of food security. The stakeholders tended to focus on big-picture concepts outlined in the Stability and Availability pillars, including government policy and changes to the economic climate, whilst those at risk spoke of their personal experience and the minutiae impacting their daily lives, such as prioritisation of income, found within the Access pillar. These diverse themes emerging from two different perspectives, the stakeholders and the AR group, are consistent with the findings reported by other Australian studies [11,23] and similar to trends found between stakeholders and food-insecure individuals in Canada [8].

Study respondents unanimously considered adequate income as an essential component for food security and that current government welfare allowances were insufficient. Indeed, poor resourcing has been documented by several studies as the principal barrier to healthy food acquisition [23–25]. However, a point of difference between the respondent groups shown here was the perception of the prioritisation of healthy food and the acknowledgement of price as an obstacle. In concordance with the findings of Hamelin, Mercier and Bédard [8] AR respondents noted both the importance of and desire to eat a healthy diet, but simultaneously perceived healthy foods to be unaffordable and beyond their reach. This concept was previously reported by Laurel, et al. [26], who found that Australians from the lowest income bracket were required to spend an estimated 50% of their income to eat in accordance with the recommended dietary guidelines. This amount is above a recently calculated marker of food stress, which occurs when 25% or more of income is spent on food [27]. Previous research has suggested that when the cost of fruit and vegetables is subsidised, the consumption of these foods increases within low-income households [28]. This implies that the perceived prohibitive cost of healthy food is a significant challenge, regardless of a person's desire or motivation. Additionally, AR respondents and other research have cited non-financial factors such as distance to shops [29] and lack of car ownership [3] that could quite literally put healthy food beyond the reach of some individuals.

A characteristic feature of food insecurity without hunger in developed nations is the dietary compromise of quantity over quality that typically results in the overconsumption of high-energy foods [30,31]. Ultimately, the AR respondents followed this trend, as they prioritised a feeling of fullness over the nutritional quality of food, resulting in a less nutritious diet. The stakeholders in this study, however, chiefly spoke about the overabundance of cheap, energy-dense products displacing the intake of nutritious foods in food-insecure people and the expense of healthy food was less frequently cited.

Another important disparity between the respondent groups was the identification of the main challenges, largely within the Utilisation pillar, to meal preparation. Barriers to cooking healthy meals reported in the literature and in this study include the expense of pantry items [32], the inability to obtain cultural foods [33] and poor access to kitchen or food storage facilities [11]. The AR respondents cited kitchen facilities as the greatest obstacle to cooking, while stakeholders focused more on food literacy (cooking and nutrition) skills.

"Food literacy is the ability of an individual to understand food in a way that they develop a positive relationship with it, including food skills and practices across the lifespan in order to navigate, engage, and participate within a complex food system" [34]. Food literacy is encompassed within the utilisation pillar and was regarded by the stakeholders as an important means to assist individuals ameliorate some the effects of food insecurity and improve their ability to navigate the complex food system [35,36]. This is in contrast with the current North American position, where nutrition interventions targeting food-insecure people are thought to be ineffective, as their limited income does not allow for the implementation of healthy eating principles [8,37,38]. In our study, only the male AR respondents believed their food literacy skills had impacted their intake of healthy food, whereas, female AR respondents felt they were very resourceful and used a large range of coping strategies to reduce the impact of a limited income on food intake. Furthermore, McLaughlin, et al. [39] found no association between food security status in Canadian women and the frequency of cooking from scratch. Food-insecure women, however, tended to prepare less complex recipes, possibly due to the expense of the ingredients rather than a lack of skills. However, the researchers in this study observed varied levels of nutrition knowledge among their AR group. For example, many AR respondents believed food needed to be organic to be considered healthy. It is therefore plausible that people with less severe food insecurity could benefit from an improved understanding of what constitutes a healthy diet. Regardless, stakeholders within this study also noted differences associated with gender; in particular food preparation, shopping and cooking primarily seemed to follow traditional gender roles and was largely the responsibility of women [31,40]. Studies have demonstrated that men living alone may lack basic cooking and nutrition skills, preventing them from adequately addressing their own eating requirements [40,41]. It is therefore possible that limited food literacy skills could be a barrier to food security for males. However, due to low representation of males in our study generalising these results should be cautioned, and more research is warranted focusing on the male perspective.

Emerging themes in our study also included the impact of poor health and the effect of the prioritisation of alcohol and drugs on food security status. Both respondent groups agreed that these issues were detrimental to a person's food security and competed with cost of medical appointments, medications and healthy food. Previous research shows positive associations between poor health, particularly mental health [17], and tobacco [42] and drug usage [43,44] with food insecurity. To date it is unclear whether these associations are causal or a symptom of low socioeconomic status.

The strength of this study was the consideration of viewpoints from both stakeholders and a variety of people at risk of food insecurity. Focus groups were conducted to code or data saturation and therefore provided a well-rounded depiction of the issues. A limitation of this study was an overrepresentation of female and tertiary student respondents and an underrepresentation of several subgroups (regional and remote, Aboriginal people). Therefore, our study population was not a representative sample of the Australian population and this limits the generalization of the results. Additionally, due to concerns about literacy skills, a food security measurement was not applied to the AR respondents. The researchers could therefore not definitively classify these individuals as "food-insecure" at the time of focus group or interview. However all participants in the AR focus group gave examples of food insecurity, which provided adequate justification for their classification.

Recommendations to Assist Stakeholders to Better Combat Household Food Insecurity

Based on the findings of this research the following recommendations have been suggested:

1. Include pantry items and culturally appropriate foods in emergency food relief packs.
2. Assist individuals to cook meals at home by subsidizing the cost of healthy foods, particularly fruit and vegetables.
3. Tailor food literacy programs to more effectively engage males.
4. Provide education for stakeholders that motivation or desire may not be the underlying reasons for overconsumption of non-nutritious foods in food-insecure people, and that other factors such as prioritization of funds or time may be an issue.

5. Conclusions

Although there was agreement on the perceived importance of the major drivers of food insecurity, such as income, there were notable differences between the AR individuals and stakeholders when it came to some factors, including time, food literacy, health policy and the price of food. These differences may in part be attributed to the varied role each group has to play in the resolution of the problem. It is understandable that stakeholders would focus their efforts on lobbying for enhanced government and industry policy as this would enact significant change at a system level. However, it is still important to acknowledge the lived experience of food-insecure individuals and recognize that a lack of motivation or desire may not be the underlying reason for poor dietary intake.

Supplementary Materials: The following are available online at http://www.mdpi.com/2072-6643/10/8/1059/s1, File S1: Interview guide and research questions.

Author Contributions: All authors were involved in the conceptualization and design of the study. Manuscript draft preparation was conducted by L.M.B. Focus groups were run by L.M.B. with assistance from M.M.R., T.A.O. and A.D. Results were transcribed and analysed by L.M.B., and J.L. assisted with figure development. All authors listened to the audio recordings for the accuracy of the transcription. A.D., M.M.R., T.A.O. and J.L. provided review, editing and supervision.

Funding: This research received no external funding.

Conflicts of Interest: The authors declare no conflict of interest.

References

1. Food and Agriculture Organization of the United Nations. *Food Security*; FAO's Agriculture and Development Economics Division (ESA), FAO Netherlands Partnership Programme (FNPP), EC-FAO Food Security Programme: Rome, Italy, 2006.
2. Carter, K.N.; Lanumata, T.; Kruse, K.; Gorton, D. What Are the Determinants of Food Insecurity in New Zealand and Does This Differ for Males and Females? Available online: https://doi-org.ezproxy.ecu.edu.au/10.1111/j.1753-6405.2010.00615.x (accessed on 8 July 2018).
3. Burns, C.; Bentley, R.; Lakar, T.; Kavanagh, A. Reduced food access due to a lack of money, inability to lift and lack of access to a car for food shopping: A multilevel study in Melbourne, victoria. *Public Health Nutr.* **2011**, *14*, 1017–1023. [CrossRef] [PubMed]
4. Australian Bureau of Statistics. Australian Health Survey: Nutrition-State and Territory Results, 2011–2012. Available online: http://abs.gov.au/AUSSTATS/abs@.nsf/mf/4364.0.55.009 (accessed on 3 March 2018).
5. Butcher, L.M.; O'Sullivan, T.A.; Ryan, M.M.; Lo, J.; Devine, A. Utilising a multi-item questionnaire to assess household food security in Australia. *Health Promot. J. Aust.* **2018**, 1–9. [CrossRef] [PubMed]

6. Grochowska, R. Specificity of food security concept as a wicked problem. *J. Agric. Sci. Technol.* **2014**, *4*, 823–831.
7. Mahadevan, R.; Hoang, V. Is there a link between poverty and food security? *Soc. Indic. Res.* **2016**, *128*, 179–199. [CrossRef]
8. Hamelin, A.-M.; Mercier, C.; Bédard, A. Perception of needs and responses in food security: Divergence between households and stakeholders. *Public Health Nutr.* **2008**, *11*, 1389–1396. [CrossRef] [PubMed]
9. Salganik, M.J.; Heckathorn, D.D. Sampling and estimation in hidden populations using respondent-driven sampling. *Sociol. Methodol.* **2004**, *34*, 193–239. [CrossRef]
10. Gallegos, D.; Ramsay, R.; Ong, K. Food insecurity: Is it an issue among tertiary students. *High. Educ.* **2014**, *67*, 497–510. [CrossRef]
11. Godrich, S.L.; Davies, C.R.; Darby, J.; Devine, A. What are the determinants of food security among regional and remote Western Australian children? *Aust. N. Z. J. Public Health* **2017**, *41*, 172–177. [CrossRef] [PubMed]
12. Bussey, C. Food security and traditional foods in remote aboriginal communities: A review of the literature. *Aust. Indig. Health Bull.* **2013**, *13*, 1–10.
13. Gallegos, D.; Ellies, P.; Wright, J. Still there's no food! Food insecurity in a refugee population in Perth, Western Australia. *Nutr. Diet.* **2008**, *65*, 78–83. [CrossRef]
14. Mark, S.; Lambert, M.; O'Loughlin, J.; Gray-Donald, K. Household income, food insecurity and nutrition in Canadian youth. *Can. J. Public Health* **2012**, *103*, 94–99. [PubMed]
15. Kenney, C.T. Father doesn't know best? Parents' control of money and children's food insecurity. *J. Marriage Fam.* **2008**, *70*, 654–669. [CrossRef]
16. Peterson, L. Food insecurity and homelessness. *Parity* **2016**, *29*, 20–21.
17. Pryor, L.; Lioret, S.; van der Waerden, J.; Fombonne, É.; Falissard, B.; Melchior, M. Food insecurity and mental health problems among a community sample of young adults. *Soc. Psychiatry Psychiatr. Epidemiol.* **2016**, *51*, 1073–1081. [CrossRef] [PubMed]
18. Naylor, R.; Maye, D.; Ilbery, B.; Enticott, G.; Kirwan, J. Researching controversial and sensitive issues: Using visual vignettes to explore farmers' attitudes towards the control of bovine tuberculosis in England. *Area* **2014**, *46*, 285–293. [CrossRef]
19. Clarke, V.; Braun, V. *Successful Qualitative Research: A Practical Guide for Beginners*; SAGE: London, UK, 2013.
20. Carter, N.; Bryant-Lukosius, D.; DiCenso, A.; Blythe, J.; Neville, A.J. The use of triangulation in qualitative research. *Oncol. Nurs. Forum* **2014**, *41*, 545–547. [CrossRef] [PubMed]
21. Creswell, J.W.; Plano Clark, V.L. *Designing and Conducting Mixed Methods Research*; SAGE Publications: Thousand Oaks, CA, USA, 2007.
22. Walker, J.L. Research column. The use of saturation in qualitative research. *Can. J. Cardiovasc. Nurs.* **2012**, *22*, 37–41. [PubMed]
23. Rosier, K. *Food Insecurity in Australia: What Is It, Who Experiences It and How Can Child and Family Services Support Families Experiencing It?* Australian Institute of Family Studies: Canberra, Australia, 2011.
24. Nolan, M.; Rikard-Bell, G.; Mohsin, M.; Williams, M. Food insecurity in three socially disadvantaged localities in Sydney, Australia. *Health Promot. J. Aust.* **2006**, *17*, 247–253. [CrossRef]
25. Gorton, D.; Bullen, C.R.; Mhurchu, C.N. Environmental influences on food security in high-income countries. *Nutr. Rev.* **2010**, *68*, 1–29. [CrossRef] [PubMed]
26. Laurel, B.; Sharon, F.; Katrin, E.; Lilian, C. The cost of a healthy and sustainable diet—Who can afford it? *Aust. N. Z. J. Public Health* **2014**, *38*, 7–12.
27. Landrigan, T.J.; Kerr, D.A.; Dhaliwal, S.S.; Savage, V.; Pollard, C.M. Removing the australian tax exemption on healthy food adds food stress to families vulnerable to poor nutrition. *Aust. N. Z. J. Public Health* **2017**, *41*, 591–597. [CrossRef] [PubMed]
28. Anderson, J.V.; Bybee, D.I.; Brown, R.M.; McLean, D.F. 5 a day fruit and vegetable intervention improves consumption in a low income population. *J. Am. Diet. Assoc.* **2001**, *101*, 195–202. [CrossRef]
29. Pollard, C.; Nyaradi, A.; Lester, M.; Sauer, K. Understanding food security issues in remote Western Australian Indigenous communities. *Health Promot. J. Aust.* **2014**, *25*, 83–89. [CrossRef] [PubMed]
30. Lee, S.; Gundersen, C.; Cook, J.; Laraia, B.; Johnson, M. Food insecurity and health across the lifespan. *Adv. Nutr.* **2012**, *3*, 744–745. [CrossRef] [PubMed]
31. Mishra, G.; Ball, K.; Arbuckle, J.; Crawford, D. Dietary patterns of Australian adults and their association with socioeconomic status: Results from the 1995 national nutrition survey. *Eur. J. Clin. Nutr.* **2002**, *56*, 687. [CrossRef] [PubMed]

32. Wright, B.; McCormack, L.; Stluka, S.; Contreras, D.; Franzen-Castle, L.; Henne, B.; Mehrle, D.; Remley, D.; Eicher-Miller, H. Pantry use predicts food security among rural, midwestern emergency food pantry users. *J. Nutr. Educ. Behav.* **2017**, *49*, S16–S17. [CrossRef]
33. Borre, K.; Ertle, L.; Graff, M. Working to eat: Vulnerability, food insecurity, and obesity among migrant and seasonal farmworker families. *Am. J. Ind. Med.* **2010**, *53*, 443–462. [CrossRef] [PubMed]
34. Cullen, T.; Hatch, J.; Martin, W.; Higgins, J.W.; Sheppard, R. Food literacy: Definition and framework for action. *Can. J. Diet. Pract. Res.* **2015**, *76*, 140–145. [CrossRef] [PubMed]
35. Vidgen, H. *Food Literacy: Key Concepts for Health and Education*; Taylor and Francis Ltd.: London, UK, 2016.
36. Vidgen, H.A.; Gallegos, D. Defining food literacy and its components. *Appetite* **2014**, *76*, 50–59. [CrossRef] [PubMed]
37. Huisken, A.; Orr, S.K.; Tarasuk, V. Adults' food skills and use of gardens are not associated with household food insecurity in Canada. *Can. J. Public Health* **2016**, *107*, E526–E532. [CrossRef] [PubMed]
38. Hamelin, A.; Beaudry, M.; Habicht, J. Charaterization of household food insecurity in Quebec: Food and feelings. *Soc. Sci. Med.* **2002**, *54*, 119–132. [CrossRef]
39. McLaughlin, C.; Tarasuk, V.; Kreiger, N. An examination of at-home food preparation activity among low-income, food-insecure women. *Am. Dietet. Assoc. J. Am. Diet. Assoc.* **2003**, *103*, 1506–1512. [CrossRef]
40. Thompson, J.; Tod, A.; Bissell, P.; Bond, M. Understanding food vulnerability and health literacy in older bereaved men: A qualitative study. *Health Expect.* **2017**, *20*, 1342–1349. [CrossRef] [PubMed]
41. Kennedy, L.A.; Hunt, C.; Hodgson, P. Nutrition education program based on EFNEP for low-income women in the United Kingdom. *J. Nutr. Educ.* **1998**, *30*, 89–99. [CrossRef]
42. Farrelly, M.C.; Shafer, P.R. Comparing trends between food insecurity and cigarette smoking among adults in the United States, 1998 to 2011. *Am. J. Health Promot.* **2016**, *31*, 413–416. [CrossRef] [PubMed]
43. Davey-Rothwell, M.A.; Flamm Laura, J.; Kassa Hilina, T.; Latkin Carl, A. Food insecurity and depressive syptoms: Compariosn of drug using and nondrug using women at risk of HIV. *J. Community Psychol.* **2014**, *42*, 469–478. [CrossRef] [PubMed]
44. McLinden, T.; Moodie, E.E.M.; Harper, S.; Hamelin, A.M.; Aibibula, W.; Cox, J.; Anema, A.; Klein, M.B. Injection drug use, food insecurity, and HIV-HCV co-infection: A longitudinal cohort analysis. *AIDS Care* **2018**, 1–7. [CrossRef] [PubMed]

nutrients

MDPI

Article

Metabolic Syndrome among Refugee Women from the West Bank, Palestine: A Cross-Sectional Study

Salwa G. Massad [1,*], Mohammed Khalili [2], Wahida Karmally [3], Marwah Abdalla [1,4], Umaiyeh Khammash [5], Gebre-Medhin Mehari [6] and Richard J. Deckelbaum [1]

1 Institute of Human Nutrition, Columbia University, New York, NY 10032, USA; ma2947@columbia.edu (M.A.); rjd20@cumc.columbia.edu (R.J.D.)
2 United Nations Relief and Works Agency for Palestine Refugees in the Near East (UNRWA), Jerusalem 972, Palestine; m.khalili@unrwa.org
3 Irving Institute for Clinical and Translational Research, Columbia University Medical Center, New York, NY 10032, USA; wk2@cumc.columbia.edu
4 Division of Cardiology, Department of Medicine, Columbia University Medical Center, New York, NY 10032, USA
5 Juzoor for Health and Social Development, Ramallah 970, Palestine; ukhammash@juzoor.org
6 Department of Women's and Children's Health, Pediatrics, University Hospital, SE-751 85 Uppsala, Sweden; Mehari.Gebre-Medhin@kbh.uu.se
* Correspondence: salwamassad@gmail.com; Tel: +1-9705-9816-1071

Received: 17 June 2018; Accepted: 16 August 2018; Published: 18 August 2018

Abstract: This study was carried out among Palestinian refugee women in the West Bank to provide data on the prevalence of metabolic syndrome (MetS) and its correlates. Data were obtained from a cross-sectional study of 1694 randomly selected refugee women from the United Nations Relief and Works Agency for Palestine Refugees in the Near East (UNRWA) health centers throughout the West Bank during June and July 2010. In this cohort, 30% of the refugee women were overweight, 39% were obese, and 7% were extremely obese. Based on World Health Organization (WHO) criteria, the age-adjusted prevalence of MetS was 19.8%. The results of the binary logistic regression analysis indicated that older age and younger marital age were significantly associated with an increased likelihood of MetS in the women. The high prevalence of obesity and MetS mandates the implementation of national policies for its prevention, notably by initiating large-scale community intervention programs for 5.2 million refugees in Palestine, Jordan, Lebanon, and Syria, to tackle obesity and increase the age at marriage.

Keywords: Obesity; metabolic syndrome; refugee; women; Palestine

1. Introduction

The post-2015 development agenda offers an opportunity to ensure a future framework that fully integrates non-communicable diseases (NCDs), which are the leading global determinants of death in adults, and cause more deaths than all other factors combined [1]. About 80% of deaths attributed to NCDs are believed to occur in emerging low- and middle-income countries [2]. In 2010, the World Economic Forum cited NCDs as one of the most important threats to economic development, alongside the current financial crisis, natural disasters, and influenza pandemics [1]. NCDs are also the leading causes of death in the Arab world, particularly in middle- and high-income countries, where is chaemic heart disease is the number one cause of death [3]. As in the rest of the world, NCDs have increased among Palestinian refugees, and are an added burden on the health care system. For example, in 2011 the prevalence of hypertension and diabetes in Palestinian refugees in the West Bank was 17.3% and 12.5%, respectively [4]. From 2001 to 2011, the number of Palestinian refugees affected by NCDs and treated at UNRWA (United Nations Relief and Works Agency for Palestine Refugees in the Near East) health centers in the West Bank, Gaza Strip, Jordan, Lebanon, and Syria was estimated to have increased from about 85,000 to approximately 212,000, with females (61%) bearing the brunt of the conditions [4].

Like NCDs, the prevalence of obesity has also increased worldwide. Obesity rates are estimated to have nearly doubled between 1980 and 2008 [1]. In the Middle East region, obesity rates are higher among women than men [5]. It is well-known that individuals with overall or abdominal obesity have an increased risk of developing metabolic syndrome (MetS) and diabetes mellitus [6]. As obesity rates continue to rise globally, the prevalence of MetS will also increase [7].

Despite the plethora of studies from other regions of the world, there is a paucity of data on MetS in Palestine in general [8–12]. In a small study conducted in the West Bank in 2001 [11], 58% of refugee women met the criteria for metabolic syndrome. However, this study was limited, as it examined women aged 40–65 years selected from only two of the 19 camps in the West Bank. More up-to-date evidence from larger studies is currently lacking. In line with the UNRWA Health Department strategy to collect systematic data on performance and management indicators, the overall aim of this study is to estimate the prevalence of MetS and its components, including obesity in Palestinian female refugees in the West Bank. Based on a review of the factors associated with MetS [6,13–16], we postulate that MetS increases with age, younger age at marriage, parity, urban living, and lower levels of education.

2. Materials and Methods

Description of Target Population and Sampling Design

The UNRWA has provided comprehensive primary health care to four generations of Palestine refugees, who lost their homes and means of livelihood as a result of the 1948 conflict. There are 58 camps in five fields of operation: the West Bank, Gaza Strip, Jordan, Lebanon, and Syria. There are 19 camps in the West Bank, with a total of 874,627 registered refugees [17]. Most of the other refugees live in towns and villages in the West Bank. Some camps are located next to major towns, and others are in rural areas.

We conducted this cross-sectional study in the 42 UNRWA health centers and mobile clinics throughout the West Bank during June and July 2010. We selected all women $\geq$15 years who reported to all 42 UNRWA primary health care centers and mobile health clinics in the designated time period. We excluded pregnant women and women in the puerperal period (up to 6 weeks following termination of labor). Data were collected during June and July 2010 by a field team of a doctor and 6 nurses.

Women visiting the health centers or mobile clinics on a day designated for data collection were interviewed and their body measurements and blood pressure were taken, and blood samples were collected the following day at the clinic laboratory to examine fasting blood glucose. A mercury sphygmomanometer was used for the measurement of blood pressure in the right arm. The participants rested quietly in a seated position for at least 15 min before the blood pressure measurement. Systolic and diastolic blood pressures were defined as the average of three readings. Using a measuring board, electric balance, and measuring tape, nurses at the clinic recorded the standing height, weight, and waist of each study index twice with light clothing. Waist circumferences measurements were taken with the measuring tape in a horizontal plane, midway between the inferior margin of the ribs and the superior border of the iliac crest. To avoid inter-subjective error, all measurements were taken by the same person. If the difference between the two measurements was more than 10%, a third measurement was obtained. Body mass index (BMI) was calculated as weight in kilograms divided by the square of height in meters, to determine a designation of underweight, normal weight, overweight, and obesity. Data on hypertension and medication for diabetes were extracted from medical records to minimize report bias. Blood was drawn after an overnight fast and analyzed for serum triglycerides, high-density lipoprotein (HDL) cholesterol, and glucose determinations. Biochemical analysis was conducted on fasting plasma samples, all blood analyses being done at the UNRWA laboratory on the day of blood collection. HDL cholesterol and triglyceride (TG) blood levels were measured using the HUMAN kit from Boehringer Mannheim, Mannheim, Germany. The UNRWA Health Department Ethics Committee, Jerusalem, Palestine, approved the study protocol in January 2010. Written informed consent (or assent) was obtained from the participants and the parents of those aged below 18 years.

3. Variables

3.1. Definition of Metabolic Syndrome

The definition of MetS is based on WHO diagnostic criteria [18]. For the purpose of comparison with other regional and international data, the prevalence of MetS is also reported based on the National Cholesterol Education Program (NCEP) Adult Treatment Panel III (ATP III) [19]. Direct standardization of prevalence was performed according to the population data published by the United Nations population division, as well as for the "WHO new world population" [20].

3.2. World Heath Organization Criteria

WHO criteria for MetS in epidemiologic studies were met if an individual had impaired fasting glucose, defined as a fasting glucose level between 110 and 126 mg/dL; diabetes (fasting glucose level $\geq$126 mg/dL); or was on diabetes treatment plus two or more of the following abnormalities: blood pressure of $\geq$140/90 mmHg or taking antihypertensive drugs, serum triglycerides of $\geq$150 mg/dL or serum HDL cholesterol of <39 mg/dL, or BMI $\geq$ 30 kg/m^2 or waist circumference >85 cm.

3.3. National Cholesterol Education Program-ATP III

ATP III criteria for MetS were met if an individual had three or more of the following criteria: waist circumference > 88 cm, fasting plasma glucose (FPG) $\geq$ 110 mg/dL, blood pressure $\geq$ 130/85 mmHg or mediation use, serum triglycerides $\geq$ 150 mg/dL, and serum HDL cholesterol < 50 mg/dL.

3.4. Individual and Household Measurements

Data collected on individual factors were age, age at marriage, social status, parity, education, employment, obesity, hypertension, impaired fasting glucose, and hyperlipidemia. The household variable was the type of residence: urban, rural, or camp. Age of participants was determined to the nearest year.

3.5. Statistical Analyses

Means, standard deviations for continuous variables, and percentages for categorical variables were used to describe the characteristics of the study sample. All analyses were performed by age. Chi-square tests were used to compare the distribution of metabolic syndrome components among women with and without obesity. MetS prevalence was adjusted to the WHO world standard for the 2000 population by direct standardization [21]. A binary logistic regression analysis was performed using the dichotomous variable MetS (1 = present, 0 = absent). The independent covariates included in the binary logistic regression analysis were age, type of residence, level of education, age at marriage, and parity. In all statistical analyses, p values less than 0.05 were considered significant. Statistical analyses were performed using Statistical Package for the Social Sciences (SPSS) v.17 (SPSS Inc., Version 17.0, Chicago, IL, USA).

4. Results

Data were collected on 1694 (98%) women visiting the health centers and mobile clinics at the time of data collection, of which 1562 (92%) had complete blood testing. The missing blood tests are for women who did not return for the blood test. The characteristics of the study sample are summarized in Table 1. The mean age was 39 years. Most women were unemployed and had completed high school education or below. Most women were married. Mean marital age was 19.6 years.

Table 1. Study sample characteristics (n = 1694) for refugee women (15–84 years), West Bank/Palestine 2010.

Variable	Mean (SD [1])
Age	38.6 (13.1)
Menarcheal Age	13.6 (1.4)
Age at Marriage	19.6 (4.3)
Marital Status	
Single	15.2%
Married	77.8%
Divorced	1.7%
Widow	5.3%
Number of children	5.4 (3.0)
Number of abortions	1.1 (1.5)
Residency	
City	26.4%
Camp	41.8%
Village	30.3%
Bedouin	1.5%
Work Status	
Employed	13.9%
Unemployed	77.2%
Student	8.9%
Education	
Illiterate	7.9%
Finished up to 12th grade	70.4%
High School Diploma	11.0%
University	10.6%

[1] Standard deviation.

4.1. Components of Metabolic Syndrome

Seventy six percent (1282 out of 1692) of the women in the study were overweight/obese (BMI $\geq$ 25) and 58% (988 out of 1694) of the women had central obesity, with a waist circumference greater than 88 cm (Table 2).

Table 2. Health status of the study sample (n = 1694) of refugee women (15–84 years), West Bank/Palestine 2010.

Variable	n (% Unless Otherwise Indicated)
Body weight [1]	
Underweight (Body Mass Index (BMI) < 18.5)	21 (1.2%)
Normal weight (BMI 18.5–24.9)	388 (22.9%)
Overweight and obesity (all)	1282 (75.9%)
Overweight (BMI 25–29.9)	512 (30.3%)
Obesity I (BMI 30–34.9)	422 (24.9%)
Obesity II (BMI 35–39.9)	231 (13.7%)
Extreme Obesity (BMI ≥ 40)	118 (7.0%)
Waist circumference above 88 cm	988 (58.3%)
Low High-density lipoprotein (<50 mg/dL)	445 (28.6%)
Triglycerides ≥ 150 mg/dL	449 (28.8%)
Mean fasting blood glucose level in patients without impaired fasting glucose or diabetes (mg/dL) (SD) [2]	87.98 (11.20)
Patients with diabetes n (%)	193 (11.4%)
On medication n (%)	177 (91.7%)
Patients with impaired fasting glucose [2]	358 (22.9%)
Fasting Blood Glucose (FBG) ≥ 110 mg/dL with/without medication	332 (21.2%)
Normal FBG (FBG < 110 mg/dL) on diabetes treatment	26 (1.7%)
Hypertension (≥140 mm Hg systolic or ≥90 mm Hg diastolic [3] and/or take medication)	200 (11.8%)
Metabolic syndrome [4]	
Based on the definition of the World Health Organization	262 (16.9%)
Based on the definition of The Adult Treatment Panel III	415 (26.6%)

[1] Data based on 1692 out of 1694 women. [2] Estimate based on 1562 out of 1694 women. [3] Estimate based on 1692 out of 1694 women. [4] Estimate based on 1552 out of 1694 women.

4.2. Metabolic Syndrome

Based on WHO criteria, the prevalence of MetS was 16.9% (Table 2). The age-adjusted prevalence rate based on the WHO standard population was 19.8%. Based on ATP III criteria, 26.6% of women had MetS, with an age adjusted prevalence rate of 28.6%. Similar to the findings on diabetes, hypertension, central obesity, and low HDL, the prevalence of MetS increased significantly with age, with sharp increases occurring after the age of 44 (Figure 1).

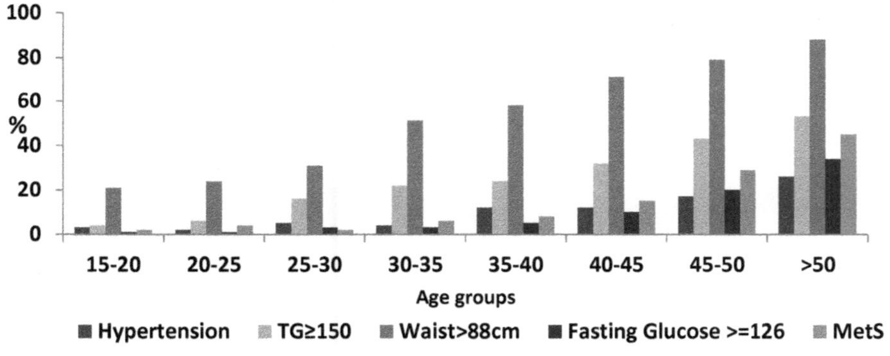

Figure 1. Prevalence of metabolic syndrome and its components by age groups. TG: triglycerides; MetS: metabolic syndrome.

The frequencies of the individual components of the metabolic syndrome were more prevalent in obese compared to nonobese women (Table 3). By the ATP III definition, large waist circumference was the most common abnormality in women with obesity. Around 18.4% of obese women and 4% of nonobese ones had four or more components for MetS. A much higher percentage of nonobese (40.9%) than obese women (3.2%) had no MetS component abnormalities. About four times the percentage of obese versus nonobese women had all five metabolic abnormalities indicative of the MetS (4.1% versus 1.1%).

Table 3. The relative frequencies of the individual components of the metabolic syndrome and the number of MetS components present in refugee women by body mass index (BMI).

Variable	BMI < 30 kg/m^2	BMI $\geq$ 30 kg/m^2	*p*-Value (BMI < 30 vs $\geq$ 30 kg/m^2)
n (%)	921 (54.4%)	772 (45.6%)	
Waist circumference > 88 cm	30.2	92	<0.0001
Blood pressure $\geq$ 130/85 mmHg or medication use	16.0	37.7	<0.0001
Triglycerides $\geq$ 150 mg/dL	18.6	40.9	<0.0001
Low High Density Lipoprotein (<50 mg/dL)	26.5	31.0	<0.027
Fasting Blood Glucose ($\geq$10 mg/dL) or medication use	12.4	31.6	<0.0001
Number of components			
$\geq$1	59.2	96.8	<0.0001
$\geq$2	27.1	71.6	<0.0001
$\geq$3	12.4	42.5	<0.0001
$\geq$4	4.0	18.4	<0.0001
5	1.1	4.1	<0.0001

4.3. Factors Associated with Metabolic Syndrome in the Study Sample

The results of the binary logistic regression analysis indicate that older age (odds ratio 1.10, 95% CI:1.09–1.12) and younger marital age (1.06, CI: 1.02–1.10) were significantly associated with an increased likelihood of MetS among the women. Based on our sample, the level of education, parity, and residency were not associated with MetS.

5. Discussion

We found a high prevalence of metabolic syndrome and its individual components is high in this group. The rate of obesity among Palestinian refugee women 15–64 years in the present study was much higher than that in Palestinian women in the same age group, based on the WHO STEPS survey from 2010–2011 (45% versus 27%, respectively) [22]. Among our cohort, 76% of the refugee women were overweight/obese (BMI > 25), a figure that is higher than in most countries in the Eastern Mediterranean Regional Office (EMRO), apart from Kuwait (79%) [1]. While the majority of those who were obese were aged 45 years and above, rates among adolescent women were also high. The prevalence of overweightness and obesity among adolescent women in our cohort was 38.2%, which is close to that in Kuwait (41.4%) [23]. The UNRWA had provided food rations to refugees living in camps in the form of oil, sugar, rice, flour, and powdered milk, distributed to needy families every three months. These food parcels contributed only a small proportion of food consumption, and the UNRWA replaced food parcels with cash cards in 2016. We believe the main factor behind the high prevalence of obesity is poverty and food insecurity in camps. People consume mostly carbohydrates and fatty foods, rather than fruit and vegetables. This is why the "double burden of under- and overnutrition" remains prevalent in Palestine, among other public health challenges. Based on our earlier published report on a random sample of children aged 6–15 years, 24% of the girls aged 14–15 years were overweight or obese, and 5% had stunting [24].

This high rate of obesity among Palestinian refugee women in this cohort is similar to figures observed in high-income Middle Eastern countries like Kuwait (47.9%), Saudi Arabia (44.0%), and Qatar (45.3%) [25]. The high rate of obesity in our cohort (46.0%) is surprising given the differences in socioeconomic status (SES) between Palestinian refugee women and those in Kuwait, Saudi Arabia, and Qatar. These findings suggest that SES alone does not explain the obesity epidemic, and other risk factors may be present, including biological, genetic, environmental, or nutritional factors that predispose Palestinian refugee women to high rates of obesity. This calls for the identification of local environmental risk factors for obesity, specifically within refugee camps and their surroundings.

Data on obesity in adult refugee women are limited. A study by Grijalva-Eternod was the first to examine obesity and undernutrition among adults residing for extended periods in refugee settings. Grijalva-Eternod et al. found a similar trend of high obesity rates in a study conducted in Western Saharan refugee camps in Algeria [26]. In that study, the prevalence of obesity among refugee women was 21.9%, a lower figure than that observed in our study population. Additionally, the authors also observed a double burden of obesity and malnutrition among the cohort in Algeria. The possible occurrence of such a status was not assessed in our study.

Only limited data are available regarding MetS in Palestine. Whatever information is available emanates from small studies conducted in the West Bank and Gaza Strip in small geographical areas, or for patients with schizophrenia or cardiovascular diseases [8,10,12,27]. To our knowledge, the present study is the first observational study focusing on obesity and related risk factors among a random sample of Palestinian refugee women in the West Bank. Our results, not previously reported, clearly point to the occurrence of silent yet massive obesity of epidemic proportions among Palestinian refugee women in the West Bank.

Given that Palestinians constitute one of the largest refugee populations in the world, with a population of more than four million distributed across several geographic areas and countries, our findings have important policy implications, both for the local population and globally among adults residing for extended periods in refugee settings. Although further investigations will be required, our findings call for the establishment of a priority NCD focus on obesity, MetS, and diabetes for refugee women. Whether these NCD priorities apply equally to men is a subject for further investigation.

Based on ATP III criteria, the age-adjusted prevalence of MetS among women 20 years old and above was highest in our study sample (27%), in comparison with similar studies among Arab women in Saudi Arabia and Oman, and among Arab-Americans in the United States, where the prevalence was 14%, 23%, and 25%, respectively [15,16,27]. In line with previous studies in Iran [13], Saudi Arabia [15], Oman [28], and Kuwait [6], the prevalence of MetS increased with age. Age-related changes in body size, fat distribution, and insulin sensitivity contribute to the prevalence of this syndrome increasing with age [16]. Overweightness and obesity were associated with MetS. However, the presence of abdominal obesity is more highly correlated with the metabolic risk factors than an elevated BMI (95% of women with MetS had waist size greater than 88 cm), which is in agreement with published reports [29]. Lower marital age was one of the factors associated with MetS in our study sample (11% were married at age 15 or below, and 35% were married before the age of 18). While Sirdah et al., report a higher incidence of MetS among married women, the link between lower marital age and MetS found in our data has not been reported previously in other Palestinian studies [9]. This link may be partially explained by early onset of childbirth, multi-parity, and an increased risk of gestational diabetes; however, these issues were not investigated further in the present study. It is essential to consider the role of non-traditional demographic risk factors, such as marital age and the link to MetS. Direct implications could include the implementation of national policies to eradicate child marriage.

Although the present study adds to the NCD and MetS literature, it has several limitations. First, this is a clinic-based rather than a population-based study, and was conducted among women attending primary health care clinics. Second, it is a cross-sectional study, and as such, causality could not be examined. Third, our study was limited only to refugee women, and whether refugee men have similar rates of MetS and obesity could not be determined. This study was carried out in one of the five regions covered by the UNRWA, but we believe that the results can be generalized to all refugees in the four remaining regions covered by the UNRWA (Gaza Strip, Lebanon, Syria, Jordan). Further gender-based comparative studies are needed. Despite these limitations, our study is the first to report a high prevalence of MetS and obesity among Palestinian refugee women who reported to all 42 UNRWA health centers and mobile health clinics in the designated time period.

6. Conclusions

Based on our study findings, the high prevalence of obesity and MetS, both of which pose a considerable burden on the middle-aged population, require national policies to be implemented for the prevention, detection, and treatment of these diseases, which are known to contribute to the rising incidence of NCDs. These measures should go hand in hand with holistic, multidisciplinary, and multi-sectorial preventive measures at the individual, community, and societal levels, and should focus on promoting healthy dietary habits and enhancing regular physically active lifestyles, particularly for children and adolescents [30]. Curbing the growing burden of NCDs among Palestinian refugees to reach the "25 by 25" global goals (reduce avoidable mortality from NCDs by 25% by 2025) is a huge challenge for society and the world community in the post-2015 Millennium Development Goals agenda. Management of people with NCDs and multi-morbidity will continue to be an increasingly demanding responsibility for the UNRWA, but is hindered by decreasing resources at its disposal. However, the situation depicted in this report leaves no room for inaction.

Author Contributions: M.K., U.K., G.-M.M. and S.M. contributed to the study design. M.K. and U.K. were responsible for data collection. W.K., S.M., R.D., G.-M.M. and M.A. contributed to the data analysis. All authors were responsible for the interpretation of the results and contributed to writing and editing the paper. All authors have read and approved the final paper for publication.

Funding: This study was supported by funding from the United Nations Relief and Works Agency for Palestine Refugees in the Near East. This work was also supported by HL117323-02S2 (MA) and T32 HL007854 (MA) from the National Heart, Lung, and Blood Institute at the National Institutes of Health (NIH). The views expressed are those of the authors and not necessarily those of NIH.

Conflicts of Interest: We declare that we have no conflicts of interest.

References

1. World Health Organization. *Global Status Report on Noncommunicable Diseases 2010*; World Health Organization: Geneva, Switzerland, 2011; ISBN 9789241564229. Available online: http://www.who.int/chp/ncd_global_status_report/en/ (accessed on 17 August 2018).
2. Di Cesare, M.; Khang, Y.-H.; Asaria, P.; Blakely, T.; Melanie, J.C.; Farzadfar, F.; Guerrero, R.; Ikeda, N.; Kyobutungi, C.; Msyamboza, K.P.; et al. Inequalities in non-communicable diseases and effective responses. *Lancet* **2013**, *381*, 585–597. [CrossRef]
3. Abdul Rahim, H.F.; Sibai, A.; Khader, Y.; Hwalla, N.; Fadhil, I.; Alsiyabi, H.; Mataria, A.; Mendis, S.; Mokdad, A.H.; Husseini, A. Non-communicable diseases in the Arab world. *Lancet* **2014**, *383*, 356–367. [CrossRef]
4. United Nations Relief and Works Agency for Palestine Refugees in the Near East. The Annual Report of the Department of Health 2011. 2012. Available online: http://www.unrwa.org/userfiles/file/publications/HealthReport2012.pdf (accessed on 17 August 2018).
5. World Health Organization. Obesity. Available online: http://www.emro.who.int/health-topics/obesity (accessed on 17 August 2018).
6. Al Zenki, S.; Al Omirah, H.; Al Hooti, S.; Al Hamad, N.; Jackson, R.T.; Rao, A.; Al Jahmah, N.; Al Obaid, I.; Al Ghanim, J.; Al Somaie, M.; et al. High prevalence of metabolic syndrome among Kuwaiti adults—A wake-up call for public health intervention. *Int. J. Environ. Res. Public Health* **1984**, *9*, 1984–1996. [CrossRef] [PubMed]
7. Grundy, S.M. Metabolic Syndrome Pandemic. *Arterioscl. Throm. Vas.* **2008**, *28*, 629–636. [CrossRef] [PubMed]
8. Abdul-Rahim, H.F.; Husseini, A.; Bjertness, E.; Giacaman, R.; Gordon, N.H.; Jervell, J. The Metabolic Syndrome in the West Bank Population. *Diabetes Care* **2001**, *24*, 275–279. [CrossRef] [PubMed]
9. Sirdah, M.M.; Al Laham, N.A.; Abu Ghali, A.S. Prevalence of metabolic syndrome and associated socioeconomic and demographic factors among Palestinian adults (20–65 years) in the Gaza Strip. *Diabetes Metab. Syndr Clin. Res. Rev.* **2011**, *5*, 93–97. [CrossRef] [PubMed]
10. Sweileh, W.M.; Zyoud, S.H.; Dalal, S.A.; Ibwini, S.; Sawalha, A.F.; Ali, I. Prevalence of metabolic syndrome among patients with schizophrenia in Palestine. *BMC Psychiatry* **2012**, *12*, 235. [CrossRef] [PubMed]

11. Rizkallah, N.; Marshall, T.; Kritz-Silverstein, D. Parity and risk factors for coronary heart disease in Palestinian women in two refugee camps in the West Bank: A population based cross-sectional survey (Abstract). *Lancet* **2010**, *382*, S28. [CrossRef]
12. Abu Sham'a, R.A.; Darwazah, A.K.; Kufri, F.H.; Yassin, I.H.; Torok, N.I. MetS and cardiovascular risk factors among Palestinians of East Jerusalem. *East. Mediterr. Health J.* **2009**, *15*, 1464–1473. [PubMed]
13. Delavari, A.; Forouzanfar, M.H.; Alikhani, S.; Sharifian, A.; Kelishadi, R. First nationwide study of the prevalence of metabolic syndrome and optimal cutoff points of waist circumference in the Middle East: The national survey of risk factors for noncommunicable diseases of Iran. *Diabetes Care* **2009**, *32*, 1092–1097. [CrossRef] [PubMed]
14. Katulanda, P.; Ranasinghe, P.; Jayawardana, R.; Sheriff, R.; Matthews, D.R. Metabolic syndrome among Sri Lankan adults: Prevalence, patterns and correlates. *Diabetol. Metab. Syndr.* **2012**, *4*, 24. [CrossRef] [PubMed]
15. Alzahrani, A.M.; Karawagh, A.M.; Alshahrani, F.M.; Naser, T.A.; Ahmed, A.A.; Alsharef, E.H. Prevalence and predictors of metabolic syndrome among healthy Saudi adults. *Br. J. Diabetes Vasc. Dis.* **2012**, *12*, 78–80. [CrossRef]
16. Jaber, L.A.; Brown, M.B.; Hammad, A.; Zhu, Q.; Herman, W.H. The prevalence of the metabolic syndrome among Arab Americans. *Diabetes Care* **2004**, *27*, 234–238. [CrossRef] [PubMed]
17. United Nations Relief and Works Agency for Palestine Refugees in the Near East (UNRWA) Department of Relief and Social Services. *Registration Statistical Bulletin Third Quarter 2014*; UNRWA: Amman, Jordan, March 2014.
18. Alberti, K.G.; Zimmet, P.Z. Definition, diagnosis and classification of diabetes mellitus and its complications. Part 1: Diagnosis and classification of diabetes mellitus provisional report of a WHO consultation. *Diabet. Med.* **1998**, *15*, 539–553. [CrossRef]
19. Expert Panel on Detection, Evaluation, and Treatment of High Blood Cholesterol in Adults. Executive Summary of the Third Report of the National Cholesterol Education Program (NCEP) Expert Panel on Detection, Evaluation, and Treatment of High Blood Cholesterol in Adults (Adult Treatment Panel III). *JAMA* **2001**, *285*, 2486–2497. [CrossRef]
20. Pan American Health Organization. Standardization: A Classic Epidemiological Method for the Comparison of Rates. *Paho Epidemiol. Bull.* **2002**, *23*, 9.
21. World Health Organization. *Age Standardization of Rates: A New WHO Standard GPE Discussion Paper Series: N 31*; World Health Organization: Geneva, Switzerland, 2001.
22. World Health Organization. Palestine (West Bank) STEPS Survey 2010–2011 Fact Sheet. 2012. Available online: http://www.who.int/chp/steps/Palestine_WestBank_FactSheet_2010-11.pdf?ua=1 (accessed on 17 August 2018).
23. Musaiger, A.O.; Al-Mannai, M.; Tayyem, R.; Al-Lalla, O.; Ali, E.Y.; Kalam, F.; Benhamed, M.M; Saghir, S.; Halahleh, I.; Djoudi, Z. Prevalence of Overweight and Obesity among Adolescents in Seven Arab Countries: A Cross-Cultural Study. *J Obes.* **2012**, *2012*, 981390. [CrossRef] [PubMed]
24. Massad, S.; Deckelbaum, R.J.; Gebre-Medhin, M.; Holleran, S.; Dary, O.; Obeidi, M.; Bordelois, P.; Khammash, U. Double burden of undernutrition and obesity in Palestinian schoolchildren: A cross-sectional study. *Food Nutr. Bull.* **2016**, *37*, 144–152. Available online: http://journals.sagepub.com/doi/pdf/10.1177/0379572116637720 (accessed on 17 August 2018). [CrossRef] [PubMed]
25. Nature Middle East. The Hidden Obesity Toll on Women in Arab States. 2013. Available online: http://www.nature.com/nmiddleeast/2013/130923/full/nmiddleeast.2013.161.html (accessed on 17 August 2018).
26. Grijalva-Eternod, C.S.; Wells, J.C.; Cortina-Borja, M.; Salse-Ubach, N.; Tondeur, M.C.; Dolan, C.; Meziani, C.; Wilkinson, C.; Spiegel, P.; Seal, A.J. The Double Burden of Obesity and Malnutrition in a Protracted Emergency Setting: A Cross-Sectional Study of Western Sahara Refugees. *PLoS Med.* **2012**, *9*, e1001320. [CrossRef] [PubMed]
27. Jamee, A.; Abed, Y.; Abutawila, H. Risk Factors of Metabolic Syndrome among Clinic Patients in Gaza-Palestine. *Am. J. Cardiovasc. Dis. Res.* **2013**, *1*, 20–24.
28. Al-Lawati, J.A.; Mohammed, A.J.; Al-Hinai, H.Q.; Jousilahti, P. Prevalence of Metabolic Syndrome Among Omani Adults. *Diabetes Care* **2003**, *26*, 1781–1785. [CrossRef] [PubMed]

29. Grundy, S.M.; Brewer, H.B.; Cleeman, J.I.; Smith, S.C.; Lenfant, C. Definition of Metabolic Syndrome. *Circulation* **2004**, *109*, 433–438. [CrossRef] [PubMed]
30. Misra, A.; Khurana, L. Obesity and Metabolic Syndrome in Developing Countries. *J. Clin. Endocr. Metab.* **2008**, *93*, s9–s30. [CrossRef] [PubMed]

nutrients

MDPI

Article

Consumption of Fruits and Vegetables by Low-Income Brazilian Undergraduate Students: A Cross-Sectional Study

Ygraine Hartmann, Raquel B. A. Botelho, Rita de Cássia C. de A. Akutsu and Renata Puppin Zandonadi *

Department of Nutrition, University of Brasília, Brasília 70910-900, Brazil; ygrainehartmann@gmail.com (Y.H.); raquelbabotelho@gmail.com (R.B.A.B.); rita.akutsu@gmail.com (R.d.C.C.d.A.A.)

* Correspondence: renatapz@yahoo.com.br; Tel.: +55-61-981-033-600

Received: 10 July 2018; Accepted: 13 August 2018; Published: 19 August 2018

Abstract: Objective: This study aimed to evaluate the consumption of fruits and vegetables (FV) by low-income students participating in the Brazilian Student Assistance Program. **Methods:** For three days, we measured participants' consumption through direct observation of food intake at the University Restaurant (UR) and 24-h recall outside the restaurant. The 174 undergraduates were divided into two groups to obtain data on FV intake at the weekend (Sunday) and two days of the week. Group 1 included low-income undergraduates who received their meals for free, and Group 2 included students who paid for their meals at the UR. **Results:** Both groups presented a very low consumption of FV. On the weekend, Group 1 consumption was equal to Group 2, but it was higher than Group 2 on weekdays, demonstrating how important the UR is for this population. The lowest contribution of the UR to the daily consumption of FV was 59%, reaching a percentage of 87.27%. Fruit supply in the restaurant menu may have positively influenced this consumption. **Conclusions:** The consumption of FV varied according to the menu offered at the UR. The UR should be a space to promote healthy eating habits including more FV in its menus.

Keywords: consumption of fruits and vegetables; low-income undergraduate students; Student Assistance Program

1. Introduction

Fruit and vegetable (FV) consumption is associated with several health advantages, such as lowered chronic diseases because of their low energy density, high fiber, bioactive compounds, vitamins, and minerals profile [1]. Studies [2–5] have shown that the population's consumption of FV does not meet the recommendations of the World Health Organization (WHO) (400 g per day) [6]. In some countries, socioeconomic disparities of diet quality are well established. Low-income and low levels of education have been associated with poor diets and poor health [7].

Multiple factors are known to influence diet quality, including economic barriers, inadequate nutrition knowledge and awareness, food preferences and attitudes, and cultural factors [7]. The decision to consume FV, mainly out of the home, can be influenced by several factors, including confidence in the hygiene of served raw products (salad), variety, attractiveness, sensory balance, and appearance [8]. Some studies have shown the association of physical distance to a supermarket or restaurant with FV intake or overall diet quality and body weight [7,9–11]. Therefore, ensuring physical access to FV suppliers has recently become the focus of public health policies designed to improve the diets and health [7,9–12] of low-income population.

Cook and Papadak [13], studying United Kingdom university students, showed that knowledge influences the FV consumption. Students with higher knowledge level tended to get involved in healthier eating practices, including higher consumption of FV [13]. Divergently, a study conducted in Tunisia with university students showed an inadequate consumption of FV, and 37% of the students were overweight, and 9% were obese [14]. The eating habits of young people can inform us about the future demand for food, as well as the possibility of certain diseases increasing. This knowledge is relevant to design nutritional policies on health promotion [15].

In Brazil, the Brazilian Family Budget Survey (POF) revealed that less than 10% of the population meets the recommendations of FV intake [16]. As part of public health policies designed to improve low-income diets and health, there is a National Program of University Student Assistance (PNAES), in which the low-income students have free access to food at the University Restaurants (URs) [12] to guarantee the social rights of feeding, consolidated by the Universal Declaration of Human Rights [17]. To participate in this Program, students of the Brazilian public universities should be primarily from public schools. Also, their average family income should be of up to 1.5 minimum wage. At the University of Brasilia, this program offers free breakfast, lunch, and dinner, from Monday to Saturday. The UR's meals should be nutritionally balanced, with a basic composition of fruits, raw vegetables, white and brown rice, baked bean, cooked vegetables, and protein dishes. Meals at the UR are free for students of the PNAES, while for other students, it has a cost of US$0.83 per meal [18].

It is essential that a UR subsidized by the government offers different options of FV to its students, to improve their FV consumption and to achieve the WHO's target [6]. Menu planning is the key point for this offer to be conducted in ways that encourage FV consumption. Nutrition education strategies are also important, for students to be not only exposed to FV, but to consume them. Therefore, this study aimed primarily to evaluate the consumption of FV by students participating in the Student Assistance Program who regularly eat at the UR of the University of Brasilia. We also aimed to compare them to a group of students who are not part of the program, as well as to assess the UR's contribution to the daily intake of FV.

2. Materials and Methods

2.1. Study Design

We conducted this study at the UR of the University of Brasilia, Brazil. We chose a matched cross-sectional epidemiological method with the allocation of two groups through the control of the variables age (± 2 years) and sex, to nullify the confounding variables. This increased the possibility of participants to present similar characteristics, as well as the power of the statistical tests to detect differences or associations with the objective to make easier interpretation of the results.

We gathered data for three months to complete the entire protocol. We observed each participant for two consecutive days (weekdays) during meals at the UR and on Sunday, we used 24-h recall for the whole day consumption assessment. The Health School Ethics Committee of the University of Brasilia approved this study (Report No. 610.774/2014).

2.2. Subjects

Group 1 consisted of low-income students who use the UR free of charge—support provided by the university to guarantee low-income student's food access, and permanence and graduation at the university. We used the UR's access control system to obtain data to set this group. Group 1 presented an average family income of up to 1.5 minimum wage (about US$435.00), one of the criteria created by the university for students to receive assistance. Criteria for inclusion of individuals in this study were to have free access to food at the UR, as part in PNAES assistance program; to have had two meals on the same day at the UR, at least once, within fifteen days prior the start of the study; the student's consent to take part in the research; to be at least 18 years old.

Group 2 included students from the university who do not participate in PNAES, but they go to the UR to have meals, either lunch or dinner, independently of the frequency. Group 2 had a family income higher than 1.5 minimum wage since they are not part of PNAES. We excluded pregnant women from this study, since they had different nutritional needs and body composition from the general population. Students from Group 2 also needed to be at least 18 years old and to agree to take part in the research.

In Group 1 (low-income assistance students), 439 individuals received our email, inviting students to be a participant and to answer a short questionnaire that contributed to the design of their socioeconomic profile. We used the SurveyMonkey® tool to gather information. All the individuals that answered the questionnaire were invited to be part of the follow-up research phase at the UR. The final sample for this group was 79 individuals that completed the two-days meals' observation and one-day 24-h recall.

In Group 2 (non-assistance students), students were randomly selected from the cafeteria line, at the entrance of the UR, who accepted to participate in the study. The size of the sample was the same as Group 1 (n = 439). However, during the research, students who accepted participating while in line on the first day, did not come to the UR to complete the three days established in our protocol. Therefore, the final sample for this group was 94 individuals. The selection criteria at the cafeteria line followed the methodology used by Godoy et al. [19], using a systematic order to approach users, one user for every 15 that entered the UR on the day of data gathering. When the researchers achieved the final sample, they did not invite more students to participate.

Group 2 answered the same questionnaire as Group 1 after acceptance to participate in the research on the first day of observation. Students from this group received information that they needed to come to the UR for a second and third day, and they should identify themselves to researchers at the area designed for data gathering.

Students from both groups who agreed to participate had their meals in an exclusive dining room. Their meals could consist of breakfast, lunch, and/or dinner, that were offered at the UR from Monday to Saturday. The UR represents six cafeterias divided into three different floors. To enter the UR, students enter a unique line, and when inside the main floor, they may choose their way to one of the cafeterias. Therefore, researchers approached students at the main floor to invite them for the study. Afterward, researchers conducted students at one of the cafeterias in other to gather all the participants in the same room. This procedure was important to observe the plate's assembly.

2.3. Variables and Instruments

The socioeconomic variables chosen for this study were: sex, age group, and income. Besides these data, we measured the weight and height for Group 1 and Group 2. For anthropometric evaluation, we collected measurements of weight (G-tech scale, model: 200 Glass of 200 Kg capacity) and height and, calculated the body mass index (BMI). We classified the BMI following the criteria adopted by the World Health Organization (WHO) [20]. Students who agreed to participate were invited to take part in this part of the study. Researchers provided different times and dates for students to come to the UR to take the measurements. To encourage this procedure, we informed the students that nutritionists would be available on the same day to give orientations.

To verify the consumption of each group, we applied 24-h recall for the weekend day and meals consumed outside the UR and direct observation for meals performed at the UR. Through the 24-h recall, it was possible to calculate the average number of meals performed by each group.

The assembly of meals was at the students' discretion, who were free to choose the amount of food that suited them. For breakfast, all the items on the menu were portioned, and students could be served, or not, one portion of each item. For lunch and dinner, students served themselves for the following items: rice, beans, cooked vegetables, raw salads, soup, bread, spices, olive oil, sauces, and cassava flour. For main course (protein dish) and fruit or sweet desserts, an employee of the UR portioned them every day for all the students. It is important to highlight that the students served vegetables (raw or cooked), and they could decide their portions for lunch and dinner. The employee of the UR portioned the fruit, and served students who wanted to get the fruit. Students were free to get the fruit served, as well as being able to reject FV. They could ask the employee to have a smaller serving of the fruit too, but they could not ask for more. This serving procedure is a limiting factor for fruit consumption, but the comparison is still important because students could refuse to get the fruit, they could ask for smaller portions, and they could consume fruits in other meals outside the UR. We compared the fruit consumption considering the whole day consumption for both groups.

This practice already occurred at the University Restaurant, and the researchers preserved it in this research because of the cost of these ingredients, and the amount of protein calculated for a balanced meal. Trained observers accompanied meals' assembly by previously classifying the portion sizes served by the students according to the methodology proposed by Savio et al. [21]. This methodology consists of prior weighing of portion sizes before the UR is open to the public. With the utensils presented to the students at the cafeteria, observers weighed three times small, medium, large, and extra-large portions. We invited students to participate, but they did not know that we were analyzing the intake of FV. Observers did not interfere in meal assembly. As a student walked through the food line, the observer classified each portion of each component of the meal.

We weighed the served meal (Filizola®, 20 kg capacity, Brazil) and the weight was recorded on the appropriate manner, containing the student's identification, the weight of the empty plate, the weight of the plate with the food, and the weight of the plate with leftovers. Other weighed items were those served out of the plate composition, such as salads and soups served separately, drinks, desserts, bread, spices, olive oil, sauces, and cassava flour. When the individual returned for a second serving, we repeated the observation and weighing procedure, and we considered them for the assessment of one's consumption. Both groups could have a second serving, except for the protein dish and fruits or desserts for lunch and dinner. For breakfast, the UR did not allow a second serving.

For meal leftovers, we discounted them proportionally by the items placed on the plate for every meal held at the UR. Therefore, plates had to be returned to a specific area in the cafeteria, and the researchers weighed them.

While eating their meals at the UR, the researchers asked the students about the food consumed outside the UR by using a 24-h recall (R24h) during the two weekdays of data collection. To evaluate food consumed on one day of the weekend (Sunday), we used the R24h to gather the individual's food consumption out of their routine. Therefore, we obtained three complete days of consumption for both groups.

To evaluate the intake of FV, we considered these foods separately; that is, those identified by direct observation at the UR and those that were described by the students with their respective amounts reported in the R24h. This separate data was important to evaluate FV intake outside and inside the UR. We excluded the consumption of starchy vegetables (potatoes, cassava) from the daily intake of vegetables. It is a methodology used by the WHO [6], that also excludes these foods from their recommendation of 400 g of FV per day. The researchers recorded all FV consumed during the day, excluding juices, smoothies (fruits blended with milk), and stewed meat with vegetables, due to the inaccuracy of measurement. In both groups, only four students consumed smoothies (not recorded data).

In the end, for each student, we had the following data to analyze and compare groups: body weight, height, body mass index, answered questionnaire, one-weekend day 24-h recall intake, two complete weekdays' intake using 24-h recall for meals outside the UR, and direct observation of meals consumed at the UR considering leftovers.

2.4. Statistical Treatment

We entered and processed data into a database specifically developed for this study using the Statistical Package for Science Program—SPSS version 20.0®. After the creation of the data input form, we checked them through frequency distribution analysis, comparing the values of each variable in the SPSS database to those of possible occurrence, preventing typos. Normality assumptions were checked (Kolmogorov–Smirnov), and we determined the measures of central tendency and sample variance. To verify the differences between the studied groups, we used the *t* test for means, Kruskal–Wallis and the Mann–Whitney tests along with Tukey's post hoc procedure for proportions. To evaluate the correlation among variables and the difference in consumption between groups by sex, we applied Pearson's chi-square test.

3. Results

The average number of meals eaten by both groups is 3.58 ± 0.96. The most common meals were breakfast, lunch, and dinner. When evaluating each group separately, Group 1 had an average number of meals of 3.51 ± 0.93, and Group 2 of 3.64 ± 0.99. Analyzing by group and sex, women from Group 2 presented the highest number of meals (3.94 ± 0.95). The lowest number of eaten meals was 3.40 ± 0.97 for men in Group 1.

Table 1 shows the *n* and the percentage of the anthropometric profile, socioeconomic, and demographic variables of the final samples in each group. Table 2 shows FV intake by sex and group of students by quartiles due to the large variance of intake, since we did not confirm normality assumptions. The consumption of FV on Sunday did not reach the 400 g recommendation in any of the groups (Table 2).

Table 1. Anthropometric profile, socioeconomic and demographic variables for both groups of students, consumers at the University Restaurants.

Variables		Group 1 (n = 79)		p	Group 2 (n = 94)		p
		n	%		n	%	
Sex	Male	45	57	0.216 ***	52	55.3	0.302 ***
	Female	34	43		42	44.7	
Age Group	<20	21	26.6	0.000 **	24	25.5	0.001 **
	20–29	54	68.4		63	67	
	30–39	3	3.8		5	5.3	
	>40	1	1.3		2	2.1	
BMI (average ± SD)	kg/m^2	21.8 ± 3.7		0,027 ****	23.2 ± 4.2		0.027 ****
BMI (classification)	Low weight	14	17.7		3	3.2	
	Normal	52	65.8		35	37.2	
	Overweight	8	10.1		12	12.8	
	Obesity 1	4	5.1		1	1.1	
	Obesity 2	-	-		2	2.1	
Income	<1.5 mw *	79	100	-	-	-	0.001 **
	>1.5–3 mw *	-	-		21	22.3	
	>3–5 mw *	-	-		10	10.6	
	>5 mw *	-	-		28	29.8	
	Not Declared, but >1.5 mw	-	-		35	37.2	

* mw—Brazilian minimum wage (US$289.00); ** Kruskal–Wallis; *** Mann–Whitney test; **** *t* test.

We had similar groups for comparison of data. All students from Group 1 had low family income as stated in the inclusion criteria. For Group 2, most of the students had an income above five minimum wages, showing better conditions to improve their diets.

In Group 1, we did not identify a correlation between BMI and the consumption of FV (p = 0.784). However, in Group 2, among women, for Day 2, consumption showed a negative correlation between the consumption of FV and BMI, with p = 0.04 and a correlation of 0.452. According to average BMI, groups mainly presented the normal classification, but means were statistically different. Group 1 presented more low weight students and no individuals classified as obesity 2.

The intake of FV on Day 2 was higher than on the weekend, but none of the groups achieved the recommendation level. On Day 3, the students of Group 1 in the third quartile, concerning both genders, exceeded the recommended level. The prevalence of consumption adequacy (≥400 g/day) is in Table 2.

Table 2. Fruit and vegetable intake by sex and group of students, consumers at the University Restaurant.

	Group 1 n = 89							Group 2 n = 94						
	Male (n = 45)			Female (n = 34)			p *	Male (n = 52)			Female (n = 42)			p *
	P25	Median	P75	P25	Median	P75		P25	Median	P75	P25	Median	P75	
	g	g	g	g	g	g		g	g	g	g	g	g	
FV intake weekend—Day 1	0	75	180	0	72.5	169.5	0.938	0	76	206	0	80	209	0.779
FV intake—Day 2	106	191	306	99.5	189.5	308	0.465	48	150	264	48	124	262	0.001
FV intake—Day 3	134	283	525	139.2	297	551.5	0.944	90	160	246.5	92.2	163.5	215.7	0.545

* Mann-Whitney U test.

Table 3 presents the prevalence of FV consumption by the group for each day of analysis. Consumption of Group 1 on Day 3 was higher than Group 2 with statistical difference (p = 0.001; Mann–Whitney U test), for Days 1 and 2, there was no statistical difference (p = 0.105—day1; p = 0.465—day2). When comparing both groups for the three days of the study, Group 1 consumed higher quantities of FV than Group 2 for all the quartiles (p = 0.001). It is important to highlight that percentiles demonstrate the data since we did not confirm normality assumptions.

Table 3. Fruit and vegetable intake by a group of students, consumers at the University Restaurant for each evaluated day.

	Group 1			Group 2			
	P25	Median	P75	P25	Median	P75	p
	g	g	g	g	g	g	
Weekend Day 1	0.0	100.0	196.0	0.0	76.0	180.0	0.465
Day 2	116.0	170.5	314.0	48.0	124.0	263.0	0.105
Day 3	207.0	370.0	626,00	44.0	173.0	353.0	0.000

There was a significant difference (chi-square) concerning the consumption proportion of FV between the groups by sex only for Group 2 on Day 2 (p = 0.002) (Table 4). Considering the average consumption of the two samples, on Day 3, only Group 1 achieved the recommendation of 400 g of FV. The average consumption of fruits (144.59 g/day) of the entire sample (n = 173) was higher than the consumption of vegetables (60.98 g/day).

Table 4. Percentage of students at the University Restaurant who consumed over four hundred grams of fruits and vegetables.

	Group 1 (n = 89)					Group 2 (n = 94)				
	Male (n = 45)		Female (n = 34)		p **	Male (n = 52)		Female (n = 42)		p **
	n	%	n	%		n	%	n	%	
Day 1 *	4	8.9	4	11.8	0.677	6	11.5	7	16.7	0.476
Day 2	5	11.1	4	11.8	0.928	11	21.2	0	0	0.002
Day 3	20	44.4	16	47.1	0.818	6	11.5	4	9.5	0.754

* Weekend day (Sunday), when the feeding did not occur at the University Restaurant (UR). ** Chi-square test.

The percentage contribution of the UR to the daily consumption of FV is in Table 5. It reveals that the contribution of the restaurant is significant, with 59.9% consumption by women of Group 1 on Day 2, and a higher contribution among men of Group 1 on Day 3, reaching 87.3%.

Table 5. The contribution of the University Restaurant to the daily intake of fruits and vegetables by sex and group of students.

	Group 1			Group 2		
	Male (n = 45)	Female (n = 33)	Total	Male (n = 32)	Female (n = 42)	Total
Fruits and vegetable intake—Day 2	70.0%	59.9%	64.9%	69.4%	74.1%	71.7%
Fruits and vegetable intake—Day 3	87.3%	81.5%	84.4%	73.9%	67.4%	70.6%

On Day 3, the UR's menu offered more FV, as shown in Table 6. On this day, fruits were the dessert during lunch, unlike Day 2, when the UR offered a sweet dessert. A larger watermelon portion (350 g) for breakfast, and the offer of an apple (126 g) as a dessert for lunch, had a positive effect on student's consumption, presenting statistical differences between groups on this day.

Table 6. The qualitative offer of fruits and vegetables at the University Restaurant menu.

Day/Meal	Salad 1	Salad 2	Garnish	Dessert
Day 2 breakfast	-	-	-	Banana
Day 2 lunch	Crisp lettuce	Raw beet	-	Sweet guava pastes
Day 2 dinner	Cucumber	-	Braised cabbage	Pineapple
Day 3 breakfast	-	-	-	Watermelon
Day 3 lunch	Chard	Raw carrot	-	Apple
Day 3 dinner	Crisp lettuce	-	Braised chayote	Papaya

4. Discussion

Both groups are similar, which allows comparing data by sex. Groups presented lower percentage of overweight (group 1–10.1%, group 2–12.8%) and obese (group 1–5.1%, group 2–3.2%) when compared to the Brazilian population (50% of overweight; 12% of obesity) [22].

The average number of daily meals eaten by both groups is 3.58, which may be negatively influencing the daily consumption of fruits. Brazilians tend to consume fruits mostly in the form of snacks during breaks, and they are often encouraged by nutritionists to eat fruits at these hours as well.

In this study, the median of FV intake was higher in the days that the participants ate at the UR than the median of FV intake on weekends for both groups. However, Group 1 consumption of FV on weekends did not differ from Group 2, whereas Group 1 consumption of FV was higher than Group 2 in one of the days that the groups ate at the UR. The prevalence of FV intake reached 39% among men on the day that the UR's menu offered fruits as dessert for lunch and dinner. Therefore, it is essential to highlight the importance of good menu planning and how the UR can positively contribute to the students' food choices. Since fruit portions are limited to students, this intake could be even higher at the UR. However, vegetable intake was much lower, and students were free to serve themselves from this group of food.

Several studies undertaken in different countries [5,8,13,14,23,24] showed a low prevalence of regular consumption of FV by undergraduates. A recent study carried out at the University of Acre in the northern region of Brazil with 863 students showed a prevalence of regular consumption of FV in just 14% of the sample [24].

Among Turkish college students, the prevalence of inadequate intake of FV reaches 66.1% for men and 63.1% for women. The eating habits of Greek students also proved to be particularly poor regarding the consumption of FV and, consequently, 68.1% of men and 53.9% of women presented a fiber consumption rate below RDA recommendations [14].

In this study, regarding only the women of Group 2, the higher the BMI, the lower the consumption of FV, which did not favor weight loss in this group.

In another survey conducted in Brazil, only 24.9% of the subjects interviewed consumed adequate amounts of FV [16]. In another study, undergraduate students with regular consumption of FV presented a mean BMI = 23.2 (SD = 4.0) and revealed inadequate consumption patterns of these products [25].

In the present study, Day 3 showed the highest consumption of FV. The prevalence of adequacy of FV consumption was of 23% among men and 31% among women in Group 1, and in Group 2, the rate was 39% and 36% among men and women, respectively.

Therefore, the percentages found in this study are consistent with the results found in studies undertaken internationally. Food choices during this stage of life can be a determining factor regarding optimal health outcomes in the future and the appearance of Noncommunicable Chronic Diseases (NCD) [25].

Students of Group 1 had a higher contribution from the UR in the daily intake of FV than on the weekends, when meals occurred outside the UR. On Sunday, the consumption of FV was very low and did not reach the recommendation level. Also, on the weekend, Group 1 consumption was as low as Group 2, demonstrating how important the UR is for this population, since less healthy and more convenient choices occur on weekends. It is noteworthy that, in Brazil, the consumption of FV at home involves the steps of cleaning and sanitizing, which are tiring and may hinder the options of undergraduate students for these foods. Furthermore, they are more perishable, and must be consumed closer to the date of their acquisition. Besides, to consume FV on weekends, students from Group 1 must pay for them. In the UR, they receive FV without expenses. Therefore, the Student Assistance Program in Brazilian URs guarantees low-income students to have access to healthier meals than the ones eaten out of the university. Probably, it is related to the cost and food access for this group.

Since it is a low-income population, it is difficult for them to get important nutrients from FV in other forms, like nutraceuticals. Studies have shown the role of nutrients from plants in decreasing the incidence of cardiovascular problems, such as the research from Giordano et al. [26] studying carotenoids in FV, and from Metzger et al. [27] studying pectin, polyphenols, and phytosterols in lipid lowering. Scicchitano et al. [28] showed in their review that cardiovascular protection by nutraceuticals needs more debate. However, studies show that nutrients in FV present important benefits for people's health, and they can be easily bought and consumed.

At the same time, we noted that by increasing exposure—i.e., the occurrence of FV in the UR menu—there is an increment on consumption, yielding a positive relation concerning intake.

In a study performed in Brazil, nutrition education actions on FV consumption that combined information and motivation were successful in impoverished environments [29]. The actions included providing knowledge about the advantages of consuming FV to achieve good health and enhancing the skills for its introduction in daily eating. It suggests that nutritional education programs would positively impact the students participating in the PNAES (Group 1).

It is noteworthy that the highest consumption of FV on Day 3 is due mainly to a higher offer of fruits and to the portion size of each of the fruits offered in the menu (banana—100 g; watermelon—350 g; apple—126 g, guava jelly—25 g).

A limiting factor in fruit consumption at the UR relates to the fact that the UR serves portioned fruits. This practice occurs because many users want to take a spare portion with them after leaving the UR. In other cases, not limiting fruit consumption can affect availability, which can lead to the lack of fruits for other students. One suggestion is that the UR improves the distribution of fruits during the week so that students receive greater portions and for all days of the week.

Another limiting factor is the number of researched days. More days could increase to verify the effect of the menu over FV consumption in both groups.

Considering that the consumption of fruits revealed to be higher than of vegetables, it is necessary to understand the reasons for the low consumption of vegetables and direct actions towards encouraging better food choices. Since it is a cross-sectional study, it has some limitations, which do not allow causal judgments among the associations.

Low confidence in food hygiene procedures may be one of the factors for the low consumption of raw vegetables offered in the menu [8]. Providing information about food cleaning procedures, implementing guided tours at the food area production, fostering the distribution of media newsletters, and implementing local campaigns at the cafeteria are actions that can increase student's confidence, and thus, encourage consumption. People's confidence is an important factor to improve good choices. Marinangeli and Jones [30] also showed that consumers would consume more nutraceuticals or functional foods if they can trust industrial procedures.

Nutrition education programs are essential for people to understand the importance of regular consumption of FV. It is necessary that the intake does not happen only at the UR, but during other meals and on weekends as well.

5. Conclusions

Based on the results, it is possible to affirm the great importance that the UR has over students' food consumption. The fact that they spend most of their time at the university leaves them vulnerable to eating whatever is offered. The Student Assistance actions in Brazil for Group 1 and the low price of meals for Group 2 favor the presence of students and, therefore, requires that the UR becomes a place that fosters the promotion of health and life quality, adopting healthy eating habits that lead to the prevention of chronic diseases.

Students consume much lower amounts of FV than the ones recommended by the WHO, but on the day that the UR served larger portions of fruits for breakfast and desserts were fruits, Group 1 showed a closer median of intake to recommendations. When individuals consume FV, fruits are the largest portions, which demonstrate that vegetable consumption deserves greater incentive. Students could serve themselves vegetables as much as they wanted, but the offer is not the only criteria to encourage vegetable intake. Consumption was similar between male and female, and it was not related to BMI.

Proper menu planning with daily offers of FV is essential. At the same time, promotion of educational nutrition and healthy eating habits actions can help improving students' food choices. It was possible to verify that, on the day, if the FV offer was more significant at the UR, the consumption was higher. The Student Assistance Program in Brazilian URs allows the low-income students to have access to healthier meals than the ones eaten out of the university. This result highlights the importance of the Food and Nutrition Policy developed by the universities through their URs.

Author Contributions: Conceptualization, Y.H., R.d.C.C.d.A.A. and R.B.A.B.; Methodology, Y.H., R.d.C.C.d.A.A., and R.B.A.B.; Formal Analysis, Y.H., R.d.C.C.d.A.A., R.P.Z., and R.B.A.B.; Investigation, Y.H.; Data Curation, Y.H., R.d.C.C.d.A.A., and R.B.A.B.; Writing—Original Draft Preparation, Y.H., R.d.C.C.d.A.A., R.P.Z., and R.B.A.B.; Writing—Review & Editing, R.B.A.B., and R.P.Z.; Visualization, R.C.C.A., R.P.Z, and R.B.A.B.; Supervision, R.B.A.B., and R.d.C.C.d.A.A.; Project Administration, Y.H., R.d.C.C.d.A.A. and R.B.A.B.

Funding: This research received no external funding.

Conflicts of Interest: The authors declare no conflict of interest.

References

1. De Vries, H.; Eggers, S.M.; Lechner, L.; van Osch, L.; van Stralen, M.M. Predicting Fruit Consumption: The Role of Habits, Previous Behavior and Mediation Effects. *BMC Public Health* **2014**, *14*, 730. [CrossRef] [PubMed]
2. Zazpe, I.; Marqués, M.; Sánchez-Tainta, A.; Rodríguez-Mourille, A.; Beunza, J.-J.; Santiago, S.; Fernández-Montero, A. Eating Habits and Attitudes towards Change in Spanish University Students and Workers. *Nutr. Hosp.* **2013**, *28*, 1673–1680. [PubMed]
3. Sánchez Socarrás, V.; Aguilar Martínez, A. Food Habits and Health-Related Behaviors in a University Population. *Nutr. Hosp.* **2014**, *31*, 449–457. [PubMed]
4. Marcondelli, P.; da Costa, T.H.M.; Schmitz, B.d.A.S. Nível de Atividade Física e Hábitos Alimentares de Universitários Do 3° Ao 5° Semestres Da Área Da Saúde. *Rev. Nutr.* **2008**, *21*, 39–47. [CrossRef]

5. Farias, S.C.; de Castro, I.R.R.; da Matta, V.M.; Castro, L.M.C. Impact Assessment of an Intervention on the Consumption of Fruits and Vegetables by Students and Teachers. *Rev. Nutr.* **2014**, *27*, 55–65. [CrossRef]
6. World Health Organization (WHO). *Fruit and Vegetable Promotion Initiative—A Meeting Report*; WHO: Geneva, Switzerland, 2003.
7. Aggarwal, A.; Cook, A.J.; Jiao, J.; Seguin, R.A.; Vernez Moudon, A.; Hurvitz, P.M.; Drewnowski, A. Access to Supermarkets and Fruit and Vegetable Consumption. *Am. J. Public Health* **2014**, *104*, 917–923. [CrossRef] [PubMed]
8. Franco, A.d.S.; de Castro, I.R.R.; Wolkoff, D.B. Impact of the Promotion of Fruit and Vegetables on Their Consumption in the Workplace. *Rev. Saude Publica* **2013**, *47*, 29–36. [CrossRef]
9. Moore, L.V.; Diez Roux, A.V.; Nettleton, J.A.; Jacobs, D.R. Associations of the Local Food Environment with Diet Quality—A Comparison of Assessments Based on Surveys and Geographic Information Systems: The Multi-Ethnic Study of Atherosclerosis. *Am. J. Epidemiol.* **2008**, *167*, 917–924. [CrossRef] [PubMed]
10. Laraia, B.; Siega-Riz, A.M.; Kaufman, J.S.; Jones, S.J. Proximity of Supermarkets is Positively Associated with Diet Quality Index for Pregnancy. *Prev. Med.* **2004**, *39*, 869–875. [CrossRef] [PubMed]
11. Jago, R.; Baranowski, T.; Baranowski, J.C.; Cullen, K.W.; Thompson, D. Distance to Food Stores & Adolescent Male Fruit and Vegetable Consumption: Mediation Effects. *Int. J. Behav. Nutr. Phys. Act.* **2007**, *4*, 35. [CrossRef] [PubMed]
12. Wang, M.C.; Cubbin, C.; Ahn, D.; Winkleby, M.A. Changes in Neighbourhood Food Store Environment, Food Behaviour and Body Mass Index, 1981–1990. *Public Health Nutr.* **2008**, *11*, 963–970. [CrossRef] [PubMed]
13. Cooke, R.; Papadaki, A. Nutrition Label Use Mediates the Positive Relationship between Nutrition Knowledge and Attitudes towards Healthy Eating with Dietary Quality among University Students in the UK. *Appetite* **2014**, *83*, 297–303. [CrossRef] [PubMed]
14. Neslişah, R.; Emine, A.Y. Energy and Nutrient Intake and Food Patterns among Turkish University Students. *Nutr. Res. Pract.* **2011**, *5*, 117–123. [CrossRef] [PubMed]
15. Amo, E.; Escribano, F.; García-Meseguer, M.-J.; Pardo, I. Are the Eating Habits of University Students Different to the Rest of the Spanish Population? Food Availability, Consumption and Cost. *Span. J. Agric. Res.* **2016**, *14*, e0103. [CrossRef]
16. Instituto Brasileiro de Geografia e Estatística (IBGE). *Pesquisas de Orçamentos Familiares*; IBGE: Brasília, Brazil, 2010.
17. General Assembly of the United Nations (Ed.) *Universal Declaration of Human Rights*; General Assembly of the United Nations: New York, NY, USA, 1948.
18. University of Brasília. Restaurante Universitário. Available online: http://www.ru.unb.br/ (accessed on 9 July 2018).
19. Godoy, K.C.; Sávio, K.E.O.; Akutsu, R.d.C.; Gubert, M.B.; Botelho, R.B.A.; Godoy, K.C.; Sávio, K.E.O.; Akutsu, R.d.C.; Gubert, M.B.; Botelho, R.B.A. Perfil e Situação de Insegurança Alimentar Dos Usuários Dos Restaurantes Populares No Brasil. *Cad. Saude Publica* **2014**, *30*, 1239–1249. [CrossRef] [PubMed]
20. World Health Organization (WHO). *Physical Status: The Use and Interpretation of Anthropometry*; WHO: Geneva, Switzerland, 2013.
21. Savio, K.E.O.; da Costa, T.H.M.; Miazaki, É.; Schmitz, B.d.A.S. Avaliação Do Almoço Servido a Participantes Do Programa de Alimentação Do Trabalhador. *Rev. Saude Publica* **2005**, *39*, 148–155. [CrossRef] [PubMed]
22. Instituto Brasileiro de Geografia e Estatística (IBGE). *Pesquisa de Orçamentos Familiares: Análise Do Consumo Alimentar Pessoal No Brasil*; IBGE: Rio de Janeiro, Brazil, 2011.
23. Cervera Burriel, F.; Serrano Urrea, R.; Daouas, T.; Delicado Soria, A.; García Meseguer, M.J. Food Habits and Nutritional Assessment in a Tunisian University Population. *Nutr. Hosp.* **2014**, *30*, 1350–1358. [PubMed]
24. Ramalho, A.A.; Dalamaria, T.; de Souza, O.F. Consumo Regular de Frutas e Hortaliças Por Estudantes Universitários Em Rio Branco, Acre, Brasil: Prevalência e Fatores Associados. *Cad. Saude Publica* **2012**, *28*, 1405–1413. [CrossRef] [PubMed]
25. Jaime, P.C.; Machado, F.M.S.; Westphal, M.F.; Monteiro, C.A. Educação Nutricional e Consumo de Frutas e Hortaliças: Ensaio Comunitário Controlado. *Rev. Saude Publica* **2007**, *41*, 154–157. [CrossRef] [PubMed]
26. Giordano, P.; Scicchitano, P.; Locorotondo, M.; Mandurino, C.; Ricci, G.; Carbonara, S.; Gesualdo, M.; Zito, A.; Dachille, A.; Caputo, P.; et al. Current Pharmaceutical Design. *Curr. Pharm. Des.* **2012**, *18*, 13.

27. Metzger, B.T.; Barnes, D.M.; Reed, J.D. A Comparison of Pectin, Polyphenols, and Phytosterols, Alone or in Combination, to Lovastatin for Reduction of Serum Lipids in Familial Hypercholesterolemic Swine. *J. Med. Food* **2009**, *12*, 854–860. [CrossRef] [PubMed]
28. Scicchitano, P.; Cameli, M.; Maiello, M.; Modesti, P.A.; Muiesan, M.L.; Novo, S.; Palmiero, P.; Saba, P.S.; Pedrinelli, R.; Ciccone, M.M. Nutraceuticals and Dyslipidaemia: Beyond the Common Therapeutics. *J. Funct. Foods* **2014**, *6*, 11–32. [CrossRef]
29. Reis, L.C.d.; Correia, I.C.; Mizutani, E.S. Stages of Changes for Fruit and Vegetable Intake and Their Relation to the Nutritional Status of Undergraduate Students. *Einstein* **2014**, *12*, 48–54. [CrossRef] [PubMed]
30. Marinangeli, C.P.F.; Jones, P.J.H. Gazing into the Crystal Ball: Future Considerations for Ensuring Sustained Growth of the Functional Food and Nutraceutical Marketplace. *Nutr. Res. Rev.* **2013**, *26*, 12–21. [CrossRef] [PubMed]

nutrients

MDPI

Article

Increased Adiposity as a Potential Risk Factor for Lower Academic Performance: A Cross-Sectional Study in Chilean Adolescents from Low-to-Middle Socioeconomic Background

Paulina Correa-Burrows [1,*], Yanina Rodriguez [1], Estela Blanco [2], Sheila Gahagan [2] and Raquel Burrows [1]

[1] Institute of Nutrition and Food Technology, University of Chile, Santiago 7830490, Chile; yanirod77@hotmail.com (Y.R.); rburrows@inta.uchile.cl (R.B.)

[2] Division of Child Development and Community Health, University of California San Diego, La Jolla, CA 92093, USA; esblanco@ucsd.edu (E.B.); sgahagan@ucsd.edu (S.G.)

* Correspondence: paulina.correa@inta.uchile.cl; Tel.: +56-22-978-1492

Received: 11 July 2018; Accepted: 16 August 2018; Published: 21 August 2018

Abstract: We explored the association between excess body fat and academic performance in high school students from Santiago, Chile. In 632 16-year-olds (51% males) from low-to-middle socioeconomic status (SES), height, weight, and waist circumference were measured. Body-mass index (BMI) and BMI for age and sex were calculated. Weight status was evaluated with 2007 World Health Organization (WHO) references. Abdominal obesity was diagnosed with International Diabetes Federation (IDF) references. Total fat mass (TFM) was measured with dual-energy X-ray absorptiometry (DXA). TFM values $\geq$25% in males and $\geq$35% in females were considered high adiposity. School grades were obtained from administrative records. Analysis of covariance examined the association of fatness measures with academic performance, accounting for the effect of diet and physical activity, and controlling SES background and educational confounders. We found that: (1) having obesity, abdominal obesity, or high adiposity was associated with lower school performance alone or in combination with unhealthy dietary habits or reduced time allocation for exercise; (2) high adiposity and abdominal obesity were more clearly related with lower school grades compared to obesity; (3) the association of increased fatness with lower school grades was more salient in males compared to females.

Keywords: adiposity markers; obesity; fat mass; abdominal obesity; adolescent health; school performance

1. Introduction

Excess weight at a young age is associated with cardiometabolic disorders [1,2], reduced quality of life [3], and the risk of obesity and its comorbidities in adulthood [4]. Biological, behavioural, and environmental factors lead to excess weight gain and contribute to the rising prevalence of obesity worldwide. National surveys measuring height and weight in individuals across Chile indicate that at least one in three Chilean adolescents are either overweight or obese [5,6]. Of the OECD (Organisation for Economic Cooperation and Development) countries, Chile ranks sixth in overweightness and obesity among children aged 11–15 years [7].

National reports also indicate that excess weight and risk factors are more prevalent among socially vulnerable groups [5,6,8,9]. According to these surveys, low-to-middle SES groups have greater access to energy-dense diets and efforts to provide safe and convenient places for physical activity, particularly for low-income populations, are still insufficient [9]. As a result, adolescents from low-to-middle SES are at increased risk of being obese than their high-SES counterparts. Several studies show that SES has its most crucial impact on health during adolescence [10,11]. The so-called 'adolescent-emergent model' suggests that the SES–health relationship is weak in early childhood but then strengthens with age, due to determinants such as peer influence, personality, and autonomous decision-making [10–12]. For instance, physical activity is more strongly correlated with SES during adolescence than earlier in childhood [11]. This model states that children begin to model the health behaviours of their parents early in life, but as they grow older, the extent to which these behaviours are internalized and pursued by the youth will be more influential to their health.

The cardiometabolic complications of childhood and adolescent obesity have been widely explored; however, its impact on cognition and educational outcomes has recently received a lot of scientific attention. Certain brain structures continue to develop throughout adolescence; therefore, whether obesity impacts the adolescent brain is highly relevant. Frontal and temporal lobe abnormalities as well as reduced hippocampal volume were found in obese adolescents [13]. Both the prefrontal cortex (PFC) and the hippocampus play pivotal roles in the cognitive abilities (i.e., learning, memory, and cognitive control) that are needed to perform well in school [14]. Also, obesity in youths is associated with poorer executive functioning skills, such as inhibitory control and working memory, which are critical for academic achievement [15]. Furthermore, obesity-associated biomarkers, including gut hormones (i.e., ghrelin, GLP-1), adipokines (i.e., leptin), and proinflammatory cytokines (i.e., TNF-α, CRP), have been linked with cognition and memory [15]. Abnormally high leptin levels, which are largely related to adiposity, limit the potential for synaptic plasticity and trafficking of neurotransmitter receptors in the hippocampus and might be responsible for some memory deficits [16]. In adolescents, hyperleptinemia was associated with lower academic performance in high school [17] and on tests for college admission [18].

Because paediatric obesity has been related to specific outcomes that are relevant for children's educational attainment, some authors have examined the association of weight status with academic attainment as measured by school grades and standardised test scores. A negative, significant association was reported for adolescent students in Finland [19], Iceland [20], Iran [21], Portugal [22], South Korea [23], the U.S. [24,25], and the United Kingdom [26].

Most studies addressing the academic implications of adolescent obesity rely on body-mass index (BMI) as the sole measure. With some exceptions [23,26,27], very few studies have used other measures of adiposity, despite evidence that fat tissue is metabolically active and produces proteins and inflammatory markers associated with learning, memory, and general cognitive function [15,28]. Furthermore, systematic reviews suggest that existing studies are not representative of developing countries [29,30], where overweight and obesity are steadily increasing in children and youths. A focus on academics might have important preventive implications as academic outcomes are linked to expectations of better college opportunities and future job status and income. In this study, we explored the association between excess body fat and academic performance in Chilean high school students. This paper aimed to explore the association between excess body fat and academic performance in high school students from Santiago, Chile. Because Chilean adolescents of low-to-middle SES are at greater risk of excessive weight gain, and because the SES effects on health status would be stronger in years where the child is making conscious decisions about physical activity and healthy eating, we concentrated on adolescents from low-to-middle socioeconomic backgrounds. We hypothesised that adolescents with obesity, abdominal obesity, or high adiposity would have lower school grades and lower grade-point average (GPA).

2. Materials and Methods

2.1. Study Design and Participants

This was a cross-sectional study within an infancy cohort. The sample was made up of 16–17-year-old adolescents living in Santiago, Chile, from low-to-middle SES. Participants were recruited at 4 months from public healthcare facilities in the southeast area of Santiago (n = 1791).

They were born at term of uncomplicated vaginal births, weighed >3.0 kg, and were free of acute or chronic health problems. At 6 months, infants free of iron deficiency anemia (n = 1657) were randomly assigned to receive iron supplementation or no added iron (ages 6–12 months). They were assessed for developmental outcomes in infancy and at 5, 10, and 15 years [31]. At 16–17 years, those with complete data in each wave (n = 679) were also assessed for obesity risk and the presence of cardiovascular risk factors in a half-day evaluation that included assessment of dietary habits and nutritional content of food intake. Of them, n = 632 (93%) entered high school and were eligible for this study. Ethical approval was obtained by the institutional review boards of the University of Michigan, Institute of Nutrition and Food Technology (INTA), University of Chile, and the University of California, San Diego. Participants and their primary caregiver provided informed and written consent, according to the norms for Human Experimentation, Code of Ethics of the World Medical Association (Declaration of Helsinki, 1995).

2.2. Measurements

2.2.1. School Grades

School grades in high school (9th to 12th) and final grade-point average (GPA) were collected from administrative records of the Ministry of Education (Chile). Since schools may have differed in grading policies, grades (on a scale of 1–7) were transformed into scores (range of 210–825), following the Ministry of Education criteria. The arithmetic average of each subject taken during each academic year was calculated and the result was compared in the conversion table provided by the Department of Assessment, Measurement and Educational Record, University of Chile, which complies with specifications on behalf of the Ministry of Education. The same procedure was used to convert the GPA into a score. Both school grades and GPA were used as continuous variables.

2.2.2. Anthropometric Assessment and Definitions

A physician used standardized procedures to measure the adolescent's height (cm) to the nearest 0.1 cm, using a Holtain stadiometer, and weight (kg) to the nearest 0.1 kg, using a scale (Seca 703, Seca GmbH & co. Hamburg, Germany). Waist circumference (WC) was measured with nonelastic flexible tape and recorded to 0.1 cm (Seca 201, Seca GmbH & co. Hamburg, Germany). Measurements were taken twice, with a third measurement if the difference between the first two exceeded 0.3 kg for weight, 0.5 cm for height, and 1.0 cm for WC. BMI and BMI for age and sex (BMIz) were calculated. Weight status was evaluated according to WHO references: normal weight (BMIz from -1 to 1 SD); excess weight (BMIz > 1 SD). Abdominal obesity was defined as WC $\geq$ 90 cm for males and $\geq$80 cm for females, according to the International Diabetes Federation (IDF). Total fat mass (TFM) was determined via dual-energy X-ray absorptiometry (DXA) (apparatus: Lunar Prodigy Corp. Software: Lunar iDXA ENCORE 2011, Version 13.60.033, Madison, WI, USA.). Because there is no generally accepted definition of obesity based on TFM, we used cutoffs by Taylor et al.: values $\geq$25% in males and $\geq$35% in females were considered high adiposity [32].

2.2.3. Dietary Assessment at Age 16 Years

Nutritional quality of diet was measured considering the amount of saturated fats and sugars in the foods consumed during breakfast, lunch, dinner, snacks at school, and snacks at home within the past three months. Assessment was performed with a food frequency questionnaire (FFQ), validated using three 24-h recalls to include weekends (Spearman's rank correlation coefficient between the FFQ and the 24-hour dietary recalls exceed 0.35 in two-thirds of the food items, and all correlation coefficients were significant) [33,34]. A list of 120 foods and beverages was used. The frequency of food consumption was assessed by a multiple response grid; respondents were asked to estimate how often a particular food or beverage was consumed. Categories ranged from 'never' to 'five or more times a week'. The electronic version of the Chilean Food Composition Tables/Database was used to assess the quality of the foods' composition [35]. Food items were classified as high in saturated fats and sugars, high in sugars although low in saturated fats, and nutrient-rich foods. We assigned adjustment weights to each food item conditioned to its nutritional quality. A continuous score ranging from 0–10 was computed by adjusting the frequency of food consumption to the nutritional quality, with higher scores representing healthier dietary habits. We applied quartile cutoffs for the Chilean adolescent population (comprising students of high-, middle-, and low-SES) to classify the nutritional quality of the overall diet of participants into three groups: unhealthy (≤4.3 or ≤25th percentile), fair (from 4.4 to 5.9 or >25th percentile and <75th percentile), and healthy (≥6.0 or ≥75th percentile) [33].

2.2.4. Physical Activity at Age 16 Years

We approached physical activity (PA) with scheduled, repetitive, and planned PA, accounting for the number of weekly hours devoted to physical education (PE) and extracurricular sports. To measure this, we used a questionnaire that was validated in a previous study using accelerometry-based activity monitors in both elementary and high school children [36]. The questionnaire was administered by a researcher to all students at the time they attended the anthropometric examination. Participants were asked: (1) On average, over the past week, how often did you engage in PE and extracurricular sports? (2) On those days, on average, how long did you engage in such activities? With this information, we estimated the average hours per week of scheduled PA. Participants having ≤90 minutes of weekly scheduled PA, which is the mandatory time for school-based PE in Chile, were considered to be physically inactive.

2.2.5. Socioeconomic Background

The present study used family structure and parental education level as proxies of SES. Parental education is an important predictor of children's educational outcomes [37]. In infancy, participants' parents reported the highest schooling level they have been enrolled in, and also the highest grade they completed at that level. Five hierarchic levels were defined: (1) no education completed, (2) first level (primary school), (3) secondary level (first phase or 9th–10th), (4) secondary level (second phase or 11th–12th), and (5) post-secondary nontertiary educations [38]. Then, we merged these categories into two: incomplete secondary education (1 + 2 + 3), and complete secondary education or higher (4 + 5). Also, because a relationship between children's educational outcomes and family structure has been described [39], we included a variable denoting whether the participant was raised in a fatherless family. This information was reported by the participant's mother or legal guardian. Last, to control for potential design biases, we used a categorical variable denoting whether the participant had received iron supplementation or no added iron at 6–12 months.

2.2.6. Type of Secondary Education

In Chile, secondary education includes academic high schools, which provide theoretical education in languages, mathematics, history, and sciences; vocational training schools; and adult schools. Data on the type of secondary education attended by participants was retrieved from publicly available records at the Ministry of Education.

2.2.7. Iron Supplementation in Infancy

Aiming to control for potential design biases, we used a categorical variable denoting whether the participant had received iron supplementation or no added iron at 6–12 months.

2.3. Statistical Analysis

Student's *t*-test and chi-squared test were used for comparison of continuous and categorical variables, respectively, in male and female participants. Due to sex differences in fatness and academic attainment, we ran separate analyses for male and female participants. To examine the association of excess weight, abdominal obesity, and high adiposity (exposure) with school performance (outcome), we conducted analysis of covariance (ANCOVA). Each fatness measure was tested against school grades (9th to 12th) and overall GPA using two models. Model 1 was unadjusted. Model 2 added parental education, family structure, age at high school completion, type of secondary education (vocational and adult school), and a variable denoting iron supplementation in infancy (no added iron at 6–12 months). Because diet and physical activity have been found to be associated with academic achievement in studies conducted in Chile [40–42], all models included interactions of fatness measures with diet as well as interactions of fatness with time allocation for PA. Last, the effect size (ES) for difference was estimated using Cohen's *d* coefficients. Data were analyzed using Stata for Windows version 15.0 (Lakeway Drive College Station, TX, US). A *p* value of 0.05 was used to test for statistical significance.

3. Results

3.1. Description of the Sample

Of the adolescents ($n = 679$) who participated in a prior obesity/cardiovascular study, 632 (93%) entered high school and were included in the present study. A comparison of the participants included in and excluded from this study is shown in the Supplementary Materials (Table S1). The final sample was comprised of adolescents (51% males) with an average age of 16.8 years (SD: 0.3). These adolescents completed high school at an average age of 18.5 years (SD: 0.8). Thirty-eight percent had excess weight, 32.6% had abdominal obesity, and 44.3% had high adiposity (Table 1). Forty percent of adolescents came from a fatherless home, and one-third had a mother with incomplete secondary education. As for participants' lifestyles, 21% were regarded as having an unhealthy diet, while 58% were considered to be physically inactive. Last, 51% of our participants attended a vocational high school.

Table 1. Descriptive statistics of male and female participants in the sample ($n = 632$).

	Total ($n = 632$)		Males ($n = 330$)		Females ($n = 302$)		p Value *
	Mean or n	(SD) or %	Mean or n	(SD) or %	Mean or n	(SD) or %	
Chronological age							
Age at assessment (year)	16.8	(0.3)	16.8	(0.3)	16.8	(0.2)	NS
Age at high school completion	18.5	(0.8)	18.5	(0.9)	18.4	(0.8)	NS
Anthropometrics							
Body-Mass Index (*z* score)	0.64	(1.2)	0.56	(1.2)	0.72	(1.1)	NS
Total Fat Mass (%)	29.0	(10.7)	22.3	(8.7)	36.2	(7.2)	<0.001
Waist circumference (cm)	81.9	(11.1)	80.9	(10.5)	81.1	(11.7)	NS
Obesity	86	13.6%	42	12.7%	44	14.6%	NS
Abdominal obesity	206	32.6%	61	18.5%	145	70.4%	<0.001 ‡
High adiposity	280	44.3%	115	34.7%	165	55.1%	<0.001 ‡
School grades §							
9th ($n = 632$)	464.5	(99.6)	453.7	(95.6)	476.2	(100.1)	0.008
10th ($n = 615$)	468.5	(98.5)	457.7	(90.9)	480.1	(100.5)	0.011
11th ($n = 576$)	482.8	(95.9)	464.1	(90.1)	502.1	(102.2)	<0.001
12th ($n = 571$)	494.2	(98.4)	475.7	(89.9)	513.1	(103.1)	<0.001
Grade-Point Average ($n = 571$)	481.1	(92.3)	466.3	(82.7)	496.3	(98.8)	<0.001
Socioeconomic background							
Mother with incomplete HS	212	33.5%	114	32.5%	98	34.5%	NS ‡
Father with incomplete HS	176	27.9%	74	22.4%	102	33.8%	0.001 ‡
Fatherless family	250	39.6%	131	39.7%	119	39.4%	NS ‡
Lifestyles							
Unhealthy diet	132	20.9%	66	20.0%	66	21.9%	NS ‡
Physically inactive	367	58.1%	147	44.6%	220	72.9%	<0.001 ‡
Type of secondary education							
Academic	179	28.3%	85	25.8%	94	31.1%	NS ‡
Vocational	330	52.2%	176	53.3%	154	51.0%	
Adult	123	19.5%	69	20.9%	54	17.8%	
Fe supplementation (6–12 months)							
No added Fe	269	42.6%	148	44.5%	121	40.1%	NS ‡

* Two-tailed Student's *t*-test was used for independent samples, except as indicated. ‡ Pearson's chi-squared test. § School grades expressed as standardized score (scale 210–825), according to the Ministry of Education (Chile). Obesity: BMIz score >2 SD. Abdominal obesity: Waist Circumference ≥90 cm (males) or ≥80 cm (females). High adiposity: Total Fat Mass ≥25% (males) or ≥35% (females). Abbreviations: NS: not significant. HS: high school.

After controlling for sex, we found that female adolescents had better school performance than males ($p < 0.001$). While the prevalence of obesity was similar in both groups, the prevalence of abdominal obesity ($p < 0.001$) and high adiposity ($p < 0.001$) was significantly higher in females. As for SES background, we found that females were more likely to have a father with incomplete higher education ($p < 0.001$). They were also more likely to be physically inactive compared to males ($p < 0.001$), although no differences were observed in relation to diet quality.

3.2. Relationship of Increased Adiposity with Academic Attainment, Accounting for the Effect of Diet Quality

When we explored the association of fatness with school grades, accounting for the effect of diet quality, we observed that in both males and females, the greatest losses in school attainment were related to the combined effect of increased fatness and poor diet quality. In a first analysis, where fatness was approached with obesity (Table 2), the combined effect of obesity and unhealthy dietary habits was associated with lower school grades across high school (grades 9th to 12th and overall GPA) in both sexes. The ES for the difference in males indicates that the combined effect of obesity and poor diet quality was moderate to large (Cohen's *d* ranging from 0.51 to 0.67) in males, whereas in females, the effect was moderate (Cohen's *d* ranging from 0.33 to 0.45). In males who had a fair-to-healthy diet, but still were obese, obesity was related to lower school attainment across high school, whereas in females who had a fair-to-healthy diet, but still were obese, obesity was associated with lower school performance only in grades 11 and 12. As for the effect of diet quality in nonobese adolescents, we observed that in males, a poor diet quality was related to lower school attainment in grades 11 and 12. A lower GPA was also observed in nonobese males who had unhealthy diets. In nonobese females, unhealthy dietary habits were associated with lower school performance only in grade 11.

Table 2. Analysis of covariance (ANCOVA) measuring the effect of obesity and diet quality on school grades in male and female adolescents.

	MALE PARTICIPANTS										
	Obesity (−)					Obesity (+)					
	Fair-to-Healthy Diet §		Unhealthy Diet			Fair-to-Healthy Diet §			Unhealthy Diet		
	Intercept	SE	Coefficient	SE	*d*	Coefficient	SE	*d*	Coefficient	SE	*d*
						Model 1 [a]					
9th (n = 330)	462.1 ***	6.2	−23.1 ‡	8.2	0.27	−39.6 *	19.6	0.49	−62.5 *	21.4	0.74
10th (n = 318)	464.8 ***	7.4	−21.9 ‡	6.6	0.25	−39.4 *	18.1	0.43	−75.6 *	28.2	0.70
11th (n = 292)	474.9 ***	6.6	−23.4 *	7.0	0.29	−47.8 *	16.3	0.59	−77.2 **	25.7	0.85
12th (n = 288)	485.0 ***	6.7	−25.9 **	4.2	0.32	−42.4 *	19.6	0.52	−56.2 **	15.9	0.77
HS-GPA (n = 288)	475.8 ***	5.5	−24.9 *	6.9	0.30	−42.7 *	17.3	0.62	−58.4 **	16.4	0.85
						Model 2 [b]					
9th (n = 330)	466.9 ***	9.2	−22.9 ‡	9.2	0.25	−35.6 *	15.3	0.32	−67.5 *	23.9	0.58
10th (n = 318)	474.9 ***	9.7	−23.1 ‡	9.6	0.24	−37.7 *	13.1	0.34	−77.9 *	28.2	0.67
11th (n = 292)	475.6 ***	10.6	−25.9 *	8.9	0.32	−49.1 *	16.3	0.44	−78.6 **	26.7	0.66
12th (n = 288)	488.2 ***	9.7	−25.9 *	8.2	0.33	−42.4 *	17.6	0.40	−57.2 **	19.3	0.51
HS-GPA (n = 288)	480.5 ***	9.3	−25.2 *	8.7	0.33	−43.1 *	17.1	0.42	−61.4 **	19.1	0.53
	FEMALE PARTICIPANTS										
	Obesity (−)					Obesity (+)					
	Fair-to-Healthy Diet §		Unhealthy Diet			Fair-to-Healthy Diet §			Unhealthy Diet		
	Intercept	SE	Coefficient	SE	*d*	Coefficient	SE	*d*	Coefficient	SE	*d*
						Model 1 [a]					
9th (n = 330)	485.9 ***	7.2	−19.8	12.2	0.15	−33.1	21.8	0.26	−50.3 *	22.4	0.57
10th (n = 318)	492.0 ***	9.1	−21.4	11.6	0.18	−35.2	20.5	0.26	−49.0 *	26.9	0.55
11th (n = 284)	513.5 ***	6.7	−26.6 *	8.8	0.33	−38.8 *	19.1	0.37	−50.4 **	19.1	0.60
12th (n = 281)	528.4 ***	8.1	−19.7 ‡	9.9	0.25	−41.4 *	19.6	0.36	−59.6 **	19.7	0.53
HS-GPA (n = 281)	507.6 ***	7.1	−24.1 *	10.9	0.30	−39.9 *	21.6	0.38	−51.5 *	18.4	0.43

Table 2. *Cont.*

						Model 2 [b]					
9th (n = 330)	485.9 ***	10.2	−20.5	12.2	0.15	−33.1	22.8	0.23	−56.3 *	18.0	0.45
10th (n = 318)	492.0 ***	9.7	−24.9 ‡	12.1	0.17	−37.9	22.5	0.25	−41.0 *	16.9	0.33
11th (n = 284)	508.2 **	8.8	−29.6 *	9.5	0.30	−41.1 *	19.0	0.37	−55.9 *	17.1	0.40
12th (n = 281)	518.5 ***	10.3	−28.1	10.2	0.15	−44.4 *	19.7	0.37	−59.6 *	18.7	0.42
HS–GPA (n = 281)	507.6 ***	10.9	−25.7	10.8	0.19	−35.9	22.6	0.26	−52.0 *	15.4	0.38

Obesity (+): BMIz > 2 SD for age and sex. School grades expressed as standardized score (scale 210–825), according to the Ministry of Education (Chile). [a] Model 1 is unadjusted. [b] Model 2 is adjusted for SES (parental education, family structure), type of secondary education, and iron supplementation in infancy. § Participants with obesity (−) (BMIz score < 2 SD) and a fair-to-healthy diet are the reference group. Coefficients are the mean difference between a given category and the reference group. ‡ Trend towards significance ($p < 0.10$). * $p < 0.05$; ** $p < 0.01$; *** $p < 0.001$. Cohen's d statistics were estimated accounting for different sample sizes. Abbreviation: HS–GPA: high school grade–point average.

When the exposure was abdominal obesity instead of obesity, we found that the combined effect of fatness and unhealthy dietary habits on school grades was large in males (d values ranging from 0.69 to 0.74) and moderate-to-large females (d values ranging from 0.51 to 0.69) (Table 3). In participants having fair-to-healthy dietary habits, but still having abdominal obesity, fatness was associated with lower school grades and lower GPA compared to peers without abdominal obesity and fair-to-heathy diets. In both males and females, abdominal obesity had a moderate effect on school grades, as d coefficients ranged from 0.33 to 0.42 and 0.33 to 0.40 in males and females, respectively. In this model, unhealthy dietary habits in participants without abdominal obesity was related to lower school attainment in males and females, but the association was significant only in grades 10 and 12 for males, grade 11 for females, and GPA for both groups. The ES for the difference indicates a small effect of diet alone on school grades.

Table 3. Analysis of covariance (ANCOVA) measuring the effect of abdominal obesity and diet quality on school grades in male and female adolescents.

	MALE PARTICIPANTS										
	Abdominal Obesity (−)					Abdominal Obesity (+)					
	Fair-to-Healthy Diet §		Unhealthy Diet			Fair-to-Healthy Diet §			Unhealthy Diet		
	Intercept	SE	Coefficient	SE	d	Coefficient	SE	d	Coefficient	SE	d
						Model 1 [a]					
9th (n = 330)	465.4 ***	6.6	−25.6 ‡	15.2	0.27	−43.6 *	13.8	0.41	−87.7 **	19.4	0.73
10th (n = 318)	468.5 ***	6.4	−32.9 *	11.7	0.41	−49.9 *	12.7	0.40	−88.9 **	18.2	0.73
11th (n = 292)	476.2 ***	6.6	−26.4 *	12.9	0.34	−52.4 *	11.0	0.53	−87.2 **	18.7	0.74
12th (n = 288)	485.5 ***	7.7	−28.5 *	12.5	0.36	−50.8 *	11.6	0.50	−86.4 **	19.1	0.73
HS–GPA (n = 288)	478.0 ***	5.7	−29.5 *	13.5	0.37	−54.3 *	13.3	0.58	−82.9 **	19.4	0.69
						Model 2 [b]					
9th (n = 330)	460.0 ***	9.6	−25.6	13.2	0.19	−44.1 *	18.8	0.39	−89.0 **	21.4	0.69
10th (n = 318)	478.0 ***	9.4	−33.5 *	12.7	0.37	−47.4 *	16.7	0.43	−88.9 **	22.2	0.69
11th (n = 292)	476.5 ***	9.6	−31.4 *	13.9	0.37	−50.4 *	15.0	0.41	−89.2 **	19.9	0.69
12th (n = 288)	488.1 ***	10.7	−30.5	16.5	0.21	−48.1 *	18.6	0.39	−87.7 **	19.1	0.67
HS–GPA (n = 288)	482.2 ***	9.3	−33.5 *	12.5	0.37	−53.9 *	13.9	0.45	−83.9 **	20.1	0.64
	FEMALE PARTICIPANTS										
	Abdominal Obesity (−)					Abdominal Obesity (+)					
	Fair-to-Healthy Diet §		Unhealthy Diet			Fair-to-HealthyDiet §			Unhealthy Diet		
	Intercept	SE	Coefficient	SE	d	Coefficient	SE	d	Coefficient	SE	d
						Model 1 [a]					
9th (n = 330)	505.5 ***	9.7	−32.8 *	12.2	0.30	−47.1 **	15.8	0.36	−74.0 ***	19.6	0.55
10th (n = 318)	503.5 ***	10.3	−36.2 ‡	15.7	0.24	−49.6 *	17.9	0.33	−69.8 ***	18.8	0.59
11th (n = 284)	532.1 ***	10.1	−31.4 ‡	14.6	0.27	−56.2 *	18.5	0.40	−88.0 ***	18.9	0.75
12th (n = 281)	545.5 ***	9.7	−32.6 *	12.8	0.37	−48.8 *	18.1	0.34	−91.4 ***	19.1	0.76
HS–GPA (n = 281)	525.0 ***	9.8	−36.9 **	11.2	0.38	−58.6 **	13.2	0.42	−84.6 ***	19.2	0.68

Table 3. *Cont.*

						Model 2 [b]					
9th (n = 330)	512.7 ***	12.7	−35.8 ‡	15.0	0.27	−49.1 *	18.8	0.33	−70.0 ***	21.6	0.51
10th (n = 318)	504.5 ***	12.5	−36.0	19.7	0.19	−51.4 *	20.9	0.33	−73.8 ***	21.9	0.52
11th (n = 284)	528.1 ***	12.1	−35.4 ‡	18.6	0.25	−58.0 *	20.5	0.39	−90.3 ***	21.9	0.69
12th (n = 281)	538.9 ***	11.7	−37.6 *	18.8	0.32	−50.3 *	19.6	0.34	−91.4 ***	20.1	0.69
HS–GPA (n = 281)	520.2 ***	11.8	−38.1 *	14.2	0.35	−60.6 **	17.2	0.40	−87.0 ***	21.2	0.64

Abdominal obesity (+): waist circumference ≥90 cm in males and ≥80 cm in females. School grades expressed as standardized score (scale 210–825), according to the Ministry of Education (Chile). [a] Model 1 is unadjusted. [b] Model 2 is adjusted for socioeconomic background (parental education, family structure), type of secondary education, age of high school completion, and iron supplementation in infancy. § Participants with abdominal obesity (−) and a fair-to-healthy diet are the reference group. Coefficients are the mean difference between a given category and the reference group. ‡ Trend towards significance ($p < 0.10$). * $p < 0.05$; ** $p < 0.01$; *** $p < 0.001$. Cohen's d statistics were estimated accounting for different sample sizes. Abbreviations: HS–GPA: high school grade–point average.

In a third model, where fatness was measured with total fat mass percentage, we found that the combined effect of high adiposity and unhealthy dietary habits was associated with lower school performance in both sexes (Table 4). Cohen's d coefficients indicate that the combined impact of diet and fatness on school grades was moderate in females and moderate to large in males. In males with high adiposity, although having fair-to-healthy dietary habits, we also observed lower school grades compared to males without high adiposity, although having fair-to-healthy diets. The ES for difference ranged from 0.36 to 0.39, denoting a moderate effect of high adiposity on school grades in males who had fair-to-healthy diets. In females with high adiposity, on the other hand, we only found a significant association of fatness with school attainment in grade 12 and GPA and a trend towards a lower school attainment in grade 11. As for the effect of unhealthy dietary habits in participants with normal adiposity, again, the association was more salient in males than in females. Males with normal adiposity and unhealthy diets significantly underperformed compared to males with normal adiposity and fair-to-healthy diets in the 10th, 11th, and 12th grades and in terms of GPA, whereas females with normal adiposity and unhealthy diets significantly underperformed compared to peers with normal adiposity and fair-to-healthy diets only in the 12th grade and in terms of GPA.

Table 4. Analysis of covariance (ANCOVA) measuring the effect of high adiposity and diet quality on school grades in male and female adolescents.

	MALE PARTICIPANTS										
	High Adiposity (−)					High Adiposity (+)					
	Fair–to–Healthy Diet §		Unhealthy Diet			Fair–to–Healthy Diet §			Unhealthy Diet		
	Intercept	SE	Coefficient	SE	d	Coefficient	SE	d	Coefficient	SE	d
						Model 1 [a]					
9th (n = 330)	462.4 ***	7.2	−29.9 *	9.2	0.35	−39.6 *	13.0	0.39	−65.7 **	22.4	0.61
10th (n = 318)	464.0 ***	6.4	−33.9 **	8.6	0.39	−46.7 *	12.7	0.41	−65.9 **	21.2	0.62
11th (n = 292)	467.8 ***	6.6	−34.4 **	9.9	0.39	−54.3 *	14.0	0.52	−77.2 **	23.7	0.64
12th (n = 288)	481.3 ***	7.7	−33.5 **	9.7	0.38	−52.3 **	11.6	0.51	−76.4 **	24.1	0.69
HS–GPA (n = 288)	473.0 ***	7.5	−33.9 *	10.9	0.37	−56.3 **	12.3	0.56	−72.9 **	20.4	0.68
						Model 2 [b]					
9th (n = 330)	466.9 ***	11.2	−25.9 ‡	14.2	0.27	−40.1 *	16.0	0.36	−66.8 **	23.4	0.58
10th (n = 318)	474.7 ***	7.4	−29.0 *	13.0	0.33	−43.7 *	16.7	0.36	−67.1 **	23.2	0.56
11th (n = 292)	469.6 ***	8.6	−31.8 *	12.9	0.33	−50.0 *	17.9	0.39	−72.2 **	23.7	0.58
12th (n = 288)	481.3 ***	7.7	−29.9 *	12.7	0.33	−47.9 **	17.6	0.39	−74.4 **	24.1	0.62
HS–GPA (n = 288)	478.4 ***	8.5	−30.1 *	12.9	0.30	−49.3 **	17.3	0.39	−75.9 **	21.4	0.65
	FEMALE PARTICIPANTS										
	High Adiposity (−)					High Adiposity (+)					
	Fair-to-Healthy Diet §		Unhealthy Diet			Fair-to-Healthy §			Unhealthy Diet		
	Intercept	SE	Coefficient	SE	d	Coefficient	SE	d	Coefficient	SE	d
						Model 1 [a]					
9th (n = 330)	501.9 ***	10.2	−39.2 *	13.2	0.40	−41.7 *	18.8	0.38	−61.3 *	19.4	0.45
10th (n = 318)	503.5 ***	11.1	−31.4 *	14.6	0.30	−40.6 *	16.5	0.39	−68.0 **	18.9	0.48
11th (n = 284)	530.4 ***	11.3	−32.0 *	13.8	0.32	−47.8 *	16.1	0.46	−72.4 **	18.1	0.49
12th (n = 281)	544.4 ***	11.4	−35.9 *	14.3	0.35	−52.4 *	18.6	0.50	−79.6 **	19.7	0.56
HS–GPA (n = 281)	524.3 ***	10.7	−37.0 **	13.2	0.39	−58.5 *	18.6	0.58	−64.6 **	19.4	0.52

Table 4. *Cont.*

						Model 2 [b]					
9th (n = 330)	509.6 ***	11.2	−30.0	18.2	0.22	−31.7	24.9	0.22	−64.0 *	22.4	0.45
10th (n = 318)	503.5 ***	12.5	−29.4	17.6	0.23	−32.6	25.5	0.22	−72.1 **	21.9	0.48
11th (n = 284)	526.8 ***	12.3	−28.0	17.8	0.24	−36.8 ‡	25.1	0.27	−73.1 **	22.1	0.47
12th (n = 281)	537.9 ***	12.4	−36.9 *	16.9	0.30	−52.4*	23.6	0.41	−78.0 **	22.7	0.50
HS–GPA (n = 281)	521.3 ***	12.7	−35.0 *	16.2	0.30	−55.5*	22.6	0.45	−67.0 **	23.7	0.43

High adiposity (+): Total Fat Mass ≥25% in males and ≥35% in females. School grades expressed as standardized score (scale 210–825), according to the Ministry of Education (Chile). [a] Model 1 is unadjusted. [b] Model 2 is adjusted for SES (parental education, family structure), type of secondary education, and iron supplementation in infancy. § Participants with high adiposity (−) and a fair-to-healthy diet are the reference group. Coefficients are the mean difference between a given category and the reference group. ‡ Trend towards significance ($p < 0.10$). * $p < 0.05$; ** $p < 0.01$; *** $p < 0.001$. Cohen's d statistics were estimated accounting for different sample sizes. Abbreviations: HS–GPA: high school grade–point average.

3.3. Relationship of High Adiposity with Academic Attainment, Accounting for the Effect of Physical Activity

When we explored the association of fatness with school grades, accounting for the effect of PA on the academic outcome, we observed that in both males and females, the greatest losses in school attainment were related to the combined effect of increased fatness and physical inactivity. When fatness was approached with obesity (Table 5), the combined effect of obesity and reduced time allocation for exercise was associated with lower school grades across high school (grades 9 to 12 and overall GPA) in both sexes. The ES for difference in males indicates that the combined effect of obesity and physical inactivity was large, whereas in females, the effect was moderate. In males who devoted >90 min/week to exercise, obesity was related to lower school attainment across high school. In females who devoted >90 min/week to exercise, on the other hand, obesity was associated with lower school performance only in grade 12 and overall GPA. As for the effect of exercise in nonobese adolescents, we observed that in both sexes, a reduced time allocation for exercise was related to lower school performance, with the exception of grade 9. Nonobese males and females who were physically inactive significantly underperformed compared to nonobese peers who were physically active. In both groups, however, the ES for difference indicates that the effect of reduced time allocation for exercise on school grades was small ($d < 0.30$).

Table 5. Analysis of covariance (ANCOVA) measuring the effect of obesity and time allocation for exercise on school grades in male and female adolescents.

	MALE PARTICIPANTS										
	Obesity (−)					Obesity (+)					
	Physically Active §		Physically Inactive			Physically Active §			Physically Inactive		
	Intercept	SE	Coefficient	SE	d	Coefficient	SE	d	Coefficient	SE	d
						Model 1 [a]					
9th (n = 330)	454.2 ***	7.2	−17.5 *	5.2	0.22	−26.4 *	10.6	0.41	−44.5 **	14.4	0.47
10th (n = 318)	469.0 ***	7.4	−20.6 *	5.6	0.22	−26.9 *	11.1	0.33	−36.0 *	13.2	0.40
11th (n = 292)	458.4 ***	7.5	−21.4 *	5.6	0.26	−20.8	11.1	0.27	−46.2 **	14.1	0.56
12th (n = 288)	470.4 ***	6.7	−21.1 *	5.2	0.29	−28.4 *	11.6	0.41	−42.6 *	14.7	0.41
HS-GPA (n = 288)	463.6 ***	6.5	−21.9 *	4.9	0.30	−21.9	10.6	0.30	−47.2 **	15.4	0.50
						Model 2 [b]					
9th (n = 330)	459.9 ***	8.6	−18.2	6.6	0.18	−28.1 *	13.1	0.30	−47.9 **	16.6	0.50
10th (n = 318)	466.0 ***	9.0	−22.1 *	7.4	0.20	−27.3 *	12.5	0.30	−44.7 **	16.1	0.47
11th (n = 292)	459.6 ***	8.5	−20.4 *	7.7	0.20	−24.1 *	11.8	0.28	−46.1 **	16.7	0.49
12th (n = 288)	468.4 ***	6.7	−21.9 *	6.3	0.28	−27.4 *	12.8	0.34	−45.6 *	17.8	0.51
HS-GPA (n = 288)	467.5 ***	7.8	−19.5 *	6.2	0.24	−28.4 *	12.6	0.30	−44.5 *	16.4	0.47

Table 5. *Cont.*

	FEMALE PARTICIPANTS										
	Obesity (−)					Obesity (+)					
	Physically Active §		Physically Inactive			Physically Active §			Physically Inactive		
	Intercept	SE	Coefficient	SE	*d*	Coefficient	SE	*d*	Coefficient	SE	*d*
	Model 1 [a]										
9th (n = 330)	473.4 ***	7.7	−18.1 *	5.3	0.22	−21.5	12.8	0.19	−48.7 **	14.4	0.58
10th (n = 318)	478.7 ***	7.6	−16.4 *	5.6	0.21	−22.7	12.0	0.19	−43.0 **	16.9	0.53
11th (n = 284)	458.4 ***	7.5	−17.3 *	5.6	0.21	−22.8 *	10.1	0.24	−40.4 **	13.1	0.43
12th (n = 281)	514.0 ***	6.7	−18.2 *	4.2	0.24	−23.8 *	10.6	0.28	−45.6 **	13.7	0.50
HS-GPA (n = 281)	494.9 ***	6.5	−20.5 *	4.9	0.24	−28.4 *	11.6	0.32	−47.6 **	14.4	0.57
	Model 2 [b]										
9th (n = 330)	480.0 ***	9.2	−17.1	5.3	0.17	−17.7	13.8	0.17	−45.7 *	17.4	0.41
10th (n = 318)	485.3 ***	9.4	−19.4 *	5.6	0.21	−20.1	13.5	0.18	−41.5 *	16.9	0.33
11th (n = 284)	504.8 ***	9.5	−18.3 *	4.7	0.21	−20.8	12.0	0.18	−44.4 **	16.4	0.36
12th (n = 281)	520.4 ***	9.7	−20.7 *	5.3	0.20	−29.4 *	12.5	0.27	−44.9 *	18.2	0.35
HS-GPA (n = 281)	501.5 ***	8.5	−19.1 *	4.9	0.20	−30.4 *	13.6	0.29	−44.6 *	17.6	0.40

Obesity (+): BMIz > 2 SD for age and sex. School grades expressed as standardized score (scale 210–825), according to the Ministry of Education (Chile). [a] Model 1 is unadjusted. [b] Model 2 is adjusted for SES (parental education, family structure), type of secondary education, and iron supplementation in infancy. § Participants with obesity (−) (BMIz score < 2 SD) and a fair-to-healthy diet are the reference group. Coefficients are the mean difference between a given category and the reference group. ‡ Trend towards significance ($p < 0.10$). * $p < 0.05$; ** $p < 0.01$; *** $p < 0.001$. Cohen's *d* statistics were estimated accounting for different sample sizes. Abbreviations: HS-GPA: high school grade-point average.

When the exposure was abdominal obesity instead of obesity, we found that the combined effect of fatness and physical inactivity on school grades was moderate in females and moderate to large in males (Table 6). In males and females with time allocation for exercise >90 min/week, obesity was related to lower school grades and the ES for difference indicates that the effect of abdominal obesity on school attainment was moderate in both sexes. In adolescents without abdominal obesity, the effect of physical inactivity on school grades was found to be significant only in the 12th grade (males) and in terms of GPA (males and females).

Table 6. Analysis of covariance (ANCOVA) measuring the effect of abdominal obesity and time allocation for exercise on school grades in male and female adolescents.

	MALE PARTICIPANTS										
	Abdominal Obesity (−)					Abdominal Obesity (+)					
	Physically Active §		Physically Inactive			Physically Active §			Physically Inactive		
	Intercept	SE	Coefficient	SE	*d*	Coefficient	SE	*d*	Coefficient	SE	*d*
	Model 1 [a]										
9th (n = 330)	460.9 ***	7.2	−18.7 *	4.2	0.22	−33.4 *	12.6	0.42	−59.2 *	11.4	0.74
10th (n = 318)	459.0 ***	7.4	−19.2 *	5.6	0.24	−33.5 *	12.1	0.42	−61.2 *	13.2	0.73
11th (n = 292)	462.8 ***	7.5	−16.3 *	5.6	0.20	−35.4 *	11.1	0.47	−60.7 *	12.8	0.73
12th (n = 288)	474.4 ***	6.7	−16.4 *	4.2	0.20	−30.4 *	7.6	0.41	−59.8 *	12.7	0.82
HS-GPA (n = 288)	468.7 ***	6.5	−18.9 *	5.9	0.24	−35.6 *	11.6	0.47	−57.6 *	12.4	0.82
	Model 2 [b]										
9th (n = 330)	465.7 ***	9.0	−15.9*	4.3	0.20	−35.4 *	13.6	0.36	−61.7 *	16.4	0.73
10th (n = 318)	470.0 ***	8.8	−17.8*	5.6	0.21	−33.5 *	13.1	0.36	−63.1 *	16.0	0.78
11th (n = 292)	462.6 ***	8.5	−15.3 ‡	5.9	0.19	−35.1 *	12.6	0.40	−60.2 *	18.0	0.77
12th (n = 288)	470.8 ***	7.7	−16.5 ‡	4.2	0.19	−28.9 *	13.6	0.31	−57.1 *	17.7	0.65
HS-GPA (n = 288)	471.6 ***	8.5	−19.5*	6.0	0.22	−37.0 *	12.6	0.40	−57.4 *	17.6	0.65

Table 6. *Cont.*

	FEMALE PARTICIPANTS										
	Abdominal Obesity (−)					Abdominal Obesity (+)					
	Physically Active §		Physically Inactive			Physically Active §			Physically Inactive		
	Intercept	SE	Coefficient	SE	*d*	Coefficient	SE	*d*	Coefficient	SE	*d*
	Model 1 [a]										
9th (*n* = 302)	482.7 ***	9.1	−15.1*	6.2	0.22	−30.5 *	9.1	0.34	−55.5 *	12.7	0.67
10th (*n* = 297)	484.3 ***	7.4	−15.4*	6.6	0.23	−31.9 *	10.9	0.35	−57.5 *	12.9	0.69
11th (*n* = 284)	511.3 ***	8.5	−11.1	7.3	0.19	−32.8 *	11.1	0.38	−54.0 *	12.1	0.60
12th (*n* = 281)	518.6 ***	7.7	−13.9‡	7.2	0.19	−40.3 *	11.6	0.41	−56.6 *	12.7	0.69
HS-GPA (*n* = 281)	502.3 ***	6.5	−15.1*	6.1	0.32	−30.6 *	12.6	0.38	−48.8 *	11.4	0.69
	Model 2 [b]										
9th (*n* = 302)	487.6 ***	10.7	−14.1	8.2	0.18	−31.5 *	13.5	0.32	−50.5 *	17.0	0.45
10th (*n* = 297)	490.3 ***	10.0	−15.4 *	6.6	0.23	−32.9 *	14.5	0.33	−54.5 *	17.9	0.53
11th (*n* = 284)	515.6 ***	10.4	−11.7	7.3	0.17	−34.3 *	14.3	0.35	−52.0 *	18.2	0.49
12th (*n* = 281)	524.5 ***	11.7	−13.0	7.2	0.17	−38.1 *	13.6	0.37	−54.1 *	18.3	0.54
HS-GPA (*n* = 281)	508.2 ***	9.9	−20.3 *	7.0	0.29	−36.5 *	14.6	0.35	−56.9 *	17.5	0.54

Abdominal obesity (+): waist circumference ≥90 cm in males and ≥80 cm in females. School grades expressed as standardized score (scale 210–825), according to the Ministry of Education (Chile). [a] Model 1 is unadjusted. [b] Model 2 is adjusted for socioeconomic background (parental education, family structure), type of secondary education, age of high school completion, and iron supplementation in infancy. § Participants with abdominal obesity (−) and a fair-to-healthy diet are the reference group. Coefficients are the mean difference between a given category and the reference group. ‡ Trend towards significance ($p < 0.10$). * $p < 0.05$; ** $p < 0.01$; *** $p < 0.001$. Cohen's *d* statistics were estimated accounting for different sample sizes. Abbreviations: HS–GPA: high school grade–point average.

Finally, when fatness was approached with total fat mass percentage, we found that the combined effect of high adiposity and physical inactivity on school grades was large in males and females (Table 7). In both sexes, for adolescents with time allocation for exercise >90 min/week, obesity was related to lower school grades; the ES for difference indicates that the effect of high adiposity on school attainment was small to moderate in females (*d* values ranging from 0.25 to 0.35) and moderate in males (*d* values ranging from 0.42 to 0.49). In adolescents with normal adiposity, the effect of physical inactivity on school grades was found to be significant only in the 12th grade (males) and in terms of GPA (males and females).

Table 7. Analysis of covariance (ANCOVA) measuring the effect of high adiposity and time allocation for exercise on school grades in male and female adolescents.

	MALE PARTICIPANTS										
	High Adiposity (−)					High Adiposity (+)					
	Physically Active §		Physically Inactive			Physically Active §			Physically Inactive		
	Intercept	SE	Coefficient	SE	*d*	Coefficient	SE	*d*	Coefficient	SE	*d*
	Model 1 [a]										
9th (*n* = 330)	459.8 ***	7.2	−20.0	7.2	0.19	−37.0 *	8.6	0.42	−52.2 **	9.4	0.62
10th (*n* = 318)	457.9 ***	7.4	−28.1 ‡	6.6	0.26	−36.5 *	6.1	0.42	−58.2 **	7.8	0.77
11th (*n* = 292)	456.8 ***	7.5	−28.7 ‡	6.6	0.27	−40.4 *	9.1	0.47	−59.2 **	6.8	0.78
12th (*n* = 288)	473.3 ***	6.7	−28.4 *	6.2	0.30	−44.4 *	7.6	0.49	−53.8 **	9.3	0.73
HS-GPA (*n*=288)	466.7 ***	6.5	−27.9 *	6.9	0.31	−42.3 *	6.6	0.49	−58.7 **	7.1	0.79
	Model 2 [b]										
9th (*n* = 330)	464.8 ***	9.7	−12.8	7.9	0.15	−43.7 *	9.0	0.33	−50.9 **	11.4	0.49
10th (*n* = 318)	469.4 ***	10.4	−17.5 ‡	6.6	0.20	−41.8 *	10.1	0.33	−55.7 **	10.8	0.55
11th (*n* = 292)	457.0 ***	10.5	−17.1 ‡	6.5	0.20	−46.0 *	9.7	0.40	−61.2 **	12.1	0.57
12th (*n* = 288)	469.7 ***	10.7	−19.4 *	6.2	0.29	−46.7 *	10.2	0.42	−59.8 **	11.0	0.57
HS-GPA (*n* = 288)	469.3 ***	9.8	−17.9 *	6.9	0.30	−43.0 *	11.9	0.42	−58.7 **	10.9	0.57

Table 7. *Cont.*

	FEMALE PARTICIPANTS										
	High Adiposity (−)					High Adiposity (+)					
	Physically Active §		Physically Inactive			Physically Active §			Physically Inactive		
	Intercept	SE	Coefficient	SE	*d*	Coefficient	SE	*d*	Coefficient	SE	*d*
						Model 1 [a]					
9th (n = 302)	482.7 ***	9.1	−14.1 ‡	7.2	0.23	−19.5	9.9	0.25	−55.5 **	10.7	0.55
10th (n = 297)	484.3 ***	7.4	−14.4 ‡	7.2	0.24	−20.9	10.3	0.25	−52.5 **	10.9	0.57
11th (n = 284)	511.3 ***	8.5	−19.1 *	6.4	0.30	−27.8 *	10.1	0.39	−54.0 **	10.1	0.55
12th (n = 281)	518.6 ***	7.7	−17.9 *	7.2	0.32	−26.3 *	9.6	0.41	−58.6 **	11.7	0.64
HS-GPA (n = 281)	502.3 ***	6.5	−15.1 *	6.1	0.30	−25.6 *	10.6	0.40	−57.8 **	10.4	0.64
						Model 2 [b]					
9th (n = 302)	491.3 ***	12.1	−16.1 ‡	7.0	0.23	−25.0	12.9	0.24	−53.1 **	13.3	0.49
10th (n = 297)	490.3 ***	13.1	−17.0 ‡	7.2	0.24	−26.9	13.9	0.23	−56.5 **	14.7	0.50
11th (n = 284)	519.3 ***	12.5	−20.5 *	7.4	0.30	−27.1	13.1	0.25	−61.0 **	15.9	0.52
12th (n = 281)	469.7 ***	10.7	−23.0 *	8.2	0.31	−34.3 *	11.2	0.34	−59.8 **	15.8	0.52
HS-GPA (n = 281)	514.1 ***	9.5	−15.1 ‡	7.5	0.23	−32.9 *	9.6	0.35	−64.7 **	14.1	0.57

High adiposity (+): Total Fat Mass ≥25% in males and ≥35% in females. School grades expressed as standardized score (scale 210–825), according to the Ministry of Education (Chile). [a] Model 1 is unadjusted. [b] Model 2 is adjusted for SES (parental education, family structure), type of secondary education, and iron supplementation in infancy. § Participants with high adiposity (−) and a fair-to-healthy diet are the reference group. Coefficients are the mean difference between a given category and the reference group. ‡ Trend towards significance ($p < 0.10$). * $p < 0.05$; ** $p < 0.01$; *** $p < 0.001$. Cohen's *d* statistics were estimated accounting for different sample sizes. Abbreviations: HS-GPA: high school grade-point average.

4. Discussion

4.1. Main Findings

We examined the association of fatness measures with school performance in adolescents of low-to-middle SES in a nonindustrialised country. We found that having obesity, abdominal obesity, or high adiposity was associated with lower school performance alone or in combination with unhealthy dietary habits or reduced time allocation for exercise. Second, the findings show that high adiposity and abdominal obesity are more clearly related with lower school grades compared to obesity. Last, the results also indicate that the association of increased fatness with lower school performance was more salient in males than in females.

A number of studies have tested the association of academic outcomes with obesity and their results are similar to ours. In a sample of 6346 adolescents from Iceland, Kristjánsson et al. found that BMI, physical activity, and dietary habits were all independently associated with academic achievement [20]. In this study, self-esteem, which correlated positively with school grades, was negatively influenced by increasing levels of BMI. In Portuguese adolescents ranging in age from 12 to 14 years, cardiorespiratory fitness and weight status were independently and combined related to academic achievement in in mathematics, language (Portuguese), foreign language (English), and sciences [22]. In a sample of high school and college students from five regions across the U.S., McCann and Roberts found that even after controlling for demographic variables, intelligence, personality, and well-being, obese students obtained significantly lower grades than normal-weight students in the eighth grade, community college, and university [43]. Among South Korean adolescents in grades 7–12, overweightness/obesity was negatively associated with academic performance in both boys and girls. In both sexes, the odds of having poor and very poor school performance were substantially and significantly higher in overweight and obese students compared to normal-weight students. These association remain significant after accounting for the effect of sociodemographic determinants as well as the impact of frequency of muscle-strengthening exercises and vigorous and moderate PA [44]. Also, it is worth noting that other studies also show that overweightness/obesity affects a range of behaviours that may affect students' performance, such as classroom behaviour [24], attendance, rate of drop-out [45,46], and academic adjustment [24]. Self-esteem, school satisfaction, and school connectedness have also been postulated as determinants of school performance and have been related with weight status in young populations [47].

A second major finding of our study has to do with the fact that abdominal obesity was the exposure showing the more clear association with school performance, followed by high adiposity and obesity. A *d* value from 0.3 to 0.6 corresponds with a moderate ES, whereas a *d* value greater than 0.6 corresponds with a large ES. Therefore, the effect of obesity on school performance tended to be moderate, yet the effect of abdominal obesity and high adiposity ranged from moderate to large. This suggests that BMI might be underestimating the true effects of obesity on the adolescent brain. Although BMI is the most commonly used method for diagnosing obesity, it has been criticized because it does not always reflect true body fatness, which may be better assessed using body fat percentage and distribution. This also seems to be the case when it comes to understanding how obesity impacts the adolescent brain, specifically the hippocampus and the prefrontal cortex. Adolescence is a period of rapid growth and maturation and is a particularly critical period for hippocampal development and for neural organisation and functional connectivity between the PFC and other brain areas. The hippocampus plays a role in the processing of short- to long-term memory, learning, and emotions, whereas the PFC is involved in executive functions, which allow conscious control, planning, time management, and organisation [11]. A reduced hippocampal and PFC size has been associated with obesity and obesity-related cardiometabolic complications, including insulin resistance and nonalcoholic steatohepatitis [8,13,48]. Excess adiposity also promotes chronic low-grade inflammation and elevated levels of proinflammatory cytokines in the brain, which have been linked with loss of hippocampal and PFC tissue [49]. Likewise, in these brain regions, obesity-induced oxidative stress prompts cell senescence, cytotoxicity, and apoptosis and inhibits the survival and growth of neurons [50]. Furthermore, excess adiposity impairs long-term potentiation (LTP), a process that enhances neural transmission and improves information processing, storage, and retrieval, and thereby promotes memory consolidation and learning [51]. Lastly, excess fat accumulation decreases the expression of hippocampal brain-derived neurotrophic factor [52], which also hampers the conversion of short-term potentiation into LTP.

The fact that excessive fatness appears to take a special toll on males in terms of school performance is also of interest. Cross-sectional and longitudinal studies conducted in adolescents report results similar to ours. In a sample of Hispanic adolescents in grades 9–11 in Texas (U.S.), obese males had lower scores in both reading and mathematics as measured by the Texas Assessment of Knowledge and Skills (TAKS) in comparison to their nonobese counterparts. However, no relationship was found between obesity and TAKS performance in females [53]. Using data from the Longitudinal Study of Australian Children, which were linked to national test scores in numeracy and literacy, obesity and BMI were negatively related to cognitive achievement in boys (aged 8–12 years), but not in girls [54]. The effect could not be explained by family income, parental education, genetic background, or past cognitive achievement and was robust to different measures of adiposity. Additionally, in preadolescents from Brazil, a negative association between skinfold thickness and performance in mathematics was reported to be significant in males, but not in females [55]. Our findings might be consistent with those of the literature showing that men bear a heavier burden following excessive weight gain. Males with increased body fat have higher risk of metabolic syndrome and insulin resistance and have higher liver fat levels than females with the same condition [56]. In a previous study conducted on the same sample, the risk of cardiovascular complications was higher in obese males compared to obese females [2]. The risk was even higher in obese males with reduced muscle mass or augmented body fat accumulation [57]. This sexual dimorphism of obesity is likely related to the differential distribution of adipose tissue in males and females and hence entails important metabolic consequences. Males tend to accrue visceral fat, which has been correlated with increased cardiovascular risk. Premenopausal females, on the other hand, accumulate more fat in subcutaneous deposits, which may protect females from some of the negative consequences of obesity. Visceral fat increases the production of proinflammatory cytokines and interferes with the hormones that regulate appetite, mood, and cognitive function.

4.2. Implications of These Results

Our findings have implications for public health and education policy and provide schools and parents with potentially significant incentives for encouraging the healthy weight of adolescents. Because academic results are a high priority for schools, educators, and parents, the relationship between students' health and school success is important to disseminate. Healthy dietary habits, physical activity, and healthy weight in adolescents are important contributors towards good school performance [58]. Thus, the promotion of healthy lifestyles and good academic outcomes might share a common ground. A second implication of these results relates to the detrimental effects of excess weight gain during critical periods of brain development. Adolescents around the world are highly exposed to risk factors for overweightness and obesity, and thus may also be at risk of cognitive deficits. The adolescent period is particularly critical for hippocampal and PFC development, so the adolescent brain might be particularly vulnerable to the effects of obesity [59]. Third, obesity-related cognitive deficits compromise the ability to learn and school performance, but also increase the risk of other unhealthy behaviours such as substance abuse, tobacco consumption, risky sex, and involvement in violence [60]. Last, but not least, many nonindustrialised countries have made an enormous effort to overcome undernutrition and preserve the full cognitive skills of their people. The transition from under- to overnutrition might be putting this achievement in jeopardy. Low-to-middle SES groups would be at higher risk of impaired expression of cognitive abilities due to greater exposure to overweight/obesity and risk factors.

4.3. Limitations and Strengths

These results support the connection between weight status and school performance. As most studies have been conducted in the developed world, one strength of the present study is that we provide evidence that is relevant for countries undergoing nutritional and epidemiological transitions. Second, we examined the relationship of adiposity markers and cognition using functional measures of cognition that were aimed at providing translational evidence that can be used for health promotion and brain protection in young populations. Furthermore, very few studies have examined the relation between weight status and school performance using adiposity markers other than BMI. Also, we used DXA to measure TFM. Yet, several limitations should be acknowledged when interpreting these results. Because our sample consisted of adolescents from low-to-middle SES, we are not able to extrapolate these results to the overall population of Chilean adolescents. Although a limitation, this SES bias makes our findings particularly relevant and thus could be taken as a strength for several reasons. The prevalence of overweightness/obesity is higher in adolescents of low-to-middle SES according to nationally conducted surveys [5,6]. Also, Chilean adolescents from these socioeconomic levels are more exposed to risk factors for excessive weight gain, such as unhealthy dietary habits and physical inactivity. Studies have shown that the negative effects of excess weight may disproportionately affect minorities and poor school children [61]. Last, the impact of SES on weight status and lifestyles could be critical during adolescence. Other limitations of this study should be mentioned and thus considered when interpreting our results. Although we controlled for sex, diet quality, PA status, family structure, and type of secondary education, we did not consider other important influences, such as school characteristics, potential learning disorders, or general motivational factors. Further studies should replicate this analysis in other populations of nonindustrialized countries. Finally, because the association between weight status and school performance does not imply causation, subsequent research should further investigate the effects of adiposity on cognitive health and educational outcomes.

5. Conclusions

In Chilean adolescents of low-to-middle socioeconomic background, we found a negative and significant association of several fatness measures with school performance, independent of other influences, including diet quality and time allocation for PA. Having obesity, abdominal obesity, or high adiposity might be a potential risk factor for lower academic performance in males, but not always in females. When increased fatness is combined with unhealthy eating and physical inactivity, it becomes a risk factor for lower school performance in both males and females.

Supplementary Materials: The following are available online at http://www.mdpi.com/2072-6643/10/9/1133/s1: Table S1: Comparison of participants included and excluded in the current analysis.

Author Contributions: Conceptualization, P.C.B. and R.B.; Methodology, P.C.B. and R.B.; Formal Analysis, P.C.B.; Investigation, P.C.B., R.B. and S.G.; Data Curation, Y.R.; Writing—Original Draft Preparation, P.C.B.; Writing—Review & Editing, E.B., S.G. and R.B.; Supervision, R.B.; Project Administration, Y.R. and E.B.; Funding Acquisition, S.G., R.B. and P.C.B.

Funding: This research was carried out with financial support from the National Heart Lung and Blood Institute (NHLBI), National Institutes of Health (USA), under grant R01HL088530, the Advanced Human Capital Program (grant code: 79140003), and the National Fund for Scientific and Technological Development (grant code: 1160240), from the National Council for Scientific Research and Technology (CONICYT) (Chile).

Acknowledgments: The authors wish to acknowledge the ongoing commitment of participants and their families. We also thank all the people who contributed to the development of this project, especially Professor Betsy Lozoff.

Conflicts of Interest: The authors declare no conflict of interest. The funders had no role in the design of the study; in the collection, analyses, or interpretation of data; in the writing of the manuscript; and in the decision to publish the results.

References

1. Botton, J.; Heude, B.; Kettaneh, A.; Borys, J.; Lommez, A.; Bresson, J.; Ducimetiere, P.; Charles, M. Cardiovascular risk factor levels and their relationships with overweight and fat distribution in children: The Fleurbaix Laventie Ville Santé II study. *Metabolism* **2007**, *56*, 614–622. [CrossRef] [PubMed]
2. Burrows, R.; Correa, P.; Reyes, M.; Blanco, E.; Albala, C.; Gahagan, S. High cardiometabolic risk in healthy Chilean adolescents: Associations with anthropometric, biological and lifestyle factors. *Public Health Nutr.* **2015**, *19*, 486–493. [CrossRef] [PubMed]
3. Pulgaron, E. Childhood obesity: A review of increased risk for physical and psychological comorbidities. *Clin. Ther.* **2013**, *35*, A18–A32. [CrossRef] [PubMed]
4. Litwin, S. Childhood obesity and adulthood cardiovascular disease: Quantifying the lifetime cumulative burden of cardiovascular risk factors. *J. Am. Coll. Cardiol.* **2014**, *64*, 1588–1590. [CrossRef] [PubMed]
5. Encuesta Global de Salud Escolar. Ministerio de Salud: Santiago de Chile, 2013. Available online: http://www.who.int/chp/gshs/2013_Chile_GSHS_fact_sheet.pdf (accessed on 18 January 2018).
6. Informe Mapa Nutricional 2017. Junta Nacional de Auxilio Escolar y Becas. Ministerio de Educación: Santiago de Chile, 2018. Available online: www.junaeb.cl/wp-content/uploads/2013/03/Mapa-Nutricionalpresentacio%CC%81n2.pdf (accessed on 18 March 2018).
7. Health Data at a Glance 2017: OECD Indicators. Organization for Economic Cooperation and Development, 2017. Available online: http://www.oecd.org/health/health-systems/health-at-a-glance-19991312.htm (accessed on 18 January 2018).
8. Ministerio de Salud. Encuesta Nacional de Consumo Alimentario. Informe Final de Resultados. Subsecretaría de Salud Pública. Santiago de Chile: Ministerio de Salud. Available online: Web.minsal.cl/sites/default/files/ENCA-INFORME_FINAL.pdf (accessed on 7 December 2017).
9. Ministerio de Educación. Informe de Resultados Nacionales de Educación Física 2015. Santiago de Chile, Chile: Ministerio de Educación; 2016. Available online: http://archivos.agenciaeducacion.cl/Informe_Nacional_EducacionFisica2015.pdf (accessed on 20 January 2018).
10. Chen, E.; Matthews, K.A.; Boyce, W.T. Socioeconomic differences in children's health: How and why do these relationships change with age? *Psychol. Bull.* **2002**, *128*, 295–329. [CrossRef] [PubMed]
11. Hungerford, T.L. The persistence of hardship over the life course. *Res. Aging* **2007**, *29*, 491–511. [CrossRef]

12. Jones, A. Race, Socioeconomic Status, and Health during Childhood: A Longitudinal Examination of Racial/Ethnic Differences in Parental Socioeconomic Timing and Child Obesity Risk. *Int. J. Environ. Res. Public Health* **2018**, *15*, 728. [CrossRef] [PubMed]
13. Yau, P.L.; Kang, E.; Javier, D.; Convit, A. Preliminary Evidence of Cognitive and Brain Abnormalities in Uncomplicated Adolescent Obesity. *Obesity* **2014**, *22*, 1865–1871. [CrossRef] [PubMed]
14. Preston, A.; Eichenbaum, H. Interplay of hippocampus and prefrontal cortex in memory. *Curr. Biol.* **2013**, *23*, 764–773. [CrossRef] [PubMed]
15. Miller, A.; Jong, H.; Lumeng, J. Obesity-Associated Biomarkers and Executive Function in Children. *Pediatr. Res.* **2015**, *77*, 143–147. [CrossRef] [PubMed]
16. Irving, A.; Harvey, J. Leptin regulation of hippocampal synaptic function in health and disease. *Philos. Trans. R. Soc. Lond. B. Biol. Sci.* **2013**, *369*, 20130155. [CrossRef]
17. Correa-Burrows, P.; Blanco, E.; Reyes, M.; Castillo, M.; Peirano, P.; Algarín, C.; Lozoff, B.; Gahagan, S.; Burrows, R. Leptin status in adolescence is associated with academic performance in high school: A cross-sectional study in a Chilean birth cohort. *BMJ Open* **2016**, *6*, e010972. [CrossRef]
18. Burrows, R.; Correa, P.; Reyes, M.; Blanco, E.; Gahagan, S. Leptin resistance is independently associated with low academic achievement in the tests for college admission in healthy Chilean adolescents. *Homone. Res.* **2014**, *82*. [CrossRef]
19. Mikkila, V.; Lahti-Koski, M.; Pietinen, P.; Virtanen, S.M.; Rimpelä, M. Associates of obesity and weight dissatisfaction among Finnish adolescents. *Public Health Nutr.* **2003**, *6*, 49–56. [CrossRef] [PubMed]
20. Kristjánsson, A.; Sigfúsdóttir, I.; Allegrante, J. Health behavior and academic achievement among adolescents: The relative contribution of dietary habits, physical activity, body mass index, and self-esteem. *Health Educ. Behav.* **2010**, *37*, 51–64. [CrossRef] [PubMed]
21. Heshmat, R.; Larijani, F.; Pourabbasi, A.; Pourabbasi, A. Do overweight students have lower academic performance than their classmates? A pilot cross-sectional study in a middle school in Tehran. *J. Diabetes Metab. Disord.* **2014**, *13*, 87. [CrossRef] [PubMed]
22. Sardinha, L.; Marques, A.; Martins, S.; Palmeira, A. Fitness, fatness and academic performance in seventh grade elementary school students. *BMC Pediatr.* **2014**, *14*, 176. [CrossRef] [PubMed]
23. Kamijo, K.; Khan, N.; Pontifex, M.; Scudder, M.; Drollette, E.; Raine, L.; Evans, E.M.; Castelli, D.M.; Hillman, C.H. The Relation of Adiposity to Cognitive Control and Scholastic Achievement in Preadolescent Children. *Obesity* **2012**, *20*, 2406–2411. [CrossRef]
24. Carey, F.; Singh, G.; Brown, H.; Wilkinson, A. Educational outcomes associated with childhood obesity in the United States: Cross-sectional results from the 2011-2012 National Survey of Children's Health. *Int. J. Behav. Nutr. Phys. Act.* **2015**, *12*, S3. [CrossRef] [PubMed]
25. Booth, J.; Tomporowski, P.; Boyle, J.; Ness, A.; Joinson, C.; Leary, S.; Reilly, J. Obesity impairs academic attainment in adolescence: Findings from ALSPAC, a UK cohort. *Int. J. Obes.* **2014**, *38*, 1335–1342. [CrossRef] [PubMed]
26. Huang, T.; Goran, M.; Spruijt-Metz, D. Associations of Adiposity with Measured and Self-Reported Academic Performance in Early Adolescence. *Obesity* **2006**, *14*, 1839–1845. [CrossRef] [PubMed]
27. Huang, T.; Tarp, J.; Domazet, S.; Thorsen, A.; Froberg, K.; Andersen, L.; Bugge, A. Associations of Adiposity and Aerobic Fitness with Executive Function and Math Performance in Danish Adolescents. *J. Pediatr.* **2015**, *167*, 810–815. [CrossRef] [PubMed]
28. Lasselin, J.; Magne, E.; Beau, C.; Aubert, A.; Dexpert, S.; Carrez, J.; Layé, S.; Forestier, D.; Ledaguenel, P.; Capuron, L. Low-grade inflammation is a major contributor of impaired attentional set shifting in obese subjects. *Brain Behav. Immun.* **2016**, *58*, 63–68. [CrossRef] [PubMed]
29. Taras, H.; Potts-Datema, W. Obesity and student performance at school. *J. Sch. Health* **2005**, *75*, 291–295. [CrossRef] [PubMed]
30. Daniels, Y. Examining attendance, academic performance, and behavior in obese adolescents. *J. Sch. Nurs.* **2008**, *24*, 379–387. [CrossRef] [PubMed]
31. Lozoff, B.; Castillo, M.; Clark, K.; Smith, J.; Sturza, J. Iron supplementation in infancy contributes to more adaptive behavior at 10 years of age. *J. Nutr.* **2014**, *144*, 838–845. [CrossRef] [PubMed]
32. Taylor, R.; Falorni, A.; Jones, I.; Goulding, A. Identifying adolescents with high percentage body fat: A comparison of BMI cutoffs using age and stage of pubertal development compared with BMI cutoffs using age alone. *Eur. J. Clin. Nutr.* **2003**, *57*, 764–769. [CrossRef] [PubMed]

33. Burrows, R.; Díaz, E.; Schiaraffia, V.; Gattas, V.; Montoya, A.; Lera, L. Dietary intake and physical activity in school age children. *Rev. Med. Chil.* **2008**, *136*, 53–63.
34. Gattas, V.; Burrows, R.; Burgueño, M. Validity Assessment of a Food Frequency Questionnaire in Chilean School-Age Children. In Proceedings of the XVI Congress of the Latin-American Society of Pediatric Research and the XXII Pan-American Meeting of Pediatrics, Santiago, Chile, 25–30 April 2007.
35. Ministerio de Salud. *Tablas Chilenas de Composición Química de los Alimentos*; Ministerio de Salud: Santiago, Chile, 2010. Available online: http://www.minsal.cl/composicion-de-alimentos/ (accessed on 14 March 2018).
36. Godard, C.; Rodríguez, M.; Díaz, N.; Lera, L.; Salazar, G.; Burrows, R. Value of a clinical test for assessing physical activity in children. *Rev. Med. Chil.* **2008**, *136*, 1155–1162.
37. Dobow, E.; Boxer, P.; Huesmann, L. Long-term Effects of Parents' Education on Children's Educational and Occupational Success: Mediation by Family Interactions, Child Aggression, and Teenage Aspirations. *Merrill Palmer* **2009**, *55*, 224–249. [CrossRef] [PubMed]
38. International Standard Classification of Education. ISCED 2011. United Nations Educational, Scientific and Cultural Organization (UNESCO): Paris, 2012. Available online: http://www.uis.unesco.org/Education/Documents/isced-2011-en.pdf (accessed on 14 September 2017).
39. Ginther, D.; Pollak, R. Family Structure and Children's Educational Outcomes: Blended Families, Stylized Facts, and Descriptive Regressions. *Demography* **2004**, *41*, 671–696. [CrossRef]
40. Burrows, R.; Correa, P.; Orellana, Y.; Lizana, P.; Almagiá, A.; Ivanovic, D. Scheduled physical activity is associated with better academic performance in Chilean school-age children. *J. Phys. Act. Health* **2014**, *11*, 1600–1606. [CrossRef] [PubMed]
41. Correa-Burrows, P.; Burrows, R.; Blanco, E.; Reyes, M.; Gahagan, S. Nutritional quality of diet and academic performance in Chilean students. *Bull. World Health Org.* **2016**, *94*, 185–192. [CrossRef] [PubMed]
42. Correa-Burrows, P.; Rodríguez, Y.; Burrows, R.; Blanco, E.; Reyes, M.; Gahagan, S. Snacking quality is associated with secondary school academic achievement and the intention to enroll in higher education: A cross-sectional study in adolescents from Santiago, Chile. *Nutrients* **2017**, *9*, 433. [CrossRef] [PubMed]
43. McCann, C.; Roberts, R. Just as smart but not as successful: Obese students obtain lower school grades but equivalent test scores to non-obese students. *Int. J. Obes.* **2013**, *37*, 40–46. [CrossRef] [PubMed]
44. Kim, J.; So, W. Association between overweight/obesity and academic performance in South Korean adolescents. *Cent. Eur. J. Public Health* **2013**, *21*, 170–183. [CrossRef]
45. An, R.; Yan, H.; Shi, X.; Yang, Y. Childhood obesity and school absenteeism: A systematic review and meta-analysis. *Obes. Rev.* **2017**, *18*, 1412–1424. [CrossRef] [PubMed]
46. Lanza, H.I.; Huang, D.Y. Is obesity associated with school dropout? Key developmental and ethnic differences. *J. Sch. Health* **2015**, *85*, 663–670. [CrossRef] [PubMed]
47. Wang, F.; Veugelers, P.J. Self-esteem and cognitive development in the era of the childhood obesity epidemic. *Obes. Rev.* **2008**, *9*, 615–623. [CrossRef] [PubMed]
48. Veit, R.; Kullmann, S.; Heni, M.; Machann, J.; Häring, H.; Fritsche, A.; Preissl, H. Reduced cortical thickness associated with visceral fat and BMI. *Neuroimage. Clin.* **2014**, *6*, 307–311. [CrossRef] [PubMed]
49. Miller, A.; Spencer, S. Obesity and neuroinflammation: A pathway to cognitive impairment. *Brain Behav. Immun.* **2014**, *42*, 10–21. [CrossRef] [PubMed]
50. Vieira, A.; Michels, M.; Florentino, D.; Nascimento, D.; Rezin, G.; Leffa, D.; Jeremias Fortunato, J.; Dal-Pizzol, F.; Barichello, T.; Quevedo, J.; et al. Obesity promotes oxidative stress and exacerbates sepsis-induced brain damage. *Curr. Neurovasc. Res.* **2015**, *12*, 147–154. [CrossRef] [PubMed]
51. Gerges, N.Z.; Aleisa, A.M.; Alkadhi, K.A. Impaired long-term potentiation in obese zucker rats: Possible involvement of presynaptic mechanism. *Neuroscience* **2003**, *120*, 535–539. [CrossRef]
52. Leal, G.; Afonso, P.; Salazar, I.; Duarte, C. Regulation of hippocampal synaptic plasticity by BDNF. *Brain Res.* **2015**, *1621*, 82–101. [CrossRef] [PubMed]
53. Effects of Obesity and Physical Fitness on Academic performance in Hispanic High School Students. Available online: http://digitalcommons.wku.edu/ijesab/vol2/iss4/55 (accessed on 20 January 2018).
54. Black, N.; Johnston, D.; Peeters, A. Childhood Obesity and Cognitive Achievement. *Health Econ.* **2015**, *24*, 1082–1100. [CrossRef] [PubMed]
55. De Almeida Santana, C.; Farah, B.; Azevedo, L.; Gunnarsdottir, T.; Hill, J.; Botero, J.; do Prado, E.C.; do Prado, W.L. Associations between cardiorespiratory fitness and overweight with academic performance in 12-year old Brazilian children. *Pediatr. Exerc. Sci.* **2016**, *6*, 1–22. [CrossRef] [PubMed]

56. Palmer, B.; Clegg, D. The sexual dimorphism of obesity. *Mol. Cell. Endocrinol.* **2015**, *402*, 113–119. [CrossRef] [PubMed]
57. Burrows, R.; Correa, P.; Reyes, M.; Albala, C.; Gahagan, S. Low muscle mass is associated with cardiometabolic risk regardless of nutritional status in adolescents: A cross-sectional study in a Chilean birth cohort. *Pediatr. Diabetes* **2017**, *18*, 895–902. [CrossRef] [PubMed]
58. Burkhalter, T.; Hillman, C. A narrative review of physical activity, nutrition, and obesity to cognition and scholastic performance across the human lifespan. *Adv. Nutr.* **2011**, *2*, 201S–206S. [CrossRef] [PubMed]
59. Khan, N.; Baym, C.; Monti, J.; Raine, L.; Drollette, E.; Scudder, M.; Moore, R.D.; Kramer, A.F.; Hillman, C.H.; Cohen, N.J. Central adiposity is negatively associated with hippocampal-dependent relational memory among overweight and obese Children. *J. Pediatr.* **2015**, *166*, 302–308. [CrossRef] [PubMed]
60. Health Risk Behaviors and Academic Achievement. Centers for Disease Control and Prevention, US Department of Health and Human Services: Atlanta (GA), 2008. Available online: http://www.cdc.gov/healthyyouth/health_and_academics/pdf/health_risk_behaviors.pdf (accessed on 12 March 2018).
61. Barriuso, L.; Miqueleiz, E.; Albaladejo, R. Socioeconomic position and childhood-adolescent weight status in rich countries: A systematic review, 1990–2013. *BMC Pediatr.* **2015**, *15*, 129. [CrossRef] [PubMed]

nutrients

Article

The Identification of the Factors Related to Household Food Insecurity among Indigenous People (Orang Asli) in Peninsular Malaysia under Traditional Food Systems

Leh Shii Law, Sulaiman Norhasmah *, Wan Ying Gan, Adznam Siti Nur'Asyura and Mohd Taib Mohd Nasir

Department of Nutrition and Dietetics, Faculty of Medicine and Health Sciences, Universiti Putra Malaysia, Serdang 43400, Malaysia; lehshii@gmail.com (L.S.L.); wanying@upm.edu.my (W.Y.G.); asyura@upm.edu.my (A.S.N.A.); nasir.jpsk@gmail.com (M.T.M.N.)

* Correspondence: norhasmah@upm.edu.my; Tel.: +60-3-8947-2461

Received: 30 August 2018; Accepted: 29 September 2018; Published: 8 October 2018

Abstract: Over the course of 16 years, a high percentage of Orang Asli (OA) households in Malaysia has been found to be burdened with food insecurity. Therefore, a study was conducted to improve the understanding of the challenges faced by the OA in Peninsular Malaysia to achieve food security under traditional food systems. In this study, in-depth interview sessions, which were assisted by an interview protocol, were conducted with 61 OA women from nine villages that were selected purposefully across three states (Kelantan, Pahang, and Perak) in Peninsular Malaysia. Furthermore, thematic analysis was performed during data analysis. As a result, four themes were identified, namely (i) the failure in agriculture (sub-themes: threats from wild animals and insufficient land supply), (ii) ineffectiveness of traditional food-seeking activities (sub-themes: exhausting, tiring, dangerous, and time-consuming journey for food-seeking activities, depletion of natural commodities, reduced demands of natural commodities, and lack of equipment), (iii) weather (sub-themes: rainy and dry seasons), and (iv) water issues (subthemes: continuity of water supply and cleanliness of water). The identified modifiable factors of this issue should be incorporated into future schemes of food security intervention in order to efficiently manage the food shortage among the OA.

Keywords: Orang Asli; food insecurity; Malaysia; challenges; in-depth interview

1. Introduction

Acknowledging food insecurity as a public health concern is a huge advancement in the chronological development of this issue. Several populations, namely children, the elderly, minorities, and low-income households have been known to possess a higher risk of facing food insecurity [1]. Furthermore, being the minority, Indigenous People are not excluded from this dilemma as the prevalence rate of food insecurity among this population has been reported to be high in some countries. Willows et al. [2] showed that 33% of Indigenous households in Canada were categorized as food-insecure. Within that total percentage, 14% of the cases were found to be severe. On the other hand, according to the Australian Institute of Health and Welfare [3], 24% of the Indigenous People in Australia, aged 15 or older, had faced food shortage in the previous 12 months from 2004 to 2005. Moreover, about 8% of the people affected by this issue claimed that they could not afford to buy food during a food shortage.

This issue was not widely explored by previous studies in Malaysia. The first research related to food security among the Orang Asli (OA) was conducted by Zalilah and Tham [4] who found that 82% of the OA households at Hulu Langat, Selangor were food-insecure. Meanwhile, Nurfahilin and Norhasmah [5] reported that 88% of OA households at Gombak, Selangor State had been food insecure until 2015. In addition, the most recent study on this matter revealed that 82.9% of the OA households (Mah Meri) at Carey Island and Tanjung Sepat (both are located in the Kuala Langat district) faced food insecurity; 29.3% household food insecurity, 23.4% individual food insecurity, and 30.2% experiencing child hunger [6]. Besides, Haemamalar et al. [7] and Chua et al. [8] found evidence related to food insecurity among the OA, which referred to the issue of the low dietary diversity (one of food insecurity indirect measures) among the OA in Pahang State, Malaysia.

Indigenous People, including the OA, are well-equipped with traditional knowledge inherited from generation to generation. This line of knowledge should have developed further with all the available natural resources offered by Mother Nature [9,10]. Therefore, the high prevalence rate of food insecurity among the Indigenous People is rather unexpected. This could be due to several challenges they encounter in practicing traditional food systems, which include the declining amount of plant and animal species, lack of transfer of cultural knowledge to youth, reduced time and energy invested for harvesting due to employment, decreased densities of species, and decreased land use. Moreover, the raising concern about environmental contamination and the increasing availability and acceptance towards new food are linked with the abandonment of traditional food systems in this community [11].

In addition, food security is closely linked with food systems. Food systems play a role in the food management process that consists of four stages including the production, processing and packaging, distribution and retail, and consumption of food. To put this simply, food systems regulate the overall process of food management [12]. Furthermore, the management of food loss and waste, which is another component under the food system, is a foundation of food security. Recently, significant food loss and waste has been reported during the harvesting, transportation, storage, packaging, wholesaling, retailing, and consumption of food [12]. Food loss and waste was estimated to be approximately one third of total food production globally (1.3 billion tons) [13]. The food loss and waste is not acceptable as millions of people are suffering food insecurity globally, yet tons and tons of food that were aimed to feed the targeted groups were wasted due to mismanagement [12]. This also implies that presence of food availability alone does not guarantee food security. The food should be made (physically, economically, and socially) accessible to the public [14]. Therefore, the primary focus of this study is the traditional food system. The traditional food system for Indigenous People is described as "being composed of items from the local, natural environment that are culturally acceptable" [11] (p. 417). An in-depth exploration of the traditional food system is necessary, provided that most of the Indigenous People worldwide depend on the food systems to obtain food and generate income [9].

Based on the data obtained from the Department of Orang Asli Development (JAKOA), the population of OA in Peninsular Malaysia was 178,197 in 2013, and this number was divided into three main ethnic groups, which were Senoi, Malay-Proto, and Negrito [15]. Orang Asli were expected to flourish under the traditional food systems attributed to their rich knowledge of their surrounding environment (forests/lakes/rivers) and food-seeking activities (farming/hunting/gathering). However, contradictive findings from other studies showed a high prevalence of food insecurity and low dietary diversity among the OA in Peninsular Malaysia. This information proves that the OA are facing hardships to obtain sufficient food through traditional food-seeking methods, namely farming, hunting, fishing, and gathering. Therefore, drastic measures are needed to curb food insecurity issues among the OA. Before any recommendations and resolutions can be planned or proposed, a thorough understanding of this issue is important. For this reason, this study was conducted to identify the factors connected with food insecurity among the OA. This study aims to find out the factors for the absence of traditional food practices as a safeguard for OA to obtain enough food.

2. Materials and Methods

This is a qualitative research study using a case study design. According to Yin [16], a case study is an empirical enquiry into answering the "how" and "why" research questions. The focus of the case study is the contemporary phenomenon in real life contexts where investigators have little to no control over real-life events. The particular case concerned in this study is the occurrence of household food insecurity, while the unit of analysis is the 'hardcore poor' OA households.

2.1. Study Location

The locations for this study were selected purposefully based on the number of the food assistant recipients under JAKOA. The list of food recipient names from each administrative region was obtained from the JAKOA state headquarters or the JAKOA administrative offices. The administrative regions were then divided into three groups, namely Senoi dominant, Proto-Malay dominant, and Negrito dominant. Then, one district was selected under each ethnic cluster. The villages from each district were also purposefully selected using the priority given to the particular villages with a high number of food assistant recipients. However, the provision of this priority was subjected to the advice given by the JAKOA staff as they were more familiar with the conditions in the villages. The selected study locations were at Gua Musang District (Kelantan State), Rompin District (Pahang State), and Gerik District (Perak State). The study locations are shown in the Figure 1 [17].

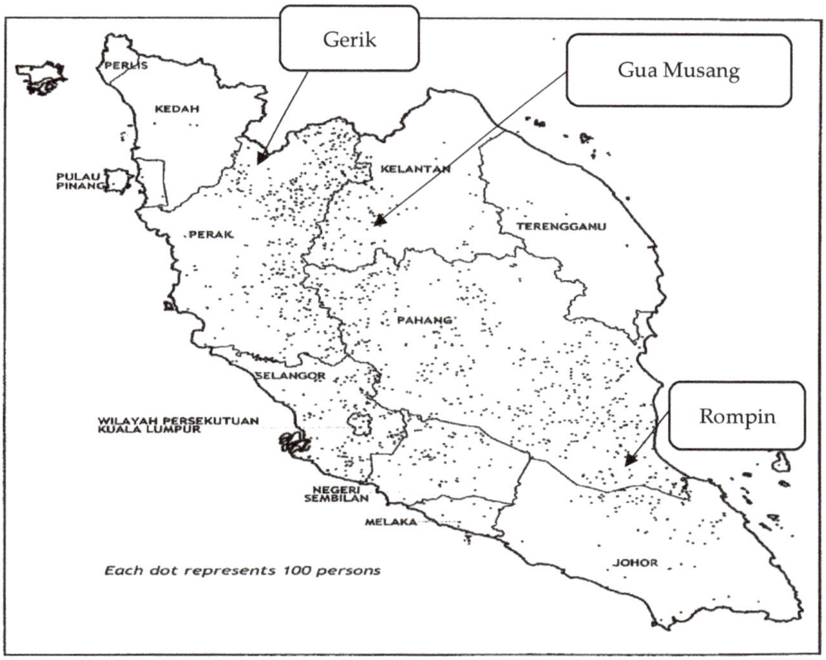

Figure 1. Distribution of *Orang Asli* in Peninsular Malaysia, 2000.

Gerik is a *mukim* (administrative division) of Hulu Perak, a district at the north of Perak State. Based on the information provided by JAKOA, a majority of the OA here are Negrito. Meanwhile, Gua Musang is a district at the southern part of Kelantan State, with Senoi as the biggest community there. Lastly, Rompin is a district located at the southeast corner of Pahang State, and Proto-Malay appears to be dominant in this region.

2.2. *Informants*

The informants consisted of 61 OA women. The inclusion criteria was that they were of child-bearing age (20–49 years old), brought along at least a single child during data collection, and lived in 'hardcore poor' households that received food assistance from JAKOA. According to JAKOA, the classification of the households as 'hardcore poor' was based on the guidelines provided by the Economic Planning Unit [18] which stated that the households which receive an income below Malaysian Ringgit (MYR) 520 per month (United States Dollar (USD) 127.45 (10 August 2018)) are classified as 'hardcore poor'. The sample size of the informants was based on the concept of saturation. A stage of saturation was achieved when no new information emerged as the interview progressed [19].

2.3. *Ethical Clearance and Permissions*

Prior to data collection, ethical clearance was obtained from the Ethics Committee for Research Involving Human Subjects (JKEUPM) of Universiti Putra Malaysia (Serdang, Malaysia) [Reference no.: FPSK(EXP15)P004]. The permission to carry out this study at the OA villages was obtained from JAKOA. At the same time, all the informants needed to sign a written consent form to prove their willingness to voluntarily participate in this study. However, they were allowed to withdraw from the study without any penalty, and all the information provided by the informants were kept confidential.

2.4. *Data Collection*

This process was conducted through several sessions of semi-structured in-depth interviews with the help from an interview protocol. The interview protocol referred to a list of questions and issues of interest that were covered during the in-depth interview. The interviews were audio-recorded with permissions from the informants. The Malay language, a national language among Malaysians regardless of their ethnic background, was used during this session. However, for informants who were not able to express themselves in this language, the services of translators were used to smooth the interview sessions, and they consisted of the local OA who were able to speak both the native OA language and the Malay language. Another instrument used in this study was a sociodemographic questionnaire that was used to assess the sociodemographic characteristics of the informants.

Each of the informants was required to go through two sessions of the in-depth interview. The primary aim of these sessions was to establish a sense of rapport between the researcher and the informants [20]. To reemphasize, this study particularly looked into the contributing factors of household food insecurity under traditional food systems. The questions which were directed to the informants were:

- Are you facing any problems in obtaining sufficient food?
- (Based on Question 1) If yes, can you elaborate the problem(s) you are facing by providing a suitable example(s)?
- (Based on Question 2) How frequent is/are the problem(s)?

2.5. *Quality Control*

In order to ensure the authenticity of the information extracted from the informants, the plan to involve the heads of the villages or renowned individuals during data collection was implemented. Based on the observation prior to the test, the presence of the Tok Batin (heads of the villages) or renowned individuals helped to get rid of suspicion of information. Furthermore, translation services also helped smooth the process of the interviews. Both approaches reduced the potential biases among the informants, be it intentional or unintentional, such as providing inaccurate information due to misinterpretation of the questions. Triangulation was another valid method used to secure the information gathered from the interviews. Data triangulation (the involvement of all three main ethnic groups of OA) and environmental triangulation (the involvement of three study locations) were incorporated into the sampling methods [21]. The information provided by all the three ethnic groups were considered to have the highest authenticity.

2.6. Data Analysis

The findings of the numeric sociodemographic characteristics were presented with medians, while the category sociodemographic variables were presented in counts and proportions. The descriptive data of the informants were analyzed using IBM SPSS Statistics version 22.0 (IBM Corp., Armonk, NY, USA). On the other hand, the extraction of the information from the interview was done through thematic analysis. This action was based on the techniques guide from Braun and Clark [22]. First, the verbal data from the interviews were transcribed verbatim. The transcription process helped researchers familiarize themselves with the data [23]. Then, the transcripts were read repeatedly in order to determine the breadth of the data. Normally, the repeated reading is followed by other processes such as note-taking and marking the ideas for the coding process that follows after. Through the familiarization of data conducted in the previous step, the coding process starts. In this study, the coding process was carried out manually using highlighters or colored pens. The codes identified from the data familiarization were matched up with the data extracted from individual transcripts. These transcripts were found to demonstrate the characteristics of the code. Each code that was identified, including the relevant data extracts, was kept in a separate computer file. Following that, the identified codes were categorized into potential themes/sub-themes, while the relevant coded data extracts were categorized into the identified themes/sub-themes.

3. Results

3.1. Characteristics of the Informants

A total of 61 informants from three districts (Gua Musang, Rompin, and Gerik), with a median age of 32 (range: 20–49) years, were recruited. Most of the informants were from big households where four or more children resided. Furthermore, a high percentage of the informants either had a low formal education or did not pursue a formal education at all. As for their socioeconomic characteristics, most of the informants were housewives, while most of their spouses were skilled agricultural, forestry, and fishery workers. Subsequently, the selected households were then categorized as 'hardcore poor' except for a single household, which was labeled as 'poor'. Further details regarding the informants' demographic and socioeconomic characteristics are presented in Table 1.

3.2. Factors Related to Household Food Insecurity

Meals of OA comprised mixtures of market and traditional food due to the variances in their food-seeking behaviors. Market food was purchased from nearby food outlets, including rice, flour, biscuits, tea, cereal, and green leafy vegetables. Traditional food was usually obtained through food-seeking activities and farming that included gathering edible fruits and vegetables (stinky bean, fern shoot, and natural herbs), fishing (local fish and prawn), hunting (wild boar, squirrel, and lizards), farming (tuber roots, rambutan, and durian), and raising poultry (chicken and duck). In brief, traditional food was obtained from their surrounding environment without involving money.

The thematic analysis revealed four potential themes which contributed to household food insecurity among the OA under traditional food systems. The aforementioned themes were the failure in agriculture, the ineffectiveness of traditional food searching methods, water issues, and weather.

3.2.1. The Failure in Agriculture

In the case of the failure in agriculture, the informants expressed their concerns of the agricultural products cultivated from their farms being under the threat from wild animals, such as wild boars, monkeys, and rats if not guarded properly. The wild animals that invaded the farms, not only stole the agricultural products, but also destroyed the plants. It was reported that this case was faced by the Senoi and Proto-Malay groups only.

Table 1. Sociodemographic characteristics of the informants (n = 61).

Variable	Count (n)	Percentage (%)	Median (Range)
Age (years)			32 (20–49)
20–29	26	42.6	
30–39	22	36.1	
40–49	13	21.3	
Ethnicity			
Senoi (Temiar)	20	32.8	
Proto-Malay (Temuan)	20	32.8	
Negrito (Jahai)	21	34.4	
Religion			
Islam	27	44.3	
Christianity	8	13.1	
Animism	26	42.6	
Marital Status			
Married	57	93.4	
Widowed	4	6.6	
Number of Children			3 (1–13)
≤2	24	39.3	
3–5	19	31.1	
6–8	13	21.3	
≥9	5	8.2	
Education Level of Informants			1.5 (0–11.0)
No formal education	25	41.0	
Primary school	21	34.4	
Secondary school	15	24.6	
Education Level of Spouses			2.5 (0–11.0)
No formal education	24	39.3	
Primary school	26	42.6	
Secondary school	10	16.4	
Do not know	1	1.6	
Occupation of Respondents			
Skilled agricultural, forestry, and fishery worker	12	19.7	
Plant and machine-operators and assembler	1	1.6	
Housewife	48	78.7	
Occupation of Spouses			
Skilled agricultural, forestry, and fishery worker	52	85.2	
Craft and related trade worker	1	1.6	
Plant and machine-operators and assembler	3	4.9	
Elementary occupation	1	1.6	
Divorced	1	1.6	
Passed away	3	4.9	
Monthly household income (MYR *)			200.0 (50.0–750.0 †)
Income per capita (MYR *)			41.7 (8.3–250.0)
Expenses of food and beverage (MYR *)			100.0 (20.0–250.0)

* USD = United States Dollar, MYR = Malaysian Ringgit; USD 1 = MYR 4.08 (10 August 2018). † A household was grouped under "poor" (monthly household income between MYR 520 and 830) due to job opportunity weeks before interview. The household was in the name list of food assistant recipient in 2014. Therefore, the household was eligible for this study.

Informant 15:

"The products were eaten by the foxes and the birds. Yes. Today, when I went there (farm), everything seemed fine. However, tomorrow or the day after, when I went there, the wild boars might have eaten the products. I guard my farm myself. I do the patrol around the farm. I find the rattans, cut the bamboos, to build a guard post. I guard it myself. There are animals out there which eat our products.

Sometimes, when we plant tuber roots, the wild boars eat it. As for pumpkins, the insects from the forest eat them. The insects eat ... the grasshoppers eat the shoots of the tuber plants until nothing is left behind."

Informant 42:

"It (wild boar) eats the tapioca. It eats the sweet potatoes. It eats the banana tree. If we plant the pineapple, it also eats the pineapple. Nowadays, there are many wild boars.

In addition, the informants were concerned with the lack of arable land for them to carry out self-sustainable agricultural activities. Orang Asli did not possess the arable lands nearby and the lands were taken to run domestic agricultural activities and mining. The Senoi and Proto-Malay were the only groups who were reported to face this issue:

Informant 3:

"For example, I really do not own any piece of land. It is not belonged to me. Whatever farms you can see here are all belonged to the other people.

Informant 50:

"Not enough land. Only have a small piece of land. Do not have new land because all have been cleared up to become the (domestic) farms."

3.2.2. The Ineffectiveness of Traditional Food-Seeking Methods

Besides the failure in agriculture, the ineffectiveness of traditional food seeking methods was found to be another theme which explained the failure of the OA to achieve household food security. This is because this method only depends on wild plants and animals from their surrounding environment. Furthermore, food gathering and hunting were described as time-consuming, dangerous, uncertain, and exhausting. Despite the hard work, traditional food-seeking activities did not always guarantee enough food. These factors were reported by all three ethnic groups involved during the interview.

Informant 7:

"(Leaves) at six o'clock in the morning, comes back at seven o'clock, or eight o'clock at night. If we travel through the forest at seven in the morning, will come back at three or four in the afternoon."

Informant 21:

"When my husband travels to the forest, there are a lot of challenges awaiting him, such as the presence of elephants, tigers, snakes, and centipedes."

Informant 13:

"Searching for food is not easy. Sometimes, the food that we wish to find is available, but sometimes it is not. Especially when we go fishing. Sometimes the fish bites, and sometimes we have to go back home with empty hands."

Informant 52:

"The road ... the road is covered with mud. We need to go through the bushes too. Sometimes, the walking path is covered by stones. Climbing up and down, up and down the hills."

Due to deforestation, the condition of the food insecurity among informants worsened due to the depletion of natural commodities in the forests. Forests provide habitat for various flora and fauna. Many species that OA depended on for food cannot survive due to loss of home. This factor was reported by all three ethnic groups (Senoi, Proto-Malay, Negrito).

Informant 2:

"It (the fern shoot) is not available here, very hard to find. Want to eat (wild) vegetables, but it is not available. (The place with fern shoots is) only reachable by a motorcycle as it is far away. Do not have (wild vegetables here), if you find at surrounding here, (you) only manage to get a few, three or four sticks. Not enough to eat."

Informant 16:

"Difficult. It was quite easy in the old days, but now, it is hard. Due to some people who conduct the mining activities, and because of that, the natural products of the forest are no longer available. At the side (of the forest) where people conduct the tin ore mining activities, the forest will be demolished."

Furthermore, the demand for natural commodities, such as herbs, was no longer popular compared to the demand for these resources from decades ago. This led to the drop in the price of the natural commodities. This factor was reported by all three ethnic groups (Senoi, Proto-Malay, Negrito).

Informant 32:

"It is not sold at high price, not very high and sometimes it is sold in low price. Take the herbs with medical value from the forest as an example, we get three Ringgit fifty cents for a kilogram. If we manage to get a few kilograms, we get a few dozen Ringgit."

Informant 57:

"Only my husband knows about the price of the natural commodities. The price was only known before though. Nowadays, no one has been requesting for natural herbs. For example, people requested Tongkat Ali (a traditional medicine) only during the old days. It is no longer requested now."

The informants were also reported to abandon hunting activities due to the lack of the equipment needed. Weapons were needed to hunt big-sized animals (e.g., wild boar and deer). This problem was found to occur among all ethnic groups, namely Senoi, Proto-Malay, and Negrito.

Informant 42:

"I do not have an equipment for fishing. How can I go fishing? (Besides that, it is) hard to get wild animals. No gun is available for hunting. (We) do not have an equipment (for the activities)."

Informant 50:

"It is because we do not have the equipment for fishing. We do not have the gun for hunting."

3.2.3. Water Issues

It was found that the *Orang Asli* in Malaysia were still burdened with the problems of obtaining sufficient clean water supply which explained the failure of the OA to achieve household food security. Water issues were labeled as the third theme under factors associated with household food insecurity among OA. To be specific, the water supply was reported to be inconsistent due to the blockage of the pipe system, especially after the rain. Besides, agricultural and logging activities became a concern as these activities contaminated the rivers or lakes which were known to be the primary water sources for the OA. The river became muddy especially after raining due to deforestation. Meanwhile, the OA were worried about the possible leakage of pesticides used for domestic agriculture activities into the rivers. This problem was reported by all ethnic groups in the present study.

Informant 56:

"For me, if I want to declare the water supply that I got is clean is not true. (The water) may be considered moderately clean. The problem is due to land clearing and logging, water is affected and is no longer clean. When it rains, water looks muddy."

Informant 59:

"Water supply? We are not satisfied with it. Because when some people performing logging activities, the water will be exposed to pollution. When it rains ... during the dry seasons, the water looks a bit clear. However, when it rains, it looks a bit muddy. Therefore, it is hard for us to get obtain a clean water supply. Water supplies cannot be continued as sometimes the pipe is blocked during the rain and we need to go repair it. Therefore, the actual problem is the blocked pipe, not the water."

3.2.4. Weather

This issue fell under the fourth theme which explained the failure of the OA to achieve household food security. To be specific, Malaysia experiences two monsoon seasons, namely the southwest monsoon (June to September) and northeast monsoon (November to March) as well as two inter-monsoon seasons (October and April to May). The southwest monsoon brings rain to the east coast while the northeast monsoon increases rainfall to the west coast of Peninsular Malaysia [24]. The extreme rainy season was found to interrupt economic activities, such as rubber tapping, mining, and searching for natural commodities in the forests. Furthermore, heavy rain also led to the occurrence of floods which destroyed the farms cultivated by the OA. This problem was found to occur among all ethnic groups in the present study.

Informant 46:

"Due to the raining season, we become jobless. It is hard to find a job. Some of the available jobs are related to farm works, such as rubber tapping. These jobs are usually pursued through contracts and recruits are unneeded due to rain. Workers are recruited only during dry seasons. This is why sometimes earning money is not an easy task for us."

Informant 52:

"A bit tough when the rainy season arrives. Cannot earn money. For example, we want to search vegetables or want to harvest the banana for sale are also restricted, people (traders) do not want the products. In addition, people (traders) do not travel here to pick up the products."

On the other hand, the extreme dry season reduced the chance of successful harvesting as crops or vegetables might die before the plants got to be full grown. This factor was also reported by all ethnic groups in the present study.

Informant 4:

"Dry season. The leaves wither instead of flourishing. The land is dry, but many still carry out agricultural works. Harvesting can be done, but the plants will not fully grow."

Informant 45:

"Water, sometimes do not have water. The water flow is slow. The tuber roots are also dying. Because of the heat."

4. Discussion

The findings provided evidence regarding the presence of household food insecurity among the OA, especially among those with the low socioeconomic background. Overall, the factors of household food insecurity under traditional food systems included the failure in agriculture, the ineffectiveness of traditional food seeking methods, water issues, and weather. Presence of challenges in conducting traditional food-seeking activities implies that food sovereignty of the OA was violated due to deforestation and pollution of the water sources. Orang Asli were found to have no control over their territories where they obtained their food (forests, rivers, lakes, and arable lands nearby their villages) from destruction as a consequence of the economic activities that were conducted by third parties [25,26]. This finding is important for a better understanding of the hardships faced by the OA so that counteracting policies can be implemented for an improved standard of living.

The first factor of household food insecurity among the OA was the failure in agriculture. Most of the OA cultivated their own farms either at the nearby forests or beside their houses. However, their farms were always under the threat of wild animals, such as wild boars. A similar finding was reported by Zakari et al. [27] as the occurrence of diseases and presence of insects in the farms were found to be related with household food insecurity among the farmers at Kollo district, Southern Niger. Besides, some informants reported that insufficient agricultural lands disrupted the OA's self-sustainable agricultural activities which should have been done to support the needs of their household members. As a result, the vulnerability to food insecurity of the households that owned no or small agricultural lands increased. This happened as the nearby lands in the villages were taken over for the development of mining sites, logging sites, or cash crop plantations, such as palm oil trees and rubber trees [28]. Similarly, insufficient agricultural land puts a limit on food availability for household members' daily consumption, and it dwindles the economic income that can be generated from the cultivation of household farms [29]. The importance of land in preventing household food insecurity by increasing the household income was reported by Kirimi et al. [30] in Kenya, who pointed out that the ownership of lands for households was found to reduce the risk of poverty (low household income to fulfil the needs of the basic food and non-food necessities) and help the households overcome food insecurity.

Naturally, OA are well-known for their capability of finding their own food from their surroundings, either from the forests, rivers, or lakes. One of the factors which was believed to have led to the obstacles faced by the OA in finding sufficient food is the depletion of food resources. This is the result of deforestation due to logging activities, either conducted legally or illegally. Furthermore, Malaysia had reported an increasing forest loss from 2000 to 2012 [31]. Not only that, insufficient proper equipment restricts the OA's from carrying out hunting activities for food. Similar challenges were also found to occur to other groups of Indigenous People worldwide. For example, a study conducted on Vuntut Gwitchin First Nation from the Old Crow and Tlingit households in Teslin, Canada found that insufficient time and limited availability of traditional food were the factors that disrupted the continuation of hunting activities. Other factors that disrupted the continuation of hunting activities included the unaffordable price of harvesting tools, cultural loss, and the concern of contamination [32]. In addition, the challenge faced by the Inuit communities at Pangnirtung, Nunavut, Canada was that their activity of food-searching around their surroundings was disrupted due to climate change, environmental degradation, market economy, globalization, acculturation, and nutrition transition [33].

There were two main issues associated with water supply, namely the disruption of the water supply and the concern for the cleanliness of the water. The disruption of the water supply was mainly due to the lack of maintenance and blockage of personal water pipes by sand or dry leaves after the rain, which prevented water from flowing to the reservoir. The reservoir is where all the villagers obtain water. In the case of the cleanliness of water, the informants voiced their concern about the pollution of the river near their area due to logging and agricultural activities [34]. A shift in the pattern of diseases among OA such as hepatitis A and B, tuberculosis, and dermatological and gastroenterological problems was related to the use of polluted water [35]. Besides, many other diseases were associated with this pollution issue, which included skin diseases, diarrhea, dysentery, respiratory illnesses, anemia, and complications in childbirth [36]. Therefore, water issues among the OA should be taken seriously in order to prevent these illnesses from spreading.

In the recent years, Malaysia faced several episodes of extreme weather events, such as floods, droughts, and heat waves [37]. Provided that the OA's quality of life is dependent on their surrounding environment, the weather is believed to be another factor which may determine the status of their household food security. Moreover, the interaction between extreme climate and the status of household food security was shown in Bahiigwa's [38] study, which demonstrated a fluctuating pattern in the prevalence rate of food insecurity in 1000 households from four geographical regions in Uganda (western, central, eastern, and northern). This was due to the lack of rainfall, pests and diseases, and excessive rain. Likewise, Niles and Salermo [39] revealed that households from 15 countries in Latin America, Africa, and South Asia that faced climate shock had a higher likelihood to experience household food insecurity. Meanwhile, the Food and Agriculture Organization [40] showed that climate had the potential to influence the quantities and types of food produced and the amount of the production-related income. At the same time, the extreme weather might have adverse impacts as it could destroy the transportation and distribution facilities, and it could increase the risk of food insecurity among the vulnerable groups within the community. Besides, unfavorable rainfall patterns and temperature were reported to lead to the decline in the availability of wild food that is needed by many families in the midst of food shortage.

There are several limitations to this study. The villages selected for this study were located where researchers could easily travel to by normal car. This indicated that the village location was connected to the nearby town by several roads. For this reason, the informants did not only depend on traditional food systems for food-seeking and gaining access to food markets. Therefore, one of the recommendations is that the OA from both remote and suburban villages should be involved in similar future studies. The other limitation of this research could be seen from the participants who were limited to female informants. In contrast, the involvement of male informants may improve the information obtained in a study through different question sets being used for male and female informants [20]. To be specific, the questions for male informants could focus on the socioeconomic activities of the households, while the questions for female informants could focus on the dietary patterns of the household members. Another limitation of this study was the use of a translation service, which might affect the validity of information obtained from the informants. In this case, translators might unintentionally provide unnecessary hints to the informants at some point in the interview. In order to prevent such biases from occurring, translators should be properly trained prior to data collection, and they need to always be reminded to not provide additional explanation to the informants.

5. Conclusions

In conclusion, the OA generally rely on the knowledge they inherit from their ancestors regarding nature for their survival. The traditional food systems are essential for the OA to obtain food for the daily consumption of the household members. However, due to the negative effects in the midst of urbanization, the availability of food in the natural environment to support their livelihood has been reduced. As a result, the OA have shifted to modern food systems, where food is purchased from the markets to fulfill their needs. According to the recent trend, the deterioration of the traditional food systems is due to five factors, which include the failure in agriculture, the ineffectiveness of traditional food-seeking methods, water issues, and weather. These are the important findings which have distinguished the contexts of the OA's household food insecurity from the contexts of the general population. Moreover, the findings of this study have proven that household food insecurity among the OA is an existing phenomenon, and a clear picture of the issue has been provided to demonstrate the unfortunate situation faced by this community. With this, it is recommended that local authorities and non-governmental organizations take this issue seriously due to the hazardous impacts it can bring to the health of its victims. Through a proper understanding of the household food insecurity among the OA, drastic measures could be taken by the responsible authorities in order to relieve the OA from this problem.

Author Contributions: Conceptualization, L.S.L., S.N., W.Y.G., A.S.N., and M.T.M.N.; Methodology, L.S.L., S.N., W.Y.G., A.S.N., and M.T.M.N.; Formal Analysis, L.S.L.; Investigation, L.S.L.; Data Curation, L.S.L.; Writing-Original Draft Preparation, L.S.L.; Writing-Review and Editing, S.N., W.Y.G., A.S.N., and M.T.M.N.; Visualization, L.S.L. and S.N.; Supervision, S.N., W.Y.G., A.S.N., and M.T.M.N.

Funding: This research received no external funding.

Acknowledgments: We appreciate the cooperation and advice provided by the staff of the Department of Orang Asli Development. Gratitude is also expressed to Tok Batin and the informants for their willingness to provide useful information.

Conflicts of Interest: The authors of this article declare that there has been no conflict of interest in this study.

References

1. RTI International. *Current and Prospective Scope of Hunger and Food Security in America: A Review of Current Research*; Center for Health and Environment Modeling: Chapel Hill, NC, USA, 2014; Available online: https://www.rti.org/sites/default/files/resources/full_hunger_report_final_07-24-14.pdf (accessed on 22 December 2017).
2. Willows, N.D.; Veugelers, P.; Raine, K.; Kuhle, S. Prevalence and sociodemographic risk factors related to household food security in Aboriginal peoples in Canada. *Public Health Nutr.* **2008**, *12*, 1150–1156. [CrossRef] [PubMed]
3. Australian Institute of Health and Welfare (AIHW). *Aboriginal and Torres Strait Islander Health Performance, 2010 Report: Detailed Analyses*; AIHW: Canberra, Australia, 2011. Available online: https://www.aihw.gov.au/reports/indigenous-australians/indigenous-health-performance-framework-2010/contents/table-of-contents (accessed 28 February 2018).
4. Zalilah, M.S.; Tham, B.L. Food security and child nutritional status among orang asli (Temuan) households in Hulu Langat, Selangor. *Med. J. Malays.* **2002**, *57*, 36–50.
5. Nurfahilin, T.; Norhasmah, S. Factors and coping strategies related to food insecurity and nutritional status among Orang Asli women in Malaysia. *Int. J. Public Health Clin. Sci.* **2015**, *2*, 55–66.
6. Chong, S.P.; Geetah, A.; Norhasmah, S. Household food insecurity, diet quality, and weight status among indigenous women (Mah Meri) in Peninsular Malaysia. *Nutr. Res. Pract.* **2018**, *12*, 135–142. [CrossRef]
7. Haemamalar, K.; Zalilah, M.S.; Neng Azhanie, A. Nutritional status of Orang Asli (Che Wang Tribe) Adults in Krau Wildlife Reserve, Pahang. *Malays. J. Nutr.* **2010**, *16*, 55–68. [PubMed]
8. Chua, E.; Zalilah, M.; Chin, Y.; Norhasmah, S. Dietary diversity is associated with nutritional status of Orang Asli children in Krau Wildlife Reserve, Pahang. *Malays J. Nutr.* **2012**, *18*, 1–13.
9. Kuhnlein, H.V.; Smitasiri, S.; Yesudas, S.; Bhattacharjee, L.; Li, D.; Ahmed, S. *Documenting Traditional Food Systems of Indigenous Peoples: International Case Studies. Guidelines for Procedures*; Centre for Indigenous Peoples' Nutrition and Environment: Anne de Bellevue, QC, Canada, 2006; Available online: https://www.mcgill.ca/cine/files/cine/manual.pdf (accessed on 23 December 2017).
10. Kardooni, R.; Fatimah, K.; Siti Rohani, Y.; Siti Hajar, Y. Traditional knowledge of orang asli on forests in Peninsular Malaysia. *Indian J. Tradit. Knowl.* **2014**, *13*, 283–291.
11. Kuhnlein, H.V.; Receveur, O. Dietary change and traditional food systems of indigenous peoples. *Annu. Rev. Nutr.* **1996**, *16*, 417–442. [CrossRef] [PubMed]
12. Capone, R.; Bilali, H.E.; Debs, P.; Cardone, G.; Driouech, N. Food system sustainability and food security: Connecting the dots. *J. Food Secur.* **2014**, *2*, 13–22.
13. Food and Agriculture Organization (FAO). SAVE FOOD: Global Initiative on Food Loss and Waste Reduction. Available online: http://www.fao.org/save-food/resources/keyfindings/en/ (accessed 12 September 2018).
14. Food and Agriculture Association (FAO). *Food Security*; Development Economic Division, FAO: Rome, Italy, 2006; Available online: http://www.fao.org/fileadmin/templates/faoitaly/documents/pdf/pdf_Food_Security_Cocept_Note.pdf (accessed 15 August 2017).
15. Department of Orang Asli Development (JAKOA). Data Banci Orang Asli. 2010; unpublished.
16. Yin, R.K. *Case Study Research. Design and Methods*; SAGE Publications: Thousand Oaks, CA, USA, 1994; ISBN 978-1-48332-224-7.
17. Department of Statistics Malaysia. *Population and Housing Census of Malaysia 2000*; Monograph Series No. 3; Orang Asli in Peninsular Malaysia, Department of Statistics: Putrajaya, Malaysia, 2008.
18. Economic Planning Unit (EPU). Perangkaan pendapatan dan kemiskinan isi rumah sepintas lalu. Available online: http://www.epu.gov.my/documents/10124/597ec4c8-2962-40de-9049-0f41d280b915 (accessed on 4 April 2016).
19. Morse, J.M. The Significance of Saturation. *Qual. Health Res.* **1995**, *5*, 147–149. [CrossRef]

20. Frongillo, E.A.; Nanama, S.; Wolfe, W.S. *Technique Guide to Developing a Direct, Experience-Based Measurement Tool for Household Food Insecurity*; Food and Nutrition Technical Assistance, Academy for Educational Development: Washington, DC, USA, 2004.
21. Guion, L.A.; Diehl, D.C.; McDonald, D. *Triangulation: Establishing the Validity of Qualitative Studies*; Department of Family, Youth and Community Sciences, Florida Cooperative Extension Service, Institute of Food and Agricultural Sciences, University of Florida: Gainesville, FL, USA, 2011; Available online: http://edis.ifas.ufl.edu/fy394 (accessed on 26 May 2014).
22. Braun, V.; Clarke, V. Using thematic analysis in psychology. *Qual. Res. Psychol.* **2006**, *3*, 77–101. [CrossRef]
23. Riessman, C.K. *Narrative Analysis*; SAGE Publications: Thousand Oaks, CA, USA, 1993; ISBN 978-0-80394-754-2.
24. Satari, S.Z.; Zubairi, Y.Z.; Hussin, A.G.; Hassan, S.F. Some statistical characteristic of Malaysian wind direction recorded at maximum wind speed: 1999–2008. *Sains Malays.* **2015**, *44*, 1521–1530. [CrossRef]
25. Knuth, L. *The Right to Adequate Food and Indigenous Peoples. How Can the Right to Food Benefit Indigenous Peoples*; Food and Agriculture Organization (FAO): Rome, Italy, 2009.
26. Martens, T.M.; Cidro, J.; Hart, M.A.; McLachlan, S. Understanding indigenous food sovereignty through an indigenous research paradigm. *J. Indig. Soc. Dev.* **2016**, *5*, 18–37.
27. Zakari, S.; Ying, L.; Song, B. Factors influencing household food security in West Africa: The case of southern Niger. *Sustainability* **2014**, *6*, 1191–1202. [CrossRef]
28. Gomes, A.G. Indigenous Peoples' Movements: The Orang Asli of Malaysia. Available online: https://iias.asia/sites/default/files/IIAS_NL35_10.pdf (accessed on 4 July 2018).
29. Food and Agriculture Organization (FAO). *Special Event on Impact of Climate Change, Pests and Diseases on Food Security and Poverty Reduction. 31st Session of the Committee on World Food Security*; FAO: Rome, Italy, 2003; Available online: http://www.fsnnetwork.org/sites/default/files/impact_of_climate_change_pests_and_diseases_on_food_security_and_poverty_reduction_-_background_document.pdf (accessed on 23 November 2017).
30. Kirimi, L.; Gitau, R.; Olunga, M. Household Food Security and Commercialization among Smallholder Farmers in Kenya. In Proceedings of the 2013 African Association of Agricultural Economists (AAAE) Fourth International Conference, Hammamet, Tunisia, 22–25 September 2013.
31. Hansen, M.C.; Potapov, P.V.; Moore, R.; Hancher, M.; Turubanova, S.A.; Tyukavina, A.; Thau, D.; Stehman, S.V.; Goetz, S.J.; Loveland, T.R.; et al. High-resolution global maps of 21st-century forest cover change. *Science* **2013**, *342*, 850–853. [CrossRef] [PubMed]
32. Schuster, R.C.; Wein, E.E.; Dickson, C.; Chan, H.M. Importance of traditional foods for the food security of two First Nations communities in the Yukon, Canada. *Int. J. Circumpolar Health* **2011**, *70*, 286–300. [CrossRef] [PubMed]
33. Egeland, G.M.; Charbonneau-Roberts, G.; kuluguqtuq, J.; Kilabuk, J.; Okalik, L.; Soueida, R.; Kuhnlein, H.V. Back to the future: Using traditional food and knowledge to promote a healthy future among Inuit. In *Indigenous People's Food Systems: The Many Dimensions of Culture, Diversity, and Environment for Nutrition and Health*; Kuhnlein, H.V., Erasmus, B., Spigelski, D., Eds.; FAO: Rome, Italy, 2009; pp. 9–22. ISBN 978-92-5106071-1.
34. Carol Yong; Sarawakians Access; Peninsular Malaysia Orang Asli Village Network. *Deforestation Drivers and Human Rights in Malaysia*; Forest Peoples Programme: Moreton-in-March, UK, 2014; Available online: https://rightsanddeforestation.org/wp-content/uploads/2018/02/Malaysia-deforestation-drivers-and-human-rights.pdf (accessed on 31 July 2018).
35. Endicott, K. *Malaysia's Original People. Past, Present and Future of the Orang Asli*; National University of Singapore Press: Singapore, 2016; ISBN 978-9971-69-861-4.
36. Halder, J.N.; Nazrul Islam, M. Water pollution and its impact on the human health. *J. Environ. Hum.* **2015**, *2*, 36–46. [CrossRef]
37. Tangang, F.T.; Liew, J.N.; Salimun, E.; Kwan, M.S.; Loh, J.L.; Mohumad, H. Climate change and variability over Malaysia: Gaps in science and research information. *Sains Malays.* **2012**, *41*, 1355–1366.
38. Bahiigwa, G.B.A. Household food insecurity in Uganda: An empirical analysis. *East. Afr. J. Rural Dev.* **2002**, *18*, 8–23. [CrossRef]

39. Niles, M.T.; Salermo, J.D. A cross-country analysis of climate shocks and smallholder food insecurity. *PLoS ONE* **2018**, *13*, e0192928. [CrossRef] [PubMed]
40. Food and Agriculture Organization (FAO). *Climate Change and Food Security: A Framework Document*; FAO: Rome, Italy, 2008; Available online: http://www.fao.org/forestry/15538-079b31d45081fe9c3dbc6ff34de4807e4.pdf (accessed on 23 December 2017).

nutrients

MDPI

Article

Strategies to Address the Complex Challenge of Improving Regional and Remote Children's Fruit and Vegetable Consumption

Stephanie L. Godrich [1,*], Christina R. Davies [2], Jill Darby [1] and Amanda Devine [1]

1 School of Medical and Health Sciences, Edith Cowan University, 270 Joondalup Drive, Joondalup, Perth 6027, Australia; j.darby@ecu.edu.au (J.D.); a.devine@ecu.edu.au (A.D.)
2 School of Population Health, University of Western Australia, Crawley 6009, Australia; christina.davies@uwa.edu.au
* Correspondence: s.godrich@ecu.edu.au; Tel.: +61-863-042-032

Received: 13 September 2018; Accepted: 24 October 2018; Published: 1 November 2018

Abstract: Fruit and vegetables (F&V) are imperative for good health, yet less than one per cent of Australian children consume these food groups in sufficient quantities. As guided by Social Cognitive Theory (SCT), this paper aimed to: (i) understand key informant perspectives of the amount, types and quality of F&V consumed by rural and remote Western Australian (WA) children; and, (ii) determine strategies that could increase F&V consumption among rural and remote WA children. This qualitative study included 20 semi-structured interviews with health, school/youth and food supply workers, focusing on topics including: quantity and type of F&V consumed and strategies to increase children's consumption. A thematic analysis was conducted using NVivo qualitative data analysis software (Version 10, 2014. QSR International Pty Ltd., Doncaster, Victoria, Australia). Key informants reported children consumed energy-dense nutrient-poor foods in place of F&V. Strategy themes included: using relevant motivators for children to increase their preference for F&V (i.e., gaming approach, SCT construct of 'expectations'); empowering community-driven initiatives (i.e., kitchen gardens, SCT construct of 'environment'); increasing food literacy across settings (i.e., food literacy skills, SCT construct of 'behavioural capacity'); developing salient messages and cooking tips that resonate with parents (i.e., parent newsletters, SCT construct of 'self-control'); increasing F&V availability, safety, and convenience (i.e., school provision); and, considering the impact of role models that extend beyond the family (i.e., relatable role models, SCT construct of 'observational learning'). Overall, a comprehensive strategy that incorporates relevant motivators for children and families, supports local initiatives, reinforces the range of role models that are involved with children and creates healthier environments, is required to increase F&V consumption among children.

Keywords: fruit and vegetables; rural children; Social Cognitive Theory

1. Introduction

Fruit and vegetables (F&V) are essential to good health, containing a vast array of indispensable nutrients and bioactive compounds, such as vitamins, minerals, electrolytes, dietary fibre, protein, and phytochemicals [1]. F&V are known for their high concentrations of specific phytochemical or 'non nutrient' properties, such as carotenoids [2], flavonoids [3,4], phytoestrogens [3], and terpenes. In addition, F&V have a relatively low energy density and a high water concentration [5].

F&V provide a myriad of health benefits, including a reduced risk of non-communicable diseases [6]. Such diseases include cancer through hormone-inhibiting roles [7,8], Type II diabetes [9], and a probable link with reduction in obesity [2,7,9]. Vegetables have been shown to have a cardio protective effect, reducing the risk of cardiovascular disease and stroke [10], namely due to containing a plethora of antioxidant compounds that repair cell damage due to oxidation [3]. The role of nitrates in vascular tone and integrity have also been recently reported [11–14]. Further, F&V have been recently shown to reduce risk of falls and fractures that are related to superior muscular strength (grip strength) and physical function in those with higher intakes and a more diverse range of vegetable intake [15]. Moreover, the benefits of vegetables on bone health include the action of nutrients, such as vitamin K, magnesium, phytoestrogens, and other active compounds on improved bone metabolism [16,17]. Given the wide-ranging health benefits that are provided by F&V, adequate consumption in childhood is critically important. This is especially important, given child eating habits track into adulthood [5].

Despite these health benefits and evidence associating poor childhood intake of F&V with subsequent low adult consumption [18], many Australian children are consuming insufficient F&V [19]. In Australia, "sufficient" consumption of F&V is two serves of fruit (i.e., two medium pieces) and five serves of vegetables for children aged 9–11 years and females aged 12–13 years [20], where one serve is equivalent to one cup of salad or half a cup of cooked vegetables [20,21]. For boys aged 12–13 years, the recommended vegetable intake is 5.5 serves [20].

National data estimates that less than one per cent of Australian children aged 9–13 years are consuming vegetables in sufficient quantities for good health [22]. A higher proportion of Australian children reportedly met fruit guidelines, with 45% of 9–11 year olds and 34% of 12–13 year old children achieving the recommended fruit serves per day [22]. Consumption of F&V is higher across Western Australia (WA), with statewide surveillance data reporting 8.8% of children met vegetable guidelines and 64% met fruit guidelines [23]. Recent research that was conducted specifically in rural and remote WA reported a slightly higher proportion of children met guidelines, with 65.8% meeting fruit and 15.4% meeting vegetable guidelines, respectively. While in rural Victoria, 97% of children aged 6–12 years consumed adequate fruit and 12% consumed adequate vegetables [24]. To date, comprehensive data outlining the difference in F&V consumption between urban, rural, and remote children is lacking, due to limitations that are associated with availability of data at a local level [25].

With respect to the classification of rural and remote Australia, the Australian Statistical Geography Standard Remoteness Structure classifies locations in relation to their access to services [26]. Covering one-third of Australia's land mass, WA spans a vast 2.5 million square kilometres [27], with much of this state being classified as remote.

National data has demonstrated that people living in remote locations are more likely to be overweight or obese than their urban counterparts, with reduced health service provision purported to be a contributing factor [25]. A number of barriers to F&V consumption have been postulated, including price, promotion, low availability, poor quality, location of outlets, and taste preferences [28]. These are particularly magnified in rural and remote communities where food availability and access issues are heightened, such as through transport disruptions [29,30]. As poor diet, such as low consumption of F&V, is a contributing factor towards overweight and obesity [6], and given the aforementioned barriers to F&V consumption in rural and remote locations, the consumption levels could be estimated to be lower in rural and remote areas.

To overcome barriers to F&V consumption among children, a number of strategies have been proposed internationally and nationally, such as a settings approach where core foods are provided or nutrition education delivered in early years and school settings [5,28]. School-based interventions have achieved moderate increases in children's intake of F&V [18]. To increase impact, suggested approaches have included extending school-based activities to the home environment, whereby parents are engaged through activities delivered by teachers and health professionals [31,32]. To increase relevance for child audiences, a focus on fun has been recommended as more salient [31] and it should be a key strategy adopted in initiatives. Incentives and rewards should also be incorporated [5], with children provided the freedom to make personal food choices [31]. In addition, goal setting, role playing, and critical thinking are advocated for [5]. Overall, longer-term, higher intensity interventions with multiple strategies have been demonstrated to be most effective in increasing children's F&V consumption [18,33].

However, there is limited evidence for successful strategies that specifically target rural and remote populations. Gaps in the literature include an understanding of high-risk and disadvantaged groups' needs, such as those living in rural and remote areas [34]. Recent research [35] has highlighted the differences in healthy food availability, access and use in rural and remote locations, and the associated impact on children's F&V consumption [33]. Therefore, these differences must be front and centre when developing strategies to increase consumption among rural and remote children.

One framework that provides a useful context in which to situate strategies to increase F&V consumption is the Social Cognitive Theory (SCT) [36]. The SCT comprises nine constructs and considers the impact of personal factors, such as food preferences, expectations of consuming particular foods, knowledge, and self-efficacy on a behavior, such as F&V consumption. In addition, the impact of environmental factors, such as availability, accessibility, parents, peers, and the media, on the behavior, are also considered [5]. Previous research has argued this theory is ideal for the examination of the impact of interventions on children's F&V intake [5].

Given there are a number of gaps in the current evidence base relating to the increased support required for rural and remote children to consume adequate F&V, this study aimed to extend existing literature to understand potential strategies to increase rural and remote children's F&V consumption. The objectives of this study were to: (i) understand key informant perspectives of the amount, types, and quality of F&V consumed by rural and remote WA children; and; (ii) determine strategies that could increase F&V consumption among rural and remote WA children, using a SCT focus.

2. Materials and Methods

2.1. Design and Sampling

The study methodology is reported elsewhere [30]; a summary is provided below. 'Key informants' were the selected participant group for this qualitative exploratory research study. These worker types included health workers (e.g., nutritionists, dietitians, health promotion officers), school/youth workers (e.g., school principals, youth, and family workers who worked with both primary school age children—junior, previously years 1–7 and currently years 1–6 in Western Australia, and secondary school age children—senior, previously years 8–12 and currently years 7–12) [28]. Food supply workers (e.g., included store managers and farmers' market managers). These key informants were involved with children's F&V consumption, such as through a breakfast or after school feeding program, delivery of health promotion programs, or owned/managed a food outlet where children and/or their parents shopped. A database was developed using contact details from professional networks (health and school/youth workers) and Google searches using the keywords "supermarket" and the town name (food supply workers).

WA is categorised by the state government into nine regions (i.e., Peel, South West, Great Southern, Wheatbelt, Goldfields-Esperance, Mid West, Gascoyne, Pilbara, Kimberley regions) [37]. It is also classified into degrees of remoteness, according to the Australian Statistical Geography Standard Remoteness Areas [26]. Key informant recruitment was conducted to ensure diversity across WA regions, degrees of remoteness, and worker type, through the development of a spreadsheet with these criteria. A total of eight out of the nine WA regions invited were represented in this study. Where possible, sampling in this study was closely representative of the population density across WA regions [37] and degrees of remoteness. Key informant locations also ranged in Socio-Economic Index for Areas Index of Relative Socio-Economic Disadvantage decile [30,38] to ensure that areas of varying socio-economic disadvantage were included.

2.2. Data Collection

Thirty potential interviewees were invited to participate in this study and were provided with an information letter and consent form. Twenty respondents provided written consent (67% response rate) and took part in a semi-structured interview, conducted either by telephone ($n = 16$) or face-to-face ($n = 4$). The interview guide was compiled by the research team and contained questions related to quantity and type of F&V consumed (i.e., "What are your thoughts around the amount of F&V kids are eating in the areas you live/work in?"); barriers to and enablers of F&V consumption among children (i.e., "What types of things make it hard for children to eat F&V in the areas you live/work in?"); motivators of intake (i.e., "What do you think are the biggest motivators for F&V consumption among WA kids?"); and, strategies (existing or proposed) to increase children's consumption (i.e., "What successful strategies have you seen, where you work?").

One pilot interview was conducted, with minor changes made before use in the wider study.

2.3. Data Analysis

Key informant interviews were transcribed verbatim and imported into QSR Nvivo 10 (NVivo qualitative data analysis Software; Version 10, 2014. QSR International Pty Ltd., Doncaster, Victoria, Australia) A thematic analysis was conducted using techniques, such as template analysis and parallel coding [39]. In addition, word clouds and matrix-coding queries provided further insight into themes determined. Inductive, data-driven codes were created as new themes were identified. Three team members verified coding of statements by co-listening to audio recordings and cross-checking the NVivo coding. Documents including a research journal and summary of work conducted outlined codes created with exemplar quotes, key themes, and other analyses undertaken in NVivo. Saturation was confirmed at 20 interviews when the team confirmed that there were no new themes or concepts that had been identified [30,40].

2.4. Ethical Approvals

All of the subjects gave their informed consent for inclusion before they participated in the study. The study was conducted in accordance with the Declaration of Helsinki. Ethics was obtained from the Edith Cowan University Human Research Ethics Committee.

3. Results

3.1. Demographics

Interviewee demographics included 16 females and four males; 12 key informants reported on regional WA, while eight reported on remote WA. A total of eight respondents were health workers (i.e., dietitian, nutritionist, health promotion officer), six were school and/or youth workers (i.e., school principal), and six were food supply workers (i.e., farmers' market manager). Key informant demographics have been tabulated in a previous publication [30]. The results below have been grouped into suggested strategies (existing or proposed) to increase children's F&V consumption. Exemplar quotes for each strategy have been included (Table 1).

3.2. Perceptions of Consumption

Key informant perspectives with respect to the quantities of F&V consumed by children included comments such as "not enough" (Food Supply Worker, Female, Regional), "low compared to the amount of 'extras' that are consumed" (Health Worker, Female, Regional), "without the schools, that would be much more of an issue" (Health Worker, Male, Remote) and "Relatively lower than what is recommended" (Health Worker, Female. Regional). Among the 16 coded statements about F&V quantities consumed, some informants reported observing parents and children buying energy dense nutrient-poor foods, such as pies and sausage rolls, or high-carbohydrate filling foods, as opposed to F&V. A view shared by a number of participants was that adequate fruit consumption was more common than adequate vegetable consumption, which key informants perceived as being poor amongst most children. In particular, children's lunchboxes were seen to be more fruit-focused, with children "going to school without any vegetables in their lunchboxes at all" (Health Worker, Female, Regional). Perceptions of F&V types that were consumed included that they were dependent on the availability within a food outlet. Other perspectives were that school canteens were providing locally-produced F&V and that school based activities supported and promoted access to them.

Table 1. Exemplar quotes for strategies to increase children's fruit and vegetable intake.

Strategy	Exemplar Quote
Strategy One: Use relevant motivators for children to increase their preference for fruit and vegetables	*"That's a motivator—"You look good, strong, fit, you look great". How do you sustain that? For young women too. Playing on that strength, that useful, you're really concerned about your appearance, playing on that strength in a positive way is a good motivator. It's the first time I've really seen teenage boys engage, when it's talking about them and their appearance"* (Health Worker)
Strategy Two: Empower local community-driven initiatives	*"Involving local people in the creation of local resources rather than depending on outside resources for health promotion"* (School and Youth Worker)
Strategy Three: Increase food literacy education across a range of settings	*"There is the occasional dietitian doing a talk for a mothers group and that sort of thing. No sort of big focus on that audience. More of a focus once kids get to school or once a child is obese and comes to see a clinician. I think prevention would be best sort of in a way, treatment for obesity in that, before a kid gets to that point"* (Health Worker)
Strategy Four: Develop salient key messages and cooking tips that resonate with parents	*"In some cases, I've suggested or parents have said to use the star charts, to try new things basically so they would get a star just trying something new"* (Health Worker)
Strategy Five: Increase fruit and vegetable availability, safety and convenience	*"Pre-packed salads, little salads, I also did something myself trying to increase the availability of snack packs through fruit and veg, I cut up capsicum, carrots and celery and put that in a little container. Again for somebody who wanted a little snack pack, it's easy, it's there, done, it's all prepared for you but it's just like having a bag of chips, it gives you the option"* (Food Supply Worker)
Strategy Six: Consider the impact of role models that extend beyond the family	*"The youth workers organised last year to have one of the big Western football teams Skype into all of the kids at the school... significant people being involved in people's lives here makes a huge difference"* (School and Youth Worker)

3.3. Strategies to Increase Consumption

3.3.1. Strategy One: Use Relevant Motivators for Children to Increase Their Preference for Fruit and Vegetables

Based on their experiences and perceptions, Food Supply and Health Workers indicated that focusing messaging on the impact of healthy eating on sporting performance might be an effective strategy to encourage children to consume more F&V. The perspectives of School/Youth Workers focused on education about healthy food choices using a strengths-based approach, i.e., "I certainly think it makes a massive difference if they have had education around healthy choices at some stage" (School/Youth Worker, Female, Regional).

Many children were believed to understand that eating F&V kept them healthy, however, messages needed to extend beyond this due to the lack of consideration many children placed on long-term health implications that are associated with suboptimal consumption. Utilising a different perspective, such as reinforcing the benefits of being strong, fit and promoting a healthy body image, was an important consideration when promoting healthy eating. This was thought to be especially effective among teenage boys, where the strengths-based focus was on being fit. Insights included the importance of reinforcing fun, creative and experiential learning around the growing and preparation of healthy food to positively influence children's attitude to F&V. According to interviewees, children and young people sought independent food choice, and thus focusing on encouraging choice of healthy foods was important. One informant discussed their approach, which focused on promoting the enjoyment of tasting fresh F&V. This was also suggested to be done in settings, such as community garden plots. Further, promoting F&V in other settings, such as through family-friendly arts events, was another avenue for promotion. Other strategies included presenting information about the negative health consequences of low F&V consumption in movies compiled in an entertaining way.

3.3.2. Strategy Two: Empower Local Community-Driven Initiatives

Key informants discussed the importance of local community spaces and activities that promoted F&V consumption, particularly for rural and remote populations. These included community gardens, communal cooking facilities, and sporting events. Further, participants in this study reported the creation and display of healthy eating posters in food outlets and community cookbooks were successful in increasing F&V consumption. Health service providers were encouraged to support existing or the start-up of local initiatives, which had a more significant and longer lasting impact. For example, local community gardens or kitchens, which could also be used to upskill participants in short courses, such as food hygiene. In addition, practitioners embraced groups' evolving interests in healthy eating skills, such as a group formed initially to focus on exercise, evolved to focus on food label reading. Key informants emphasized the importance of a place-based approach with respect to supporting local preferences and needs, as well as showcasing local role models who were often better placed to upskill fellow community members, rather than relying on service delivery or resource creation from 'outsiders', i.e., "In terms of the women making healthy eating posters ... I just think local stuff has a huge impact as people are obviously learning through the making of the stuff as well as with the sharing" (School/Youth Worker, Female, Remote).

3.3.3. Strategy Three: Increase Food Literacy Education across Settings

A number of key informants were concerned that inequitable health education and support services resulted in certain life stages being disadvantaged. For example, the early years sector, an area that is cited as a critical life stage in which lifelong healthy habits could be initiated, and subsequently consolidated upon entry into the school setting. A number of stakeholders believed that school education could be the catalyst for health-promoting behaviours across the lifespan, i.e., "You don't always have a break through but sometimes you have a spark that goes and they will keep that with them for the rest of their lives" (Food Supply Worker, Female, Regional). The application of knowledge gained through curriculum activities was reportedly supported through experiential programs combining food production and preparation, with produce tasting a critical element. One stakeholder reiterated the importance of F&V provision through the school setting, such as through morning recess. Two stakeholders recounted the success of 'meet the farmer' or farm visits that had been held with the local school children. This approach to education reportedly increased awareness of the food system.

3.3.4. Strategy Four: Develop Salient Key Messages and Cooking Tips That Resonate with Parents

Practical strategies for parents to incorporate F&V into their family's diet were suggested, including disguising these foods into meals and snacks, i.e., "Making kebabs out of fruits, using the dips, putting pureed vegetables into things, like bolognaise sauces. Making rissoles with grated vegetables so they can disguise them to a degree" (Health Worker, Female, Regional). Other strategies included the provision of easily accessible produce, such as having chopped F&V within easy reach on the kitchen bench when children were hungry. Another informant suggested allowing the child to choose a novel fruit or vegetable each week, and making a new, in-season fruit the 'treat'. Exposure to new preparation methods and recipes through family, friends, local stores or the school environment was also recommended.

3.3.5. Strategy Five: Increase Fruit and Vegetable Availability, Safety and Convenience

One informant recommended interactive strategies, such as consumer engagement through food tastings in-store, or pairing recipes next to ingredients that could be used to make the meal. One participant reflected on her own practice to support healthy eating in her store, through the preparation of F&V snack trays. Others believed that offering mid-week farmers' markets or increasing the percentage of F&V within takeaway outlets would improve food availability in rural areas. i.e., "Get the fast takeaways with a greater percentage of vegetables and fruit in there and it may become more popular" (School/Youth Worker, Female, Remote). Another informant criticized the significant proportion of high quality produce that is exported to other countries, and commented that Australia should be prioritising the best quality F&V for local outlets instead. A number of informants underscored the importance of schools providing nutritious food to children, particularly with an emphasis on F&V.

3.3.6. Strategy Six: Consider the Impact of Role Models that Extend Beyond the Family

Key informants discussed the importance of role models outside of the family unit. For example, family friends who may have prepared meals using unfamiliar F&V, cooking methods, or food preparation skills, i.e., "being introduced to foods you might not have at home, just in different ways" (Health Worker, Female, Regional). This approach was suggested to improve their amenability to tasting less familiar foods. Elite athletes were admired in rural and remote areas, with their influence apparent when they participated in school communication projects.

4. Discussion

The objectives of this research were to understand key informant perspectives of amounts, types and the quality of F&V consumed by children; perceived motivating factors for consumption; and, effective strategies for increasing children's F&V consumption. Key findings included increasing children's preference for F&V through the utilisation of strategies using relevant motivators, empowering local community-driven initiatives, increasing food literacy in early childhood and school settings, developing salient messages for parents, increasing availability, safety, and convenience of F&V in outlets, and considering the impact of role models that extend beyond the family.

Key informants in this study reflected on their experiences that were associated with children's F&V consumption. These included that fruit consumption was higher than vegetable consumption and substantially and positively influenced by the school environment. This was previously reported in a study conducted in rural and remote WA where schools were thought to facilitate consumption through breakfast or lunch programs [28]. Previous research has also reported F&V in food outlets is inconsistent in regards to availability, quality, and promotion [30].

This study highlighted the importance of using relevant motivators to increase children's food preference for F&V. Interviewees (health, school/youth, and food supply workers) reflected on their own successful experiences where they had utilised more personalized strategies to increase F&V consumption. Examples included reinforcing the benefits of being strong, fit, and promoting a healthy body image. The use of fun, creative, and experiential learning was found to positively influence children's attitude to F&V. This supports our previous work that found attitude was a key driver of F&V consumption among WA children [28]. In their study of children in rural New Zealand, Dresler et al. recommended child-focused F&V campaigns should utilize the compelling techniques that are used by large companies to emphasise fun, energy, and colour of the produce [41]. In addition, cartoons depicting characters choosing healthy food have demonstrated a shift in children's food choices to healthier options [42]. An after-school nutrition intervention that was underpinned by the SCT with the aim of improved dietary self-efficacy, included activities focusing on exposure to healthy food, taste testing, and the link between diet and physical activity [43]. Younger children (aged 5–10 years) demonstrated a significant improvement in dietary self-efficacy because of the intervention [43]. However, the intervention had no effect on older children and adolescents [43]. Family-friendly arts events were suggested in this study as an avenue for message delivery. WA evidence corroborated this suggestion, with a significant association between nutrition messages and arts engagement being found [44].

Empowerment of local community-driven initiatives was a key theme in the current study. The focus on local community spaces promoting F&V consumption, such as community gardens, communal cooking facilities, and sporting events, were reportedly highly successful vehicles for promoting consumption of these food groups, based on key informant perceptions and experiences. Further, the creation of health promotion posters displayed in food outlets and cookbooks were reported upon favourably, with particular value being placed on the development of these initiatives by people within the community. Locally developed initiatives reportedly had a more significant and longer lasting impact than those "brought in" by outside service providers. This is of particular importance in rural areas, where service providers sometimes facilitate unsustainable programs that do not consider the local context [28]. Interest in the notion of 'co design' has increased in recent years, with benefits of collaborative design of projects reportedly including more meaningful service provision and increased consumer satisfaction [45]. Community support, such as through the provision of community knowledge and local leadership, is central to successful public health nutrition interventions. Community organisation and action can ensure communities being about health changes that they identify as priorities [46]. Extending this further, the development of social capital by initiatives is a vital success factor; those initiatives that facilitate collective social capital increase community competence in addressing issues [47,48], and ultimately, improve their health [46].

Increasing food literacy across key settings such as early years settings, schools, and workplaces emerged as an important theme in this research. Some informants commented that inadequate service provision resulted in certain life stages missing out on food literacy education. Curriculum activities which focused on experiential learning through food production, preparation and tasting were celebrated. Farm visits were also well-regarded as a powerful educational experience, and they are a unique vehicle for education in rural areas where there is a closer connection to food producers [28]. Food literacy education can increase children's understanding of how to choose healthy foods, not only for themselves, but their family [49]. In the early years sector, a recent umbrella review that examined 12 systematic reviews of 101 studies reported that healthy eating approaches embedded within services improved healthy eating in children aged 2–5 years [32]. The review found the most successful interventions were delivered by nutrition and health experts, targeted both the centre environment and the individual, included a mix of strategies that were addressed through the curricula, food and the physical environment, staff practice and policy, and engagement with parents [32]. Within a school setting, specific strategies have included designated F&V breaks or activities, such as taste testing [33] and using core food groups for curriculum activities instead of discretionary foods [50]. A WA school-based F&V program found that significantly more children brought vegetables to school as a result of targeted curriculum and parent resources [51]. However, many children have been reported to possess limited food literacy skills, including poor awareness of what constitutes healthy food choices and limited preparation skills. School programs should be linked with the curriculum, utilise media [41], and include experiential learning to enhance skills [28]. The development and possession of food skills among children and adolescents translates to favourable health behaviours, and thus, improved dietary quality [52] and has been shown to decrease children's requests for energy dense nutrient poor foods, which contribute to obesity [52]. Further, food literacy among children and adolescents can increase their beliefs regarding the "social value of food, food system issues and relationships between the food system and environmental sustainability" [49].

It is critical that health promotion projects aiming to improve healthy food consumption among children, include salient key messages and cooking tips that resonate with household gatekeepers; parents. Parental nutrition knowledge and cooking skills are essential factors to consider in the investigation of barriers and enablers of children's F&V consumption, such that specific skills in planning, decision-making, purchasing, preparing, and understanding the impact of food on health are required to meet dietary needs [53]. Adults have been suggested to lack important food purchasing and preparation skills, which reduced their children's consumption of F&V [54,55].

Messages to improve food planning, purchasing, and preparation should be clear, specific, and focus on behavior change [56]. Messaging should also focus on increasing F&V in the home environment, with resources such as newsletters utilising increasing parental engagement and understanding [33]. Importantly, messages must consider the rural or remote context in which they are being delivered, such as tailoring messaging about F&V purchasing to reflect availability, cost, and quality considerations [56].

The current research emphasized the importance of increasing fruit and vegetables availability and convenience. Strategies that were recalled by informants included food tastings in-store, or presenting ingredients to comprise a meal in the same location of a store. One store owner prepared F&V snack trays to prompt increased purchasing, while other informants recommended offering mid-week farmers' markets or increasing the percentage of F&V within takeaway outlets as strategies to increase the availability of these core food groups. These findings concur with other research, which has emphasised the importance of changing environments to include more F&V. Recent WA evidence has cited the limited availability of fresh vegetables in rural areas as problematic to support interventions, in comparison to urban environments [35]. Evidence highlighted the success that is associated with increasing provision of a range of vegetables, improving their presentation, changing the order in which they were served or changing their location. These actions resulted in increased selection and consumption of these foods in children [1]. Further, other researchers have demonstrated that provision through settings such as schools can increase consumption of fruit by 0.27 servings per day and combined F&V servings of 0.28 servings per day [57]. The inclusion of salad bars in U.S schools have encouraged increased F&V consumption among children and youth, with particular success being observed in increased fruit consumption. Further, including locally-produced F&V in the salad bar coupled with nutrition education, could be an additional strategy [58]. Moreover, policy-level interventions, such as subsidised vegetables in rural areas, have been requested [35].

The important influence of role models that extend beyond the family was highlighted in this study. Key informants underscored the importance of role models, including family friends and elite athletes. Previous evidence has concurred that role modeling of health-promoting behaviours, such as consuming F&V, has a positive correlation with intake of these foods among children. These results suggest that children are conscious of their parents' participation in these behaviours, which, in turn, have a positive impact on their own behaviour [59]. Previous WA evidence suggests that parents in rural locations may be more likely to support F&V interventions in school settings, which suggests this could be a core area to focus on in future interventions. The same study also found more rural participants recommended resources to increase child and parental knowledge about vegetables, in comparison to urban locations [35]. Recommendations arising from this research support previous evidence, which includes a multi-pronged approach to increase F&V intake among children.

Using relevant motivators that are salient to children align with the 'expectations' construct of the SCT. While skill development and taste testing [5] align with the behavioural capacity element, self-control, such as through role modelling, has been shown to be an effective strategy to increase consumption [5]. This latter activity can be adapted across settings, such as the early years settings and transition into the school years.

Strategies to empower community-based initiatives to focus on the environmental construct of the SCT need to be considered. These include increasing availability of F&V across settings and supporting initiatives like community gardens in locations close to early years services and schools.

When supporting food literacy development across settings, focusing on the behavioural capacity construct of the SCT, a focus could include skill development through the provision of recipes and an educational component. Again, these initiatives are translatable in settings such as childcare, school, food outlets, as well as in the home environment.

Developing salient messages for parents, through a focus of the self-control construct of the SCT, could incorporate cooking tips in local newsletters or developing collaborative cook books with parents [5]. This could also develop self-efficacy, an important element to increase F&V consumption through targeted messaging [5].

Increasing F&V availability, through the environment domain of the SCT, could include strategies such as placing F&V posters up in neighbourhoods [60] or F&V subscription programs in early years and school settings [61].

Recommendations for capitalizing on the power and impact of role models includes using relatable role models, humor, such as through comic books and home-based assignments to be conducted between children and their parents [5].

Strengths of this study included perspectives of a range of key informant types, such as health, school/youth, and food supply workers. In addition, sampling occurred across WA regions, degrees of remoteness, and levels of socio-economic disadvantage. This approach facilitated the inclusion of key informants who represented a range of locations with varying levels of disadvantage, and a range of work disciplines. In addition, this study had a strengths-based focus, and as such captured positive perspectives regarding potentially successful approaches to increasing rural and remote children's F&V intake. Further, the use of the SCT is useful to investigate health behavior constructs and not only considers the impact of personal factors, such as food preferences, on behavior, but also the impact of environmental factors, such as food availability, on the behavior. This study also has some limitations that must be acknowledged. This study included the views of key informants and did not incorporate parent's or children's views, which were captured in another study aspect. Therefore, in relation to potentially effective strategies to increase children's F&V consumption, a lack of child perspectives for the strategies proposed is a clear limitation. In addition, this study did not specifically focus on proposing strategies for increased F&V consumption among particular population groups, such as Culturally and Linguistically Diverse or Aboriginal and Torres Strait Islander people. Further, although attempts were made to ensure every worker type was represented across each region, this was not the case.

5. Conclusions

Overall, a comprehensive range of strategies has been recommended as an effective approach to increase F&V consumption among children [5,61]. Strategy components incorporating curriculum-based education programs, a focus on parental provision in the home environment, and F&V provision in other settings are essential [5,61].

Author Contributions: Conceptualization, S.L.G., C.R.D., J.D. and A.D.; Formal analysis, S.L.G.; Funding acquisition, S.L.G.; Investigation, S.L.G.; Methodology, S.L.G.; Project administration, S.L.G.; Resources, S.L.G.; Supervision, C.R.D., J.D. and A.D.; Writing—original draft, S.L.G.; Writing—review & editing, S.L.G., C.R.D., J.D. and A.D.

Funding: This research was supported by the Western Australian Health Promotion Foundation (Healthway), through research grant 24233.

Acknowledgments: The authors sincerely thank each of the participants involved in this study, and the reviewers of this manuscript.

Conflicts of Interest: Potential perceived conflict of interest: Stephanie L. Godrich is a consultant of Foodbank WA, a food relief organisation that delivers nutrition education and cooking sessions with WA schools and communities.

References

1. Appleton, K.M.; Hemingway, A.; Saulais, L.; Dinnella, C.; Monteleone, E.; Depezay, L.; Morizet, D.; Armando Perez-Cueot, F.J.; Bevan, A.; Hartwell, H. Increasing vegetable intakes: Rationale and systematic review of published interventions. *Eur. J. Nutr.* **2016**, *55*, 869–896. [CrossRef] [PubMed]
2. Slavin, J.; Lloyd, B. Health benefits of fruit and vegetables. *Adv. Nutr.* **2012**, *3*, 506–516. [CrossRef] [PubMed]
3. Brown, J.E. *Nutrition Now*, 5th ed.; Thomson Wadsworth: Belmont, CA, USA, 2008.
4. Panche, A.N.; Diwan, A.D.; Chandra, S.R. Flavonoids: An overview. *J. Nutr. Sci.* **2016**, *5*, 1–15. [CrossRef] [PubMed]
5. Gaines, A.; Turner, L.W. Improving fruit and vegetable intake among children: A review of interventions utilising the social cognitive theory. *Calif. J. Health Promot.* **2009**, *7*, 52–66.
6. World Health Organization. Increasing Fruit and Vegetable Consumption to Reduce the Risk of Noncommunicable Diseases. Available online: http://www.who.int/elena/titles/fruit_vegetables_ncds/en/ (accessed on 25 November 2017).
7. National Health and Medical Research Council. Fruit. Available online: https://www.eatforhealth.gov.au/food-essentials/five-food-groups/fruit (accessed on 21 June 2017).
8. World Cancer Research Fund/American Institute for Cancer Research. Continuous Update Project Expert Report 2018. In *Recommendations and Public Health and Policy Implications*; World Cancer Research Fund/American Institute for Cancer Research: London, UK, 2018.
9. Astrup, A.; Dyerberg, J.; Selleck, M.; Stender, S. Nutrition transition and its relationship to the development of obesity and related chronic diseases. *Obes. Rev.* **2008**, *9*, 48–52.
10. Van Duyn, M.S.; Pivonka, E. Overview of the health benefits of fruit and vegetable consumption for the dietetics professional: Selected literature. *J. Am. Diet Assoc.* **2000**, *100*, 1511–1521. [CrossRef]
11. Blekkenhorst, L.C.; Bondonno, C.P.; Lewis, J.R.; Devine, A.; Woodman, R.J.; Croft, K.D.; Lim, W.H.; Beilin, L.J.; Prince, R.L.; Hodgson, J.M. Association of dietary nitrate with atherosclerotic vascular disease mortality: A prospective cohort study of older adult women. *Am. J. Clin. Nutr.* **2017**, *106*, 207–216. [CrossRef] [PubMed]
12. Blekkenhorst, L.C.; Bondonno, C.P.; Lewis, J.R.; Devine, A.; Zhu, K.; Lim, W.H.; Woodman, R.J.; Beilin, L.J.; Prince, R.L.; Hodgson, J.M. Cruciferous and Allium Vegetable Intakes are Inversely Associated With 15-Year Atherosclerotic Vascular Disease Deaths in Older Adult Women. *J. Am. Heart Assoc.* **2017**, *6*, 1–15. [CrossRef] [PubMed]
13. Bondonno, C.P.; Blekkenhorst, L.C.; Prince, R.L.; Ivey, K.L.; Lewis, J.R.; Devine, A.; Woodman, R.J.; Lundberg, J.O.; Croft, K.D.; Thompson, P.L.; et al. Association of vegetable nitrate intake with carotid atherosclerosis and ischemic cerebrovascular disease in older women. *Stroke* **2017**, *48*, 1724–1729. [CrossRef] [PubMed]
14. Blekkenhorst, L.C.; Sim, M.; Bondonno, C.P.; Bondonno, N.P.; Ward, N.C.; Prince, R.L.; Devine, A.; Lewis, J.R.; Hodgson, J.M. Cardiovascular Health Benefits of Specific Vegetable Types: A Narrative Review. *Nutrients* **2018**, *10*, 595. [CrossRef] [PubMed]
15. Blekkenhorst, L.C.; Hodgson, J.M.; Lewis, J.R.; Devine, A.; Woodman, R.J.; Lim, W.H.; Wong, G.; Zhu, K.; Bondonno, C.P.; Ward, N.C.; et al. Vegetable and fruit intake and fracture-related hospitalisations: A prospective study of older women. *Nutrients* **2017**, *9*, 511. [CrossRef] [PubMed]
16. Lanham-New, S.A. Fruit and vegetables: The unexpected natural answer to the question of osteoporosis prevention? *Am. J. Clin. Nutr.* **2006**, *83*, 1254–1255. [CrossRef] [PubMed]
17. Sim, M.; Blekkenhorst, L.C.; Lewis, J.R.; Bondonno, C.P.; Devine, A.; Zhu, K.; Woodman, R.J.; Prince, R.L.; Hodgson, J.M. Vegetable Diversity, Injurious Falls, and Fracture Risk in Older Women: A Prospective Cohort Study. *Nutrients* **2018**, *10*, 1081. [CrossRef] [PubMed]
18. Evans, C.E.L.; Christian, M.S.; Cleghorn, C.L.; Greenwood, D.C.; Cade, J.E. Systematic review and meta-analysis of school-based interventions to improve daily fruit and vegetable intake in children aged 5 to 12 years. *Am. J. Clin. Nutr.* **2012**, *96*, 889–901. [CrossRef] [PubMed]
19. Australian Bureau of Statistics. Table 17.3. Children's Daily Intake of Fruit and Vegetables and Main Type of Milk Consumed, Proportion of Persons. Available online: http://www.abs.gov.au/AUSSTATS/abs@.nsf/DetailsPage/4364.0.55.0012014-15?OpenDocument (accessed on 25 October 2016).

20. National Health and Medical Research Council. Recommended Number of Serves for Children, Adolescents and Toddlers. Available online: https://www.eatforhealth.gov.au/food-essentials/how-much-do-we-need-each-day/recommended-number-serves-children-adolescents-and (accessed on 24 August 2017).
21. National Health and Medical Research Council. *Healthy Eating for Children*; National Health and Medical Research Council: Canberra, Australia, 2013.
22. Australian Bureau of Statistics. *Australian Health Survey: Consumption of Food Groups from the Australian Dietary Guidelines 2011–12*; Australian Bureau of Statistics: Canberra, Australia, 2016.
23. Tomlin, S.; Radomiljac, A.; Kay, A. *Health and Wellbeing of Children in Western Australia in 2014, Overview and Trends*; Department of Health: Perth, Australia, 2014.
24. Ervin, K.; Nogare, D.; Orr, J.; Soutter, E.; Spiller, R. Fruit and vegetable consumption in rural Victorial school children. *Primary Health Care* **2015**, *5*, 1–6.
25. Australian Institute of Health and Welfare. *Australia's Health 2018*; Australian Institute of Health and Welfare: Canberra, Australia, 2018.
26. Australian Bureau of Statistics. Australian Statistical Geography Standard (ASGS). Available online: http://www.abs.gov.au/websitedbs/d3310114.nsf/home/australian+statistical+geography+standard+(asgs) (accessed on 2 January 2017).
27. Australian Bureau of Statistics. Western Australia at a Glance. 2014. Available online: http://www.abs.gov.au/ausstats/abs@.nsf/mf/1306.5 (accessed on 28 January 2017).
28. Godrich, S.L.; Davies, C.R.; Darby, J.; Devine, A. Which ecological determinants influence Australian children's fruit and vegetable consumption? *Health Promot. Int.* **2016**, 1–10. [CrossRef] [PubMed]
29. Pollard, C.; Landrigan, T.; Ellies, P.; Kerr, D.; Lester, M.; Goodchild, S. Geographic Factors as Determinants of Food Security: A Western Australian Food Pricing and Quality Study. *Asia Pac. J. Clin. Nutr.* **2014**, *23*, 703–713. [PubMed]
30. Godrich, S.L.; Davies, C.R.; Darby, J.; Devine, A. What are the determinants of food security among regional and remote Western Australian children? *Aust. N. Z. J. Public Health* **2017**. [CrossRef] [PubMed]
31. Thomas, J.; Sutcliffe, K.; Harden, A.; Oakley, A.; Oliver, S.; Rees, R.; Brunton, G.; Kavanagh, J. *Children and Healthy Eating: A Systematic Review of Barriers and Facilitators*; EPPI-Centre, Social Science Research Unit, Institute of Education, University of London: London, UK, 2003.
32. Matwiejczyk, L.; Mehta, K.; Scott, J.; Tonkin, E.; Coveney, J. Characteristics of Effective Interventions Promoting Healthy Eating for Pre-Schoolers in Childcare Settings: An Umbrella Review. *Nutrients* **2018**, *10*, 293. [CrossRef] [PubMed]
33. Department of Health. *Getting Children Aged 5–12 Years to Eat More Fruit and Vegetables: An Evidence Summary*; Prevention and Population Health Branch, Department of Health: Melbourne, Australia, 2010.
34. McNaughton, S.; Crawford, D.; Campbell, K.; Abbott, G.; Ball, K. *Eating Behaviours of Urban and Rural Children from Disadvantaged Backgrounds*; Centre for Physical Activity and Nutrition Research, Deakin University: Melbourne, Australia, 2010.
35. Sharp, G.; Pettigrew, S.; Wright, S.; Pratt, I.S.; Blane, S.; Biagioni, N. Potential in-class stategies to increase children's vegetable consumption. *Public Health Nutr.* **2017**, *20*, 1491–1499. [CrossRef] [PubMed]
36. Bandura, A. Social Cognitive Theory: An Agentic Perspective. *Annu. Rev. Psychol.* **2001**, *52*, 1–26. [CrossRef] [PubMed]
37. Department of Regional Development. Our WA Regions. Available online: http://www.drd.wa.gov.au/regions/Pages/default.aspx (accessed on 13 September 2018).
38. Australian Bureau of Statistics. Socio-economic Indexes for Areas (SEIFA) Data Cube, 2011, Table 3: State Suburb (SSC) Index of Relative Socio-economic Disadvantage, 2011. In *cat. no. 2033.0.55.001*; Australian Bureau of Statistics: Canberra, Australia, 2013.
39. King, N. Using Templates in the Thematic Analysis of Text. In *Essential Guide to Qualitative Methods in Organizational Research*; Cassell, C., Symon, G., Eds.; Sage Publications Ltd.: London, UK, 2004; pp. 256–270.
40. Guest, G.; Bunce, A.; Johnson, L. How Many Interviews are Enough? An Experiment with Data Saturation and Variability. *Field Methods* **2006**, *18*, 59–82. [CrossRef]
41. Dresler, E.; Whitehead, D.; Mather, A. The experiences of New Zealand-based children in consuming fruits and vegetables. *Health Educ.* **2017**, *117*, 297–309. [CrossRef]

42. Goncalves, S.; Ferreira, R.; Conceicao, E.M.; Silva, C.; Machado, P.P.P.; Boyland, E.; Vaz, A. The impact of exposure to cartoons promoting healthy eating on children's food preferences and choices. *J. Nutr. Educ. Behav.* **2018**, *50*, 451–457. [CrossRef] [PubMed]
43. Rinderknecht, K.; Smith, C. Social cognitive theory in an after-school nutrition intervention for urban native American youth. *J. Nutr. Educ. Behav.* **2004**, *36*, 298–304. [CrossRef]
44. Mills, C.; Knuiman, M.; Rosenberg, M.; Wood, L.; Ferguson, R. Are the arts an effective setting for promoting health messages? *Perspect. Public Health* **2013**, *133*, 116–121. [CrossRef] [PubMed]
45. Steen, M.; Manschot, M.; De Koning, N. Benefits of Co-design in Service Design Projects. *Int. J. Des.* **2011**, *5*, 53–60.
46. Hughes, R.; Margetts, B.M. *Practical Public Health Nutrition*; Wiley-Blackwell: Hoboken, NJ, USA, 2010.
47. Kim, D.; Subramanian, S.V.; Kawachi, I. Social Capital and Physical Health. In *Social Capital and Health*; Kawachi, I., Subramanian, S., Kim, D., Eds.; Springer: New York, NY, USA, 2008.
48. Kumanyika, S.K.; Obarzanek, E.; Stettler, N.; Bell, R.; Field, A.E.; Fortmann, S.P.; Franklin, B.A.; Gillman, M.W.; Lewis, C.E.; Poston, W.C.; et al. Population-Based Prevention of Obesity. The Need for Comprehensive Promotion of Healthful Eating, Physical Activity, and Energy Balance. *Am. Heart Assoc. J.* **2008**, *118*, 428–464.
49. Nanayakkara, J.; Margerison, C.; Worsley, A. Importance of food literacy education for senior secondary school students: Food system professionals' opinions. *Int. J. Health Promot. Educ.* **2017**, *55*, 284–295. [CrossRef]
50. Wallace, R.M.; Costello, L.N.; Devine, A. Over-provision of discretionary foods at childcare dilutes the nutritional quality of diets for children. *Aust. N. Z. J. Public Health* **2017**, *41*, 1. [CrossRef] [PubMed]
51. Myers, G.; Wright, S.; Blane, S.; Pratt, I.S.; Pettigrew, S. A process and outcome evaluation of an in-class vegetable promotion program. *Appetite* **2018**, *125*, 182–189. [CrossRef] [PubMed]
52. Chung, L.M.Y. Food Literacy of Adolescents as a Predictor of Their Healthy Eating and Dietary Quality. *J. Child Adolesc. Behav.* **2017**, *5*, e117.
53. Vidgen, H.A.; Gallegos, D. Defining food literacy and its components. *Appetite* **2014**, *76*, 50–59. [CrossRef] [PubMed]
54. Goh, Y.; Bogart, L.; Sipple-Asher, B.; Uyeda, K.; Hawes-Dawson, J.; Olarita-Dhungana, J.; Ryan, G.; Schuster, M. Using community-based participatory research to identify potential interventions to overcome barriers to adolescents' healthy eating and physical activity. *J. Behav. Med.* **2009**, *32*, 491–502. [CrossRef] [PubMed]
55. Niklas, T.; Jahns, L.; Bogle, M.; Chester, D.; Giovanni, M.; Klurfield, D.; Laugero, K.; Liu, Y.; Lopez, S.; Tucker, K. Barriers and Facilitators for Consumer Adherence to the Dietary Gudelines for Americans: The HEALTH Study. *J. Acad. Nutr. Diet.* **2013**, *113*, 1317–1331. [CrossRef] [PubMed]
56. Godrich, S.L.; Lo, J.; Davies, C.R.; Darby, J.; Devine, A. Which food security determinants predict adequate vegetable consumption among rural Western Australian children? *Int. J. Environ. Res. Public Health* **2017**, *14*, 40. [CrossRef] [PubMed]
57. Micha, R.; Karageorgou, D.; Bakogianni, I.; Trichia, E.; Whitsel, L.P.; Story, M.; Peñalvo, J.L.; Mozaffarian, D. Effectiveness of school food environment policies on children's dietary behaviors: A systematic review and meta-analysis. *PLoS ONE* **2018**, *13*, e0194555. [CrossRef] [PubMed]
58. Bruening, M.; Adams, M.A.; Ohri-Vachaspati, P.; Hurley, J. Prevalence and Implementation Practices of School Salad Bars Across Grade Levels. *Am. J. Health Promot.* **2018**, *32*, 1375–1382. [CrossRef] [PubMed]
59. Draxten, M.; Fulkerson, J.A.; Friend, S.; Flattum, C.F.; Schow, R. Parental role modeling of fruits and vegetables at meals and snacks is associated with children's adequate consumption. *Appetite* **2014**, *78*, 1–7. [CrossRef] [PubMed]
60. Sacks, R.; Yi, S.S.; Nonas, C. Increasing Access to Fruits and Vegetables: Perspectives from the New York City Experience. *Am. J. Public Health* **2015**, *105*, e29–e37. [CrossRef] [PubMed]
61. Blanchette, L.; Brug, J. Determinants of fruit and vegetable consumption among 6–12 year old children and effective interventions to increase consumption. *J. Hum. Nutr. Diet.* **2005**, *18*, 431–443. [CrossRef] [PubMed]

nutrients

MDPI

Article

Does Village Chicken-Keeping Contribute to Young Children's Diets and Growth? A Longitudinal Observational Study in Rural Tanzania

Julia de Bruyn [1,*], Peter C. Thomson [2], Ian Darnton-Hill [3,4], Brigitte Bagnol [3,5,6], Wende Maulaga [7] and Robyn G. Alders [2,3,6]

1 Natural Resources Institute, University of Greenwich, Kent ME4 4TB, UK
2 School of Life and Environmental Sciences, University of Sydney, Sydney NSW 2006, Australia; peter.thomson@sydney.edu.au (P.C.T.); robyna@kyeemafoundation.org (R.G.A.)
3 Charles Perkins Centre, University of Sydney, Sydney NSW 2006, Australia; ian.darnton-hill@sydney.edu.au (I.D.-H.); bagnolbrigitte@gmail.com (B.B.)
4 The Boden Institute of Obesity, Nutrition, Exercise & Eating Disorders, University of Sydney, Sydney NSW 2006, Australia
5 Department of Anthropology, University of Witwatersrand, Johannesburg 2000, South Africa
6 International Rural Poultry Centre, Kyeema Foundation, Brisbane QLD 4000, Australia
7 Tanzania Veterinary Laboratory Agency, Dar es Salaam 11000, Tanzania; wendesamanga@gmail.com
* Correspondence: j.m.debruyn@greenwich.ac.uk; Tel.: +44-1634-883-214

Received: 11 September 2018; Accepted: 16 November 2018; Published: 19 November 2018

Abstract: There is substantial current interest in linkages between livestock-keeping and human nutrition in resource-poor settings. These may include benefits of improved diet quality, through animal-source food consumption and nutritious food purchases using livestock-derived income, and hazards of infectious disease or environmental enteric dysfunction associated with exposure to livestock feces. Particular concerns center on free-roaming chickens, given their proximity to children in rural settings, but findings to date have been inconclusive. This longitudinal study of 503 households with a child under 24 months at enrolment was conducted in villages of Manyoni District, Tanzania between May 2014, and May 2016. Questionnaires encompassed demographic characteristics, assets, livestock ownership, chicken housing practices, maternal education, water and sanitation, and dietary diversity. Twice-monthly household visits provided information on chicken numbers, breastfeeding and child diarrhea, and anthropometry was collected six-monthly. Multivariable mixed model analyses evaluated associations between demographic, socioeconomic and livestock-associated variables and (a) maternal and child diets, (b) children's height-for-age and (c) children's diarrhea frequency. Alongside modest contributions of chicken-keeping to some improved dietary outcomes, this study importantly (and of substantial practical significance if confirmed) found no indication of a heightened risk of stunting or greater frequency of diarrhea being associated with chicken-keeping or the practice of keeping chickens within human dwellings overnight.

Keywords: undernutrition; food security; nutrition security; village chickens; livestock; animal-source food; Tanzania; sub-Saharan Africa; resource-poor settings

1. Introduction

To achieve lasting impact in enhancing food and nutrition security in resource-poor settings, there is a need for strategies which align with local priorities and address context-specific constraints. Mixed crop-livestock farming is widely practiced throughout sub-Saharan Africa [1] and has been shown to strengthen the resilience of smallholder farmers to climate change [2,3]. A growing body of literature explores linkages between livestock ownership and human nutrition. Livestock-keeping is posited to offer the benefits of improved dietary quality, through access to nutrient-rich animal-source foods (ASF) [4,5] and nutritious food purchases enabled by livestock-derived income [6], but with the possible hazards associated with exposure to livestock feces in rural settings [7].

Potential risks of contact with livestock feces relate both to pathogenic bacteria, responsible for infectious diarrhea [8], and to non-pathogenic bacteria, as a cause of environmental enteric dysfunction (EED) [9]. In EED, chronic damage to the gastrointestinal tract may reduce nutrient absorption and cause low-level immune stimulation, restricting children's growth and development [10,11]; however, evidence of the causal pathways between EED and child stunting is limited, and the condition is likely to be more complex than previously conceived [12]. A systematic review examining relationships between livestock ownership and child health identified a predominant focus on diarrhea as the primary health outcome [8]. Impaired height-for-age (stunting) is advocated as a more objective measure which reflects the cumulative effect of multiple influences, such as dietary quality and recurrent diarrhea, on children's growth over an extended period of time [13].

Village chickens are an accessible and versatile form of livestock, kept in small flocks by many vulnerable households in low- and middle-income countries (LMICs). Indigenous-breed birds roam freely during the day, scavenging for food, and are often housed within human dwellings overnight to reduce risks of predation or theft [14,15]. Their contribution to income and diets is made significant by the inherently low requirements for capital, labor and other inputs [15–17]. These benefits may be further enhanced by the central role of women in raising village chickens [18–20], with income and resources managed by women shown to have disproportionately strong effects on health and nutrition [21,22]. While previously promoted as an opportunity to sustainably enhance food and nutrition security in LMICs, free-ranging chickens have faced recent scrutiny as a source of fecal contamination in rural areas.

Recent efforts to determine the net impact of chicken-keeping on children's growth and health have largely reported on the analysis of existing datasets [23–26]. These multi-purpose surveys have the advantage of large sample sizes, but offer a limited opportunity to understand specific management practices which may carry benefits and risks to human health and nutrition. In Ethiopia, the practice of keeping chickens indoors overnight was reported to counteract any positive effects of poultry ownership on children's height-for-age Z-scores (HAZ) [27]. A multi-country study found animal feces in the homestead environment to be negatively associated with children's HAZ in Bangladesh and Ethiopia, but not in Vietnam [24].

Appropriate source data is vital to draw meaningful conclusions amidst the complexity of different livestock production systems, sociocultural influences, and seasonal variation. Some studies have employed the Tropical Livestock Unit as a quantitative measure to evaluate livestock ownership as a predictor of nutrition outcomes [24,28]. This unit represents smallholder livestock holdings—of mixed species, breeds and ages—based on the approximate metabolic weight of each. This unit was developed to quantify production levels and relate livestock numbers to human populations or land resources [29,30]. There are clear limitations in its use in situations where the "amount" of livestock may not equate, for example, to their sociocultural value or to the incidence of stunting, wasting or illness in children.

The concept of the "livestock ladder" has been used to describe livestock ownership as an opportunity for rural households to accumulate assets and rise from poverty [31–33]. Beyond their economic value, however, there are notable distinctions in the roles of different livestock in resource-poor settings. Village chickens, considered the lowest step on the livestock ladder, offer a readily-accessible source of income, an opportunity to engage in social customs, and access to nutritious food items [20,34,35]. By contrast, larger livestock such as cattle are associated with wealth and social status, and provide longer-term savings, insurance, and draught animal power, but are infrequently used to meet immediate household needs [32,36,37].

This paper presents analytical approaches and results from an observational study in eight rural communities in Tanzania. Alongside other forms of livestock ownership, it includes a specific focus on village chicken-keeping to evaluate longitudinal associations with (a) diets of young children and their mothers, (b) HAZ and the probability of stunting in children, and (c) the occurrence of diarrhea in children. The study is nested within a larger investigation assessing the impact of community-based vaccination programs against Newcastle disease in village chickens and interventions to improve crop diversity, management, and storage on maternal and child health outcomes [38]. Analyses have used a range of livestock-associated predictor variables, and both short-term (i.e., diets and diarrhea) and longer-term (i.e., HAZ) outcome variables, to optimize the understanding of how domestic animal ownership has influenced children's nutrition and health over a two-year period in this setting.

2. Materials and Methods

2.1. Study Area and Population

This longitudinal study of 503 children was conducted in eight rural villages in Manyoni District, Singida Region in the semi-arid Central Zone of Tanzania. Unimodal rainfall is expected between November and April, with mean annual rainfall of 624 mm (SD = 179 mm) and a mean of 49 rain days per year (SD = 15) at a district level [39]. Project sites were selected in consultation with government partners at national, regional and district levels, guided by the prevalence of childhood stunting and the absence of existing nutritional interventions.

A ward census was conducted by the project in April 2014 in Sanza Ward and October 2014 in Majiri Ward, with local enumerators visiting all households in each community to record the age and gender of all members, based on information provided by a household representative. Two-stage sampling was used to enroll a total of 240 households in Sanza Ward and 280 in Majiri Ward, by first enrolling all households with a child under 12 months of age (mo), and then using random selection to enroll additional households with a child aged 12–24 mo. The terms "enrolled child" and "enrolled household" are used to describe participants in this study, with a single child followed within each household (the youngest child, where more than one child under 24 mo was present).

Baseline data collection was completed for 229 households from Sanza Ward in May 2014, and 274 households from Majiri Ward in November 2014, as part of the staged implementation within the larger project design [38]. A small number of enrolled children (n = 6) were identified to be above the intended maximum age of 24 months at this time (range of 24.2–28.1 mo), but were retained within the study sample.

2.2. Ethical Approval

Study design, protocols and research tools were approved by the Tanzanian National Institute for Medical Research ethics committee (NIMR/HQ/R.8a/Vol.IX/1690), and by the University of Sydney's Human Research Ethics Committee (2014/209) and Animal Ethics Committee (2013/6065). Participants' informed consent was given via a signature or thumb print at the time of data collection, for each questionnaire and set of anthropometric measurements. A participant information statement was provided to all participating households at the commencement of the study. To accommodate linguistic diversity and varying levels of literacy, all documents were read aloud to study participants by trained enumerators, using local languages where appropriate.

2.3. Data Collection

2.3.1. Questionnaires

Male and female enumerators were recruited from the community in consultation with local leaders and trained to administer two semi-structured questionnaires. One questionnaire, directed to mothers at six-monthly intervals, encompassed maternal education, household water sources and toilet facilities, and maternal and child diets (24-h dietary recall, using the "open recall" method [40]). A second questionnaire, applied annually to an intended equal number of male and female household members (actual sample comprised 60.5% female respondents of 1354 completed questionnaires) encompassed demographic data, household assets, livestock ownership and chicken-keeping practices, including the location of overnight housing for chickens. Printed survey questions and training sessions were in Swahili, but enumerators were encouraged to make use of the languages of the two predominant language groups (*Kigogo* and *Kisukuma*) where appropriate.

2.3.2. Household Visits

Male and female representatives from each village were employed as "Community Assistants" to collect ongoing data. Households were visited twice-monthly to record the number of chickens owned (categorized by age, i.e., under or over two months), the breastfeeding status of the enrolled child (exclusively breastfed, receiving both breast milk and complementary foods, or non-breastfed), and the occurrence of diarrhea in the enrolled child during the previous two weeks. Diarrhea was defined as the passage of three or more loose or liquid stools per day, or more frequent passage than is normal for the individual child [41].

2.3.3. Anthropometry

Child length or height measurements were recorded to the nearest 1 mm by trained personnel using UNICEF portable baby/child length-height measuring boards. Recumbent length was measured for children up to 24 mo, and standing height for children over 24 mo. Where this protocol was not followed, to minimize distress and maximize measurement accuracy (6.0% measurements), a standard adjustment was applied [42]. Birthdates were verified against health clinic records where available (80.7%). Measurements were taken at six-monthly intervals from May 2014 in Sanza and November 2014 in Majiri until May 2016 in both wards.

2.3.4. Rainfall Data

Daily rainfall data were recorded by trained community representatives from a rain gauge with 1 mm graduations, located at a village office in each ward.

2.4. Data Analysis

2.4.1. Defining Variables

Descriptions and data sources for predictor and outcome variables are provided in Appendix A (Table A1). Emergency Nutrition Assessment for SMART software was used to calculate child HAZ, based on World Health Organization (WHO) child growth standards [42]. Z-scores below −6 or above +6 were identified as extreme or potentially incorrect values, and were excluded from analyses [43]. Z-scores of less than −2 for height-for-age were classified as stunting. A "diarrhea score" was calculated for each six-month period preceding anthropometry, from a ratio of the number of positive records of diarrhea to the total number of records per child. This allowed for variability in the number of data points per child, due to absence during data collection visits.

For mothers, dietary diversity (DD) scores were based on the Minimum Dietary Diversity for Women of Reproductive Age (MDD-W) indicator [40] and for children, using the Infant and Young Child Minimum Dietary Diversity (IYCMDD) indicator [44]. To achieve consistency in the longitudinal evaluation of children's diets, the IYCMDD indicator was used beyond its intended age range of 6–23 months, as has been done elsewhere [45]. Results for breastfed and non-breastfed children are reported separately. Consumption of ASF, overall and in the categories of eggs, chicken meat, other meat and fish, and milk, was also evaluated.

A household was defined as a group of people living together and sharing food from the same pot, with members having lived in the household at least three days of each week for the previous six months [46]. This definition seeks to encompass individuals who share common resources and make common budget and expenditure decisions. Given the close linkages between livestock and wealth in agropastoralist communities, multiple approaches were employed to assess the influence of livestock-keeping while controlling for variation in wealth.

Socioeconomic status was represented using several variants of an index developed for use in sub-Saharan Africa, which assigns a weight to livestock and non-livestock assets according to their relative value [47]. Information on the development and validation of this index is not readily-available, but it is recommended for all projects receiving funding from the Bill and Melinda Gates Foundation. Guided by Tanzanian research partners and time in the study sites, the authors judged this tool to provide an adequate estimation of wealth in this setting. The index was modified to accommodate available data, and a weighting was applied to 11 household assets (radio, television, refrigerator, mobile phone, mosquito net, table, sewing machine, bicycle, motorcycle, car, and ox-cart) and six forms of livestock (cattle, sheep, goats, donkeys, pigs and poultry). Three variants of this index were used, as outlined in Table 1.

Table 1. Indicators to represent household socioeconomic status in this study.

Indicator	Definition	Use
Household Domestic Asset Index (HDAI)	A weighted sum of material and livestock assets	To characterize households' socioeconomic status in descriptive summaries of the study population.
HDAI excluding cattle and chickens	A weighted sum of material and selected livestock assets (sheep, goats, donkeys, pigs)	To control for variation in socioeconomic status in models for maternal and child diets, where the influence of cattle and chicken ownership was tested separately.
Non-Livestock Asset Index (NLAI)	A weighted sum of material assets only	To control for variation in socioeconomic status in models for child stunting and diarrhea, where multiple livestock-associated variables were tested separately.

Information on the first language spoken by both of the enrolled child's parents was collated with the gender of the household head to determine the dominant language group of each household, as a proxy for a range of cultural and agricultural practices [48,49]. Toilet facilities and sources of drinking water were classified as improved or unimproved [50].

To address the complex linkages between livestock, health and nutrition, multiple variables based on livestock ownership were assembled (Table A1). For each major category of animals, variables were constructed to reflect ownership:

(a) as a bivariate categorical variable (i.e., yes/no);
(b) relative to the median number of animals in this population (i.e., $</\geq$ median number); and,
(c) in terms of the number of animals owned.

A "livestock ladder" variable was also calculated, which assigned households to four categories based on the animal species owned:

(a) no livestock;
(b) chickens only;
(c) small ruminants, with or without chickens; and,
(d) cattle, with or without other livestock.

Variables were constructed to reflect ownership for the six month period preceding each round of anthropometry. Information on ruminant ownership was drawn from the annual household questionnaire, but variables relating to chicken ownership were based on twice-monthly household visits. This reflects the substantial fluctuations in chicken ownership and flock size in village settings due to short reproductive cycles, sales to meet household needs, and losses due to predation or seasonal disease outbreaks. To evaluate contributions to diets, income and household environments, chicks were excluded from measures of chicken flock size. A summary of the construction of chicken-associated variables is shown in Figure 1.

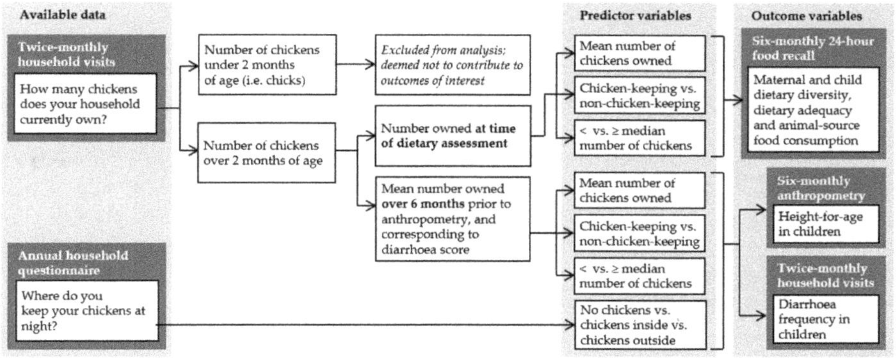

Figure 1. Construction of predictor variables to test associations between chicken-keeping and maternal and child diets, child anthropometry and diarrhea frequency (alongside other livestock and non-livestock variables). Small chicks have been excluded from chicken flock size, and consideration given to the time period over which ownership is measured.

To test associations with diets, chicken ownership during the month of dietary assessment was used. For the longer-term outcomes of children's HAZ and diarrhea, a broader assessment of chicken ownership was considered more relevant than a single point-in-time count of chicken numbers, therefore, the mean number of chickens owned during the six-month period preceding each measurement was calculated. Households were classified as "chicken-keeping" if the mean number of chickens owned was one or greater for a six-month period, and "non-chicken-keeping" if less than one.

2.4.2. Descriptive Statistics

Descriptive analyses were used to characterize the study population, explore variation between the two wards, and evaluate intended predictor and outcome variables. Percentages were determined for categorical variables, and means and standard deviations or medians and interquartile ranges calculated, for normally and non-normally distributed continuous variables, respectively. Inter-group comparisons for the two wards were performed using *t*-tests and chi-square tests for continuous and bivariate categorical variables, respectively.

2.4.3. Univariable and Multivariable Models

All analyses were conducted in the form of linear mixed models or generalized linear mixed models, using Genstat Release 18 software. Consideration was given to the potential for spatial clustering by including ward, village, and sub-village locations as random effects, along with household identifiers to account for repeat-measures data. Three broad components of the study evaluated:

(a) maternal and child dietary diversity, dietary adequacy and the consumption of ASF;
(b) child HAZ and probability of the stunting; and,
(c) children's "diarrhea score".

In each case, predictor variables of interest were collated for six-month periods corresponding to outcome variables. For livestock numbers and asset scores, log-transformations were used to minimize the excessive influence of very large numbers. Univariable models were first used to test unconditional associations between predictor and outcome variables. Multivariable models were constructed using variables of suggestive significance ($p < 0.1$) based on univariable models, and stepwise backward elimination was used to manually remove variables with p-values greater than 0.1 to reach the final models. Both significant ($p < 0.05$) and suggestive ($0.05 \leq p < 0.1$) associations have been reported.

3. Results

3.1. Characterizing the Population

Of a total of 513 children randomly selected to participate in the study, adequate baseline data were available for inclusion of 503 children in this analysis. An attrition rate of 16.9% was seen at the time of final data collection in May 2016, due to relocation outside the study area (n = 39), withdrawal from the study (n = 5), and child deaths (n = 6). Table 2 presents an overview of individual and household characteristics at the time of baseline data collection, by ward and in the overall sample. At enrolment, the mean age of children was 8.6 mo (range of 0.6–28.1 mo). Almost one-third of mothers (32.5%) reported having had no formal education, and only a small number (3.4%) indicated a level of education beyond primary school.

Table 2. Overview of study population according to baseline questionnaire responses, by ward and overall.

Location	Sanza Ward	Majiri Ward	Overall
Baseline data collection	May 2014	Nov 2014	
Enrolled households (n)	229	274	503
Sex of child, female (%)	55.5	47.4	51.1
Child age in months			
Mean (SD)	9.9 (6.1) [a]	7.6 (4.3) [a]	8.6 (5.3)
Range	1.2–28.1	0.6–22.5	0.6–28.1
Maternal age in years			
Mean (SD)	28.5 (7.5) [a]	26.8 (7.5) [a]	27.7 (7.6)
Range	15–50	13–54	13–54
Age unknown (%)	9.2 [b]	23.7 [b]	17.1
Maternal education (%)			
No formal education	22.7 [b]	40.5 [b]	32.4
Some primary school	68.6 [b]	56.6 [b]	62.0
Some secondary school	5.7 [b]	1.5 [b]	3.4
Unspecified level	3.1	1.5	2.2
Primary language of household (%)			
Kigogo	78.2 [b]	74.8 [b]	76.3
Kisukuma	6.1 [b]	14.6 [b]	10.7
Other	4.4	2.6	3.4
Unspecified	11.4 [b]	8.0 [b]	9.5
Parents of same language group (%)	92.1	95.6	94.1
Number of household members			
Mean (SD)	5.6 (2.0)	5.5 (2.3)	5.5 (2.2)
Range	2–16	2–21	2–21
Female-headed households (%)	30.2 [b]	16.4 [b]	22.7
Socioeconomic status, median (IQR)			
Non-livestock and livestock assets, HDAI	12 (5–51)	26 (7–115)	19 (7–76)
Non-livestock assets only, NLAI	7 (3–11)	9 (3–13)	9 (3–12)
Livestock ownership (%)			
Cattle	26.7 [b]	36.2 [b]	31.8
Sheep or goats	27.1 [b]	47.8 [b]	38.3
Chickens	51.1 [b]	42.1 [b]	46.3
Number of livestock, median (IQR) [c]			
Cattle	4 (2–17) [a]	10 (4–20) [a]	7 (4–20)
Sheep or goats	14 (7–20)	12 (5–25)	12 (6–24)
Chickens	7 (2–13)	8 (5–13)	8 (4–13)
Improved water source (%)	2.6	2.2	4.9
Improved toilet facilities (%)	3.1 [b]	0.4 [b]	1.6

Significant differences between wards ($p < 0.05$), as determined by [a] t-tests and [b] chi-square tests. [c] Amongst households owning livestock, by category.

Of approximately 120 language groups within Tanzania [51], 22 were represented within the study population. *Kigogo* was the primary language for 75.7% of households and *Kisukuma* the primary language for 9.1%. For a large majority of enrolled children, both parents shared their first language (94.1%). Households included a mean number of 5.5 members (range of 2–21), and 22.7% reported a female head of household. Less than 5% of households reported accessing an improved water source at the time of baseline data collection, less than 2% used improved toilet facilities, and almost three-quarters (72.7%) shared toilet facilities with one or more other households.

3.2. Livestock and Household Wealth

The index of livestock and non-livestock assets (HDAI) varied widely across the study sample, with a markedly positively-skewed distribution. The median HDAI in Majiri Ward was more than twice that in Sanza Ward (26 vs. 12), while wealth assessments based on non-livestock assets varied less prominently. Ruminants were more commonly kept in Majiri than in Sanza (36.2% vs. 26.7%, $p = 0.024$ for cattle; 47.8% vs. 27.1%, $p < 0.001$ for sheep and goats), and cattle numbers significantly greater (median herd size of 10 in Majiri vs. 4 in Sanza, $p = 0.012$). Baseline data suggested chicken-keeping to be more common in Sanza than in Majiri, however the differing months of data collection and seasonal variation in chicken numbers prevents conclusions being drawn using these data.

Based on data collated over the entire study period, 70.8% of households owned some form of livestock, with chickens kept by 55.0%, sheep and goats by 38.4% and cattle by 31.5%. Almost two-thirds of chicken-keeping households (64.2%) reported chickens to be kept inside their home overnight, rather than in a chicken house or left to roost in trees. Categorizing livestock ownership according to the "livestock ladder", around one-quarter of participating households (25.3%) kept only chickens; 14.0% kept sheep or goats, with or without chickens but without cattle; and 31.5% kept cattle, with or without other livestock.

Accounting for geographic clustering and individual household effects, the non-livestock index (NLAI) was positively associated ($p < 0.001$) with the probability of owning each category of animals—however the extent of this association varied between species (Figure 2). Households in the lowest quintile were identified to have a 0.44 probability of owning chickens, compared with a 0.12 probability of owning sheep or goats and a 0.07 probability of owning cattle. The comparative increase in the likelihood of animal ownership with increasing non-livestock wealth also varied between livestock categories. A household in the highest quintile had 21.2 times greater odds of owning cattle, 9.6 times greater odds of owning sheep or goats, and 4.1 times greater odds of owning chickens, compared to a household in the lowest quintile.

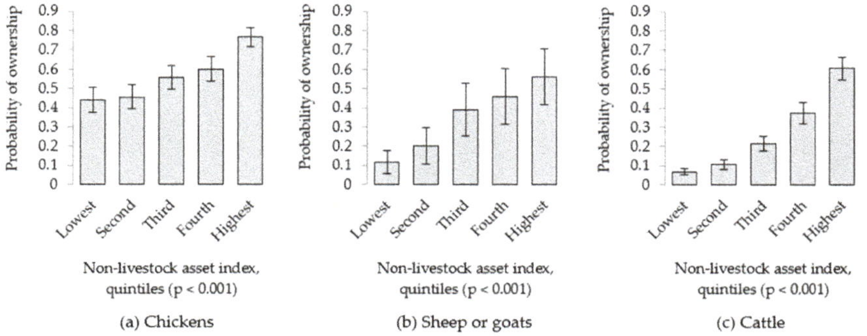

Figure 2. Probability of owning livestock, according to quintiles of the non-livestock asset index (NLAI). For all categories of animals—(**a**) chickens, (**b**) sheep and goats, and (**c**) cattle—the NLAI was positively associated with the probability of ownership ($p < 0.001$). Standard errors are shown.

Positive associations were also found between the livestock ladder and the NLAI ($p < 0.001$). Model-based means show markedly greater non-livestock wealth amongst households in the highest tier of the livestock ladder (i.e., those owning cattle), compared to other groups (Figure 3a). Ownership of chickens, small ruminants and cattle was associated with substantially higher mean non-livestock wealth scores, compared to not owning each form of livestock (Figure 3b).

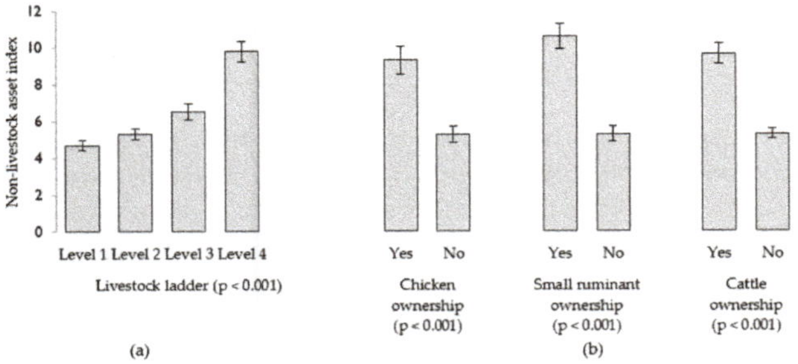

Figure 3. Model-based mean non-livestock asset index scores according to: (**a**) levels on the livestock ladder, and (**b**) ownership of chickens, sheep or goats, and cattle. Standard errors are shown.

3.3. Maternal and Child Diets

3.3.1. Dietary Diversity and Animal-Source Food Consumption

The mean DD score across all data collection periods was 3.8 (SD 1.4) for mothers, 3.0 (SD 1.3) for breastfed children and 3.7 (SD 1.1) for non-breastfed children (Figure 4). Despite similarity in the number of food groups eaten, the percentage of non-breastfed children meeting cut-offs for an "adequately diverse" diet (55.6%, based on $\geq$ 4 of 7 food groups) was double that of their mothers (27.1%, $\geq$ 5 of 10 food groups). Dietary adequacy amongst women increased across successive data collection periods, from 18.4% in November 2014 to 39.4% in May 2016. Similar increases for breastfed (21.3% to 66.7%) and non-breastfed children (34.7% to 68.6%) were noted.

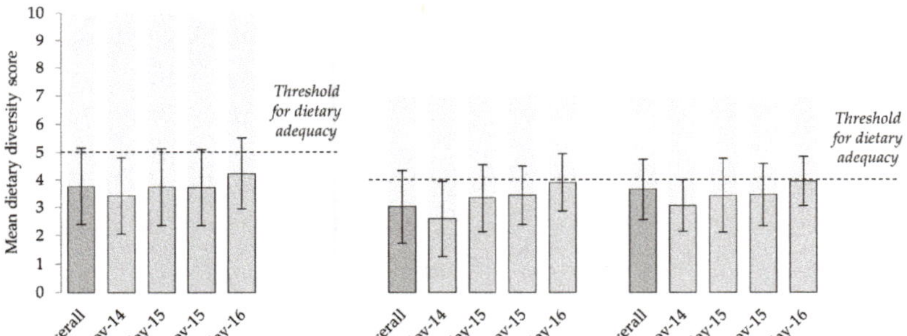

Figure 4. Mean dietary diversity scores of (**a**) mothers (using MDD-W indicator); and (**b**) breastfed and (**c**) non-breastfed children (both using IYCMDD indicator), overall and for each six-monthly data collection. Light grey shading indicates the number of food groups. Standard errors are shown.

Consumption of eggs and chicken meat was very uncommon (2.1% mothers for each item, across all records), and markedly less common than other forms of meat or fish (25.4%) and milk (19.7%). Milk consumption varied prominently between data collection periods. With the exception of the small number of breastfed children in May 2016 ($n = 21$), records indicate milk to be more commonly consumed during May than in November (Figure 5).

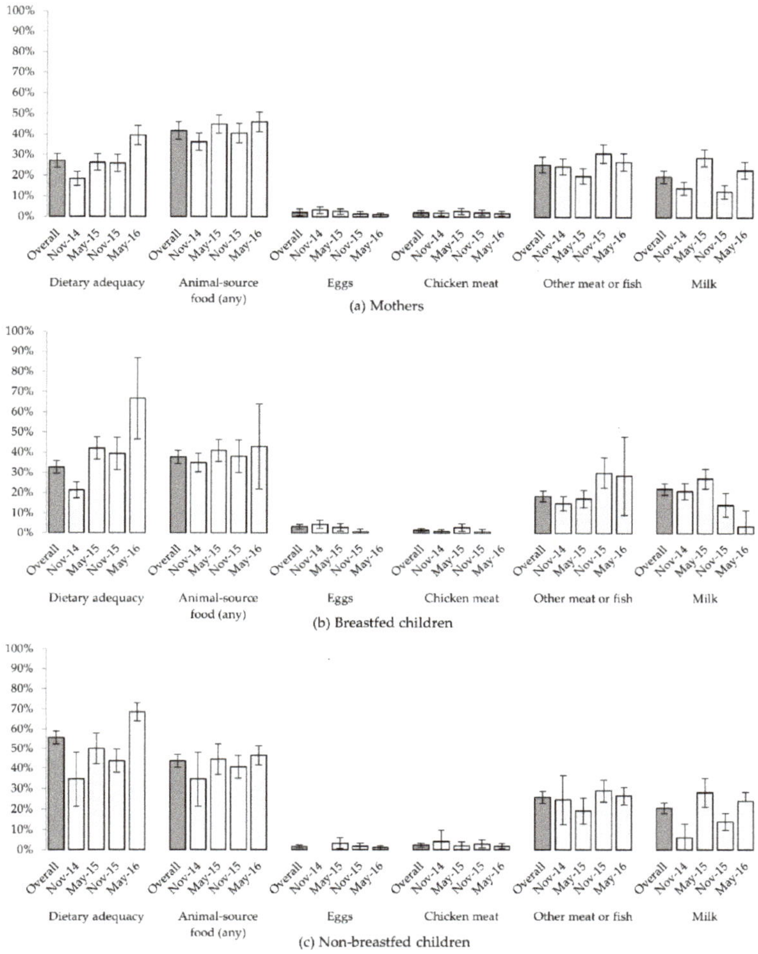

Figure 5. Percentage of (**a**) mothers, (**b**) breastfed children, and (**c**) non-breastfed children with adequate diets (according to MDD-W and IYCMDD, respectively) and consuming animal-source foods, based on six-monthly 24-h food recall, overall and for each six-monthly data collection. 95% confidence intervals are shown. Low numbers of non-breastfed children during early data collection periods, and of breastfed children later in this longitudinal study, have resulted in wide confidence intervals for some percentages reported.

3.3.2. Univariable and Multivariable Models

Unconditional associations between predictor variables of interest and dietary outcomes are included in Appendix B (Table A2). Several measures of chicken ownership were significantly associated with positive dietary outcomes in univariable models; however, a majority of these were not significant in multivariable models (Table 3). For example, despite positive unconditional associations ($p < 0.001$) between the number of chickens owned by a household and DD scores for mothers and breastfed children, no significant associations were identified when controlling for household wealth. One notable exception to this pattern was the consumption of ASF by women, which was positively associated with both the number of chickens ($p = 0.009$) and cattle ($p = 0.005$) owned, but not with measures of wealth based on other assets ($p = 0.190$).

Table 3. Multivariable models [a] for maternal and child dietary adequacy, dietary diversity and ASF consumption, showing *p*-values and the direction of significant ($p < 0.05$) and suggestive ($0.05 \leq p < 0.1$) associations. Grey shading indicates significant and suggestive associations in univariable models (Table A2), and "NS" denotes non-significant associations in final multivariable models.

Predictor Variables	Dietary Adequacy	DD Score [b]	ASF Consumption			
			Any	Chicken	Egg	Milk
(a) Mothers						
Month of dietary assessment, May	<0.001 (+)	<0.001 (+)	0.006 (+)	NS	NS	<0.001 (+)
Maternal age	NS	0.067 (−)	NS	NS	0.092 (−)	NS
Maternal formal education, yes	NS	NS	NS	NS	NS	NS
Breastfeeding, yes	NS	NS	NS	NS	NS	NS
Sex of household head, female	NS	0.068 (+)	NS	NS	<0.001 (+)	0.014 (−)
Number of household members	NS	NS	NS	NS	NS	NS
Language group, Sukuma	NS	NS	0.032 (+)	NS	NS	<0.001 (+)
Household domestic asset index [c,d]	0.002 (+)	< 0.001 (+)	NS	0.058 (+)	0.005 (+)	NS
Chickens owned, yes	NS	NS	NS	NS	NS	NS
Chickens, above median number	0.023 (+) [e]	NS	NS	NS	NS	NS
Chickens, number owned [c]	0.032 (+) [e]	NS	0.009 (+)	0.053 (+)	NS	NS
Cattle owned, yes	NS	NS	NS	NS	NS	NS
Cattle, above median number	NS	NS	NS	NS	NS	NS
Cattle, number owned [c]	NS	NS	0.005 (+)	NS	NS	<0.001 (+)
(b) Breastfed children						
Month of dietary assessment, May	0.002 (+)	0.057 (+)	NS	NS	NS	0.028 (+)
Child age	<0.001 (+)	<0.001 (+)	NS	NS	NS	NS
Sex of child, female	NS	NS	NS	NS	NS	NS
Maternal formal education, yes	NS	NS	NS	NS	NS	NS
Sex of household head, female	NS	NS	NS	NS	0.032 (+)	NS
Number of household members	NS	NS	NS	NS	NS	NS
Language group, Sukuma	0.046 (+)	NS	0.014 (+)	NS	NS	0.002 (+)
Household domestic asset index [c,d]	NS	0.002 (+)	< 0.001 (+)	NS	<0.001 (+)	NS
Chickens owned, yes	NS	NS	NS	NS	NS	NS
Chickens, above median number	NS	0.039 (+)	NS	NS	NS	NS
Chickens, number owned [c]	NS	NS	0.083 (+)	0.016 (+)	NS	NS
Cattle owned, yes	NS	NS	NS	NS	NS	0.010 (+) [f]
Cattle, above median number	NS	NS	NS	NS	NS	<0.001 (+) [f]
Cattle, number owned [c]	<0.001 (+)	NS	NS	NS	NS	<0.001 (+) [f]
(c) Non-breastfed children						
Month of dietary assessment, May	<0.001 (+)	<0.001 (+)	0.003 (+)	NS	NS	<0.001 (+)
Child age	NS	NS	NS	NS	NS	NS
Sex of child, female	0.045 (−)	0.066 (−)	0.014 (−)	NS	NS	NS
Maternal formal education, yes	NS	NS	NS	NS	NS	NS
Sex of household head, female	NS	NS	NS	NS	NS	NS
Number of household members	NS	NS	NS	0.080 (+)	0.059 (−)	NS
Language group, Sukuma	NS	NS	0.002 (+)	NS	NS	<0.001 (+)
Household domestic asset index [c,d]	NS	NS	NS	NS	0.023 (+)	NS
Chickens owned, yes	NS	NS	NS	NS	NS	NS
Chickens, above median number	NS	NS	NS	NS	NS	NS
Chickens, number owned [c]	NS	0.038 (+)	NS	NS	NS	NS
Cattle owned, yes	NS	NS	NS	NS	NS	0.003 (+)
Cattle, above median number	NS	NS	NS	NS	NS	0.050 (+)
Cattle, number owned [c]	NS	NS	NS	NS	NS	<0.001 (+)

[a] Generalized linear mixed models using binomial distribution, allowing for geographic clustering and longitudinal data; [b] Binomial totals of 10 for women (MDD-W) and 7 for children (IYCMDD); [c] log-transformed variables used to minimize excessive influence of large numbers; [d] Cattle and chickens excluded from HDAI, evaluated as separate predictor variables; [e] Two alternative models were constructed, one using the number of chickens owned and one using above-/below-median flock size, each together with the month of dietary assessment and HDAI (for which *p*-values remained unchanged); [f] Three alternative models were constructed, one using cattle ownership as a dichotomous variable, one using above-/below-median cattle herd size and one using the number of cattle owned, each with the month of dietary assessment and language group (for which *p*-values remained unchanged).

In final multivariable models (Table 3), across all participant groups, no significant differences in dietary outcomes were detected between categories of chicken-keeping and non-chicken-keeping households. In two models, one assessing the probability of dietary adequacy for mothers and one evaluating DD scores amongst breastfed children, positive associations were identified with ownership of greater than the median number of chickens (i.e., more than four birds). The number of chickens owned by a household, tested as a continuous variable, was also positively associated with DD scores for non-breastfed children ($p = 0.038$), and chicken consumption by breastfed children ($p = 0.016$), and suggested to be positively associated with chicken consumption by mothers ($p = 0.053$).

In all three participant groups, egg consumption was not associated with chicken ownership, but rather with the adjusted HDAI. Despite infrequent egg consumption across the study population, mothers in the highest wealth quintile were identified to have 16.5 times greater odds of consuming eggs than those in the lowest quintile (0.038 probability vs. 0.002), and breastfed children in the highest quintile to have 17.9 times greater odds than those in the lowest quintile (0.053 vs. 0.003). In contrast to the lack of association between chicken ownership and egg consumption, cattle numbers were a strong predictor of milk consumption for all groups ($p < 0.001$), allowing for the influence of season and language group (with households identifying as Sukuma significantly more likely to consume milk ($p < 0.001$ for mothers and non-breastfed children, $p = 0.002$ for breastfed children)).

For all groups, significant variation in DD scores, dietary adequacy and milk consumption were seen between months of dietary assessments. Diets were more diverse and more likely to meet thresholds for dietary adequacy, and milk more likely to be consumed in May (shortly after the end of the rain season) than in November. No significant associations were detected between household size or mothers' formal education and diets.

Both women and breastfed children were more likely to consume eggs in a female-headed household compared with a male-headed one ($p < 0.001$ and $p = 0.032$, respectively). While model-based predictions were low across all groups, breastfed children in female-headed households were determined to have 2.6 times greater odds of consuming eggs, compared to those in male-headed households (0.041 probability vs. 0.016). Being part of a female-headed household was also suggested to be associated with higher DD scores for women (mean of 3.90 vs. 3.74 for male-headed households, $p = 0.068$), but a lower likelihood of consuming milk ($p = 0.011$), controlling for variation in cattle ownership and language group.

Increasing child age was significantly associated with higher DD scores ($p < 0.001$) and a higher probability of an adequately diverse diet ($p < 0.001$) for breastfed children, but not for non-breastfed children. Across the range of dietary outcomes evaluated, gender-based differences were only evident amongst the non-breastfed group. Male children were significantly more likely to meet the cut-off for dietary adequacy ($p = 0.045$) and to consume ASF ($p = 0.014$), and suggested to have higher DD scores ($p = 0.066$), compared to female children.

3.4. Height-for-Age and Diarrhea in Children

3.4.1. Prevalence of Stunting

Summaries of anthropometric data were disaggregated by ward and by time period (Table 4). The prevalence of stunting increased from 36.8% to 49.5% over the first three data collection periods in Sanza Ward, reducing to 39.8% at the time of the final data collection. In Majiri Ward, where the mean age of children was lower at enrolment (7.6 mo vs. 9.9 mo; $p < 0.001$), a continuing increase in the prevalence of stunting was seen over successive data periods, from 28.3% to 53.0%.

3.4.2. Univariable and Multivariable Models

As for dietary outcomes, univariable models were first used to test unconditional associations between demographic, socioeconomic and livestock-associated variables and (a) HAZ, (b) probability of stunting, and (c) diarrhea in children. Variables relating to the consumption of ASF by children during the day prior to anthropometry were also included. These short-term dietary indicators are unlikely to be associated with long-term outcomes such as HAZ; however, the potential for patterns to be identified at a population level was considered adequate to warrant their consideration. Unconditional associations based on univariable analysis are included in Appendix B (Table A3).

Table 4. Overview of height-for-age Z-scores (HAZ) and the percentage of stunting amongst enrolled children, by ward and by data collection period.

	Mean HAZ (SD)	% Stunting	*n*
Sanza Ward			
May 2014	−1.52 (1.13)	36.8	220
Nov 2014	−1.63 (1.18)	34.5	200
May 2015	−2.02 (1.14)	49.5	202
Nov 2015	−1.98 (1.05)	48.2	191
May 2016	−1.77 (1.05)	39.8	201
Majiri Ward			
Nov 2014	−1.45 (1.21)	28.3	272
May 2015	−1.86 (1.05)	41.4	261
Nov 2015	−1.99 (0.98)	49.6	234
May 2016	−2.16 (1.00)	53.0	217

Children's age, gender, diarrhea frequency, household language group and NLAI quintiles were significantly associated with HAZ within univariable linear mixed models (Table A3), and remained significant at the 5% level in a multivariable model (Table 5). Height-for-age Z-scores were negatively associated with increasing child age, the male gender, more frequent diarrhea, language groups other than Sukuma, and lower NLAI scores. Of the livestock and dietary variables identified as being significantly or suggestively associated with HAZ in univariable models, none were significant in multivariable models. These included the number of chickens owned by a household ($p = 0.960$ in multivariable model), livestock ownership as a bivariate categorical variable ($p = 0.409$), and children's consumption of milk ($p = 0.802$) or meat or fish ($p = 0.236$) during the previous day.

Similar associations were found when evaluating stunting as a binary outcome, with a higher probability of stunting linked to increasing age, male children, language groups other than Sukuma and lower asset scores, and no significant associations with any livestock or dietary variables. Univariable analysis indicated a suggestive association with the HDAI (livestock and non-livestock assets), but it was the NLAI (non-livestock assets only) which was highly significantly associated ($p < 0.001$) with the probability of stunting in both uni- and multivariable models (Tables 5 and A3). Particularly poor outcomes were associated with the lowest NLAI quintile, including 2.1 times greater odds of stunting compared to children in the middle quintile, and 3.1 times greater odds than those in the highest quintile (Figure 6).

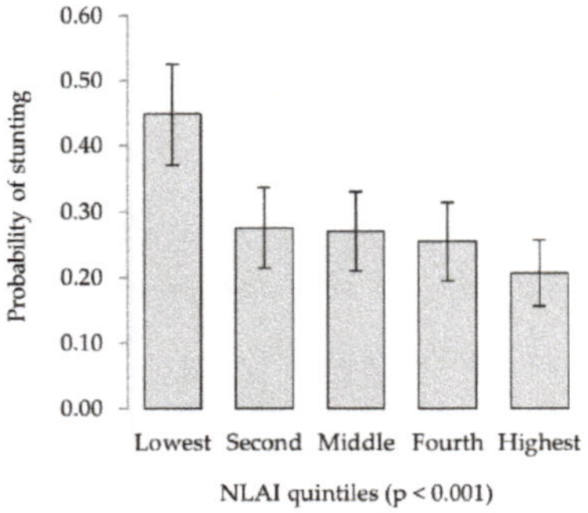

Figure 6. The non-livestock asset index was significantly associated with the probability of child stunting, with a significantly higher likelihood identified amongst the lowest wealth quintile ($p < 0.001$).

Table 5. Multivariable models for height-for-age Z-scores (HAZ) [a], probability of stunting (HAZ < −2) [b] and diarrhea frequency [b] in children, showing *p*-values and the direction of significant ($p < 0.05$) and suggestive ($0.05 \leq p < 0.1$) associations. Grey shading indicates significant and suggestive associations in univariable models (Table A3), and "NS" denotes non-significant associations in final multivariable models.

Predictor Variables	HAZ	Stunting	Diarrhea
Child age	<0.001 (−)	<0.001 (+)	<0.001 (−)
Sex of child, female	0.022 (+)	0.002 (−)	NS
Diarrhea frequency	<0.001 (−)	NS	N/A
Height-for-age Z-score	N/A	N/A	NS
Month of data collection, May [c]	NS	NS	NS
Sex of household head, female	NS	NS	NS
Number of household members	NS	NS	NS
Maternal formal education, yes	NS	NS	NS
Household language group, Sukuma	<0.001 (+)	0.002 (−)	NS
Improved water source	NS	NS	NS
Improved toilet facility	NS	NS	NS
Household domestic asset index			
Livestock and non-livestock assets [d]	NS	NS	NS
Non-livestock assets only [d]	NS	<0.001 (−) [f]	NS
Non-livestock assets only, quintiles	0.009 (+)	<0.001 (−) [f]	NS
Livestock			
Livestock owned, yes	NS	NS	NS
"Livestock ladder" [e]	NS	NS	NS
Chickens owned, yes	NS	NS	NS
Chickens, above median	NS	NS	NS
Chickens, number owned [d]	NS	NS	NS
Chickens, location of overnight housing	NS	NS	NS
Sheep or goats owned, yes	NS	NS	NS
Sheep or goats, above median	NS	NS	NS
Sheep or goats, number owned [d]	NS	NS	NS
Cattle owned, yes	NS	NS	0.014 (−)
Cattle, above median	NS	NS	NS
Cattle, number owned [d]	NS	NS	NS
Children's diet, previous 24 h			
ASF consumption, yes	NS	NS	NS
Chicken meat consumption, yes	NS	NS	0.059 (−)
Other meat or fish consumption, yes	NS	NS	NS
Egg consumption, yes	NS	NS	NS
Milk consumption, yes	NS	NS	0.007 (+)

[a] Linear mixed models, allowing for geographic clustering and longitudinal data; [a] Generalized linear mixed models using binomial distribution, allowing for geographic clustering and longitudinal data; [c] log-transformed variables used to minimize excessive influence of large numbers; [d] Two data collection months: May and November. Rainfall typically occurs between November and April in this area.; [e] Levels of livestock ownership (the "livestock ladder"): (1) none, (2) chickens only, (3) small ruminants +/− chickens, no cattle, (4) cattle +/− chickens and small ruminants; [f] Two alternative models were constructed, one using the NLAI as a continuous variable and one using the NLAI as quintiles, each together with the age and sex of child and household language group (*p*-values for these latter variables remained unchanged).

Multivariable models revealed a significantly lower likelihood of diarrhea with increasing child age ($p < 0.001$). Ownership of cattle was associated with a small but significant reduction in the probability of child diarrhea ($p = 0.021$), with a 0.036 probability of diarrhea in a given fortnight for a child in a cattle-owning household, compared to a 0.045 probability in a household without cattle (Figure 7a). Controlling for child age and cattle ownership, however, milk consumption was linked to an increased probability of diarrhea ($p = 0.007$), based on a single 24-h dietary assessment conducted in each six-month period of diarrhea records (Figure 7b). There was also a suggestive association ($p = 0.059$) between consumption of chicken meat and a lower probability of child diarrhea. When variables related to chicken-keeping were tested in the same model, no significant difference in the number of records of child diarrhea was evident according to chicken ownership ($p = 0.305$), chicken flock size ($p = 0.498$), or the practice of keeping chickens inside the home overnight ($p = 0.550$).

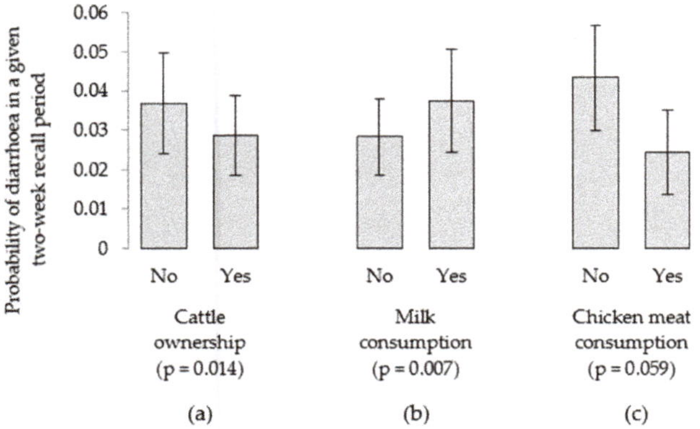

Figure 7. Probability of child diarrhea being reported in a given two-week period, according to (**a**) household cattle ownership, and (**b**) children's consumption of milk or (**c**) chicken meat the previous day.

4. Discussion

4.1. Seasonal and Temporal Variation in Diets

The opportunity to detect seasonal influences on diets has been limited by the two-year span of data. Seasonality is a key determinant of dietary adequacy in many vulnerable rural households, yet is sometimes overlooked in dietary assessments [52]. In this setting, where rain-fed agriculture is the predominant source of income and food, there is a risk of food shortage between the depletion of one year's cereal stocks and the following year's harvest. Poultry mortality due to disease outbreaks, with signs consistent with Newcastle disease, are most common between July and November in this area [53] and may also contribute to seasonal fluctuations in the availability of food resources and assets.

Of the months when dietary assessments were conducted, May would typically be a time of greater food availability (due to recently-harvested crops and associated income, and a lower risk of chicken mortality) and November a time of food scarcity for less resilient households (when crop supplies have been depleted, income-earning opportunities are scarce, and losses due to Newcastle disease likely amongst unvaccinated chicken flocks). However, daily rainfall records indicate the 2014–2015 rain season to have been particularly poor, with a total rainfall of 447 mm (30 days) in Sanza Ward and 275 mm (21 days) in Majiri Ward, substantially lower than the long-term mean annual rainfall of 624 mm (49 days) for the district [39]. A poor harvest is likely to have resulted in lower dietary diversity in May 2015 than would be common at this time of year.

While graphical summaries suggest increasing levels of dietary adequacy over time (Figure 5), this is likely to reflect diversification of children's diets with age ($p < 0.001$). Increasing age was associated with higher DD scores and a higher probability of dietary adequacy amongst breastfed children, but this did not continue beyond the point of weaning. Multivariable models, controlling for children's age, confirm the month of assessment to be highly significantly associated with dietary diversity scores, dietary adequacy and milk consumption for children and their mothers (Table 3) reflecting the expected improved diets in May compared to November.

4.2. Chicken-Keeping and Diets

Egg consumption was documented in only 3.2% of all records for breastfed children, 2.1% for women and 1.6% for non-breastfed children—even lower than the 5.2% reported amongst children under two years in the most recent national dietary assessment [54]. Associations between egg consumption and household wealth, but not chicken-keeping, suggest it is the financial capacity to purchase eggs through markets—rather than access to eggs from their own hens—which determined consumption frequency during this period. This supports findings elsewhere in African communities accustomed to high levels of mortality in scavenging chicken flocks, where households prioritize the hatching of eggs for replacement stock and retention of chickens for sale in times over home consumption [55,56]. Previous qualitative work in the study setting found no currently-held beliefs or cultural constraints to explain provide other explanations for infrequent egg consumption [57].

A significant increase in the likelihood of breastfed children consuming chicken meat with increasing chicken flock size, and a suggestive increase in the case of women, is encouraging. It is likely that initial unconditional associations between larger chicken flocks and improved dietary outcomes (such as higher DD scores) are due to flock size acting as a proxy for socioeconomic status. The significance of this association disappeared in a majority of the multivariable models, as alternative measures of household wealth were included. One exception to this was the finding of a greater likelihood of women consuming ASF with increasing numbers of chickens and cattle, but not with wealth estimation based on other assets.

In the case of cattle, this effect is likely to reflect access to milk (as shown in the specific model for milk consumption). Based on low levels of chicken meat and egg consumption, however, alternative mechanisms through which women's ASF consumption might benefit from chicken ownership should be considered. Motivations for chicken-keeping in resource-poor settings include opportunities to store wealth in a form which is readily-accessible to meet immediate household needs, including education and medical expenses, and items such as cooking oil, soap or clothing for children [55]. It may also be the case that, even if poultry products are rarely eaten at home, the sale of chickens may facilitate access to other forms of ASFs—fresh or dried fish, other forms of meat, or milk—through local markets.

4.3. Livestock and Child Growth

For 39.6% of study participants, livestock constituted more than three-quarters of their household's wealth, yet none of the measures of livestock-keeping tested were associated with children's height-for-age. It was notable that a reduced probability of stunting was associated with the non-livestock asset index, but not with the combined measure of livestock and non-livestock wealth. The concept of the "livestock ladder" emphasizes the role of livestock-keeping in poverty alleviation [32], and posits that increasing economic benefits are derived from keeping larger livestock species [58]. Since no negative associations between animal ownership and stunting were found, the observed dilution effect of including livestock in estimations of wealth indicate that these suggested economic benefits have not translated to improved growth outcomes for children in this setting during the study period.

Livestock-keeping in resource-poor settings is often not oriented towards production for market [6]. Animals represent financial savings and, particularly in the case of cattle, social status. Animal numbers may increase through the retention of offspring, adding to household wealth, but such assets may contribute little to children's diets and growth. In this study, the non-livestock asset index was based on items such as mobile phones, radios, and bicycles, which demonstrate past expenditure and may serve as a better proxy for households' purchasing behavior. A demonstrated association between this index and lower levels of stunting may reflect the utilization of economic resources to address underlying determinants of nutritional status, through nutritious food purchases, medical expenses or an improved home environment.

This argument is countered by the finding of increased milk consumption by children with increasing numbers of cattle, signifying greater access to a food item which has been shown to improve linear growth amongst stunted children [59]. Quantitative dietary assessments were not conducted, but the volume of milk consumed is likely to be relatively low in this setting, particularly in times of limited feed and water availability for cattle, and perhaps insufficient to influence growth. It is also possible that the lack of significance of cattle ownership for child height-for-age may signify the net effect of nutritional benefits of increased milk consumption being counteracted by undocumented adverse impacts, such as EED.

4.4. Livestock and Child Diarrhea

Twice-monthly records of child diarrhea and information on chicken numbers and housing location have provided an opportunity to explore associations more deeply than has been possible through analyses based on multi-purpose national surveys [24,27]. Keeping chickens inside human dwellings overnight is a common practice in this project setting, reported by over two-thirds (64.2%) of chicken-keeping households and more than a third (35.3%) of all those with a child enrolled in this study. Chicken houses may be damaged or destroyed by heavy rainfall during the wet season, and there is often little incentive to construct or repair these facilities when rates of chicken mortality are high and poultry-keeping is not a priority livelihood activity.

When relationships were tested between longitudinal child diarrhea records and households' ownership of chickens, chicken flock size and the location of overnight chicken housing, no significant associations were identified. In the case of cattle, ownership was associated with a small but significantly lower probability of diarrhea; however, milk consumption the previous day was linked to an increased incidence of child diarrhea. The potential for milk contamination with zoonotic pathogens or aflatoxins [60–62] to have negatively affected linear growth [24], cannot be excluded and, although highly speculative within this study, warrants closer investigation.

In a setting where infants and young children commonly accompany their mother to agricultural plots or are left in the care of older siblings, neighbors or relatives, opportunities for exposure to poultry feces within the homestead or broader environment are frequent, and not restricted to those households keeping chickens. It is therefore possible that free-ranging village chickens present an opportunity for "community-wide" adverse child health impacts which have not been detected in this study.

4.5. Gender and Nutrition

Much attention is given to the role of women as key mediators of agriculture-nutrition linkages. Consideration of the gender of the "household head" has attracted some criticism, because of the ambiguity in defining this role, its implication of a hierarchical relationship, and the common gender bias whereby the oldest male household member is taken as the "head" [63,64]. Assumptions about vulnerability based on this concept have also been questioned, with female-headed households at very low levels of income in Kenya shown to adopt successful coping strategies and achieve higher weight-for-age of preschool-aged children than wealthier male- and female-headed households [65]. In the present study, both women and their breastfed children were more likely to consume eggs in households identifying as female-headed. This may reflect women's greater autonomy in decision-making or differing priorities for resource allocation, compared to male-headed households.

There were no significant gender-based differences in breastfed children's diets; however, amongst non-breastfed children, boys were more likely than girls to receive an adequately diverse diet and to consume ASF. Preferential treatment of sons over daughters has been commonly reported in ethnographic and demographic research [66]. Studies in South Asia indicate that biased food allocation which favors male children is more apparent amongst higher wealth groups, and least evident amongst the very poor [67]. A puzzling situation exists in this study where male children were associated with some improved dietary indicators, and also with lower HAZ and a higher probability of stunting, compared with female children.

Gender-based differences in stunting, with poorer growth amongst boys, have been reported in several studies in sub-Saharan Africa [68–70]. The cause of this disparity is not well understood, particularly given that cases of female-biased parental investment have been rarely documented [66].

A meta-analysis of 60 national surveys from sub-Saharan Africa found no evidence of gender-based differences in breastfeeding duration or maternal health-seeking behaviors, based on rates of vaccination and the use of oral rehydration therapy [71]. The authors contended that biological differences (a concept not further elaborated in the review) may account for gender-based inequalities in the prevalence of stunting. The current study's finding of improved growth outcomes for girls, despite evidence of dietary practices which favor male children, appears to support this theory.

4.6. Limitations of This Study

Low and abnormally-timed rainfall over two consecutive rain seasons resulted in an unforeseen level of mobility amongst participating households, with a drastically reduced harvest prompting some to relocate outside the area to pursue alternative livelihood strategies. This contributed to an attrition rate of 16.9% over the study period. The potential for attrition-related bias, in which the characteristics of those lost to follow-up is associated with the outcome of interest, has been suggested as a consideration for losses of between 5–20% of participants [72]. With increasing weather variability in the future, studies of populations reliant on rain-fed agriculture should adjust sample size calculations in recognition of the potential for increased participant drop-out, and consider the implications of more vulnerable, resource-poor segments of a population being lost from the study.

A further limitation of this study has been the reliance on self-report of diarrhea. Recall periods of longer than two days have been associated with under-reporting of diarrhea, particularly milder episodes and amongst older children [73]. Given the regularity of data collection over an extended period in this study, the influence of respondent or enumerator fatigue is possible. However, the potential biases of inaccurate recall and recording are considered to be systemic and unlikely to influence associations between diarrhea frequency and livestock ownership. The use of well-regarded community members for ongoing data collection and monthly field visits by the Tanzanian research team are hoped to have contributed to maintaining positive relationships with study participants, and avoiding the pitfalls of "parachute research" [74].

5. Conclusions

The potential for livestock-keeping to sustainably improve food and nutrition security has long been recognized, yet (as for other agricultural interventions [75]) impact has been notoriously difficult to demonstrate. To address the key question of whether chicken-keeping has an impact on the growth of young children in this setting, use of height-for-age as an outcome measure sought to encompass multiple dimensions of children's health, development, and environment. On balance, there were no significant associations between HAZ and chicken ownership, when the latter was defined (a) as a dichotomous categorical variable, (b) using a threshold approach, (c) in terms of chicken flock size, and (d) accounting for overnight housing location. While the potential for community-wide effects related to free-roaming poultry cannot be ruled out, this study importantly (and of substantial practical significance if confirmed) found no indication of a heightened risk of stunting or greater frequency of diarrhea being associated with chicken ownership or the practice of keeping chickens within human dwellings overnight.

Livestock ownership was closely linked to socioeconomic status in this population; however, controlling for other forms of wealth, analyses have detected no influence of any categories of livestock on children's growth. This raises questions as to whether the economic benefits of climbing the "livestock ladder" translate into nutritional benefits for children, yet methodological constraints and challenging weather patterns during the study period must be acknowledged. Alongside two years of poor rainfall and dramatic crop losses, it is likely that the multiple and diverse household needs met by livestock-keeping have not included adequate ASF consumption or dietary diversification to influence children's growth during this time.

Chicken ownership was significantly associated with more frequent consumption of ASF by women and chicken meat by young children. Although chicken-keeping was not a significant determinant of additional dietary outcomes, contributions to socioeconomic status and resilience should not be overlooked. Improved water, sanitation and hygiene practices are central to efforts to reduce stunting; however, there is a need for careful consideration before warning against livestock ownership by vulnerable households or proposing substantial changes in livestock management practices. For example, confining chickens to enclosures will increase production costs and labor inputs, particularly for women, and will reduce their accessibility to poor families.

As efforts to support rural households to enhance dietary quality continue, questions about the complex and multiple linkages between livestock and human nutrition will endure. In this study, findings of no net benefit of cattle ownership on child growth despite a strong positive association with milk consumption warrant further investigation using mixed-methods approaches. While contributions of chicken-keeping to diets were limited during the study period, it is encouraging that no adverse impacts have been found. Integrated, multi-sectoral approaches will be central to increasing chicken flock size in vulnerable households, building resilience in the face of increasing weather variability, and developing nutritional messaging to promote home consumption of chicken meat and eggs, in order to harness the nutritional potential of chicken-keeping in support of children's growth and development.

Funding: This study was funded by the Australian Centre for International Agricultural Research (ACIAR; project FSC/2012/023). Financial support for open-access publication was provided by the Natural Resources Institute of the University of Greenwich, United Kingdom.

Acknowledgments: The authors gratefully acknowledge the support of the Government of Tanzania, and all partners involved in the development and implementation of this research. Particular thanks is given to those involved in the study design and research tool development, including Judy Simpson, Mu Li and Robyn McConchie (University of Sydney); and project implementation, including Geofrey Kiswaga (Manyoni District Council), Elpidius Rukambile and Msafiri Kalloka (Tanzania Veterinary Laboratory Agency), Elizabeth Lyimo (Tanzania Food and Nutrition Centre) and Deorinidei Mng'ong'o (Manyoni District Hospital). We would especially like to thank the women, children and households participating in this research, as well as local leaders and enumerators.

Conflicts of Interest: The authors declare no conflict of interest. The founding sponsors had no role in the design of the study; in the collection, analyses, or interpretation of data; in the writing of the manuscript, and in the decision to publish the results.

Abbreviations

EED	environmental enteric dysfunction
HAZ	height-for-age
mo	months of age
DD	dietary diversity
MDD-W	Minimum Dietary Diversity for Women of Reproductive Age
IYCMDD	Infant and Young Child Minimum Dietary Diversity
HDAI	Household Domestic Asset Index
NLAI	Non-Livestock Asset Index
LMIC	low- to middle-income country

Appendix A

Table A1. Descriptions for predictor and outcome variables evaluated.

	Variable(s)	Description
Child	Age	• From maternal recall; verified against clinic health records if available
	Gender	• Male or female
	HAZ	• From six-monthly length or height measurements [41]
	Diarrhea score	• From ratio of positive records of diarrhea, as reported by child's mother or primary caretaker, to total number of records per child
Mother and child	Dietary diversity	• Number of food groups reported as consumed by mothers (of 10 groups [40]) and children (of 7 groups [43]) during day or night prior to interview
	Dietary adequacy	• Dichotomous variable, based on minimum cut-offs for women (≥5 of 10 food groups [40]) and children (≥4 of 7 groups [43])
	ASF consumption	• Dichotomous variables, according to reports of food consumed during the day or night prior to interview. Categories considered are eggs, chicken meat, other meat and fish, and milk.
Household demographics	Maternal age	• Based on mother's recall, or calculated from self-reported date of birth if age unknown
	Maternal formal education	• Dichotomous variable for no formal education vs. some level of primary or secondary school education
	Household size	• Total number of household members, with a household defined as people living together and sharing food at least three days of each week for the previous six months [45].
	Household head	• Male or female, as reported by questionnaire respondent (any household member > 16 years of age; intended even numbers of men and women).
	Household language group	• Dichotomous variable distinguishing the *Kisukuma* language group from other groups; determined from the first language ("mother tongue") of both parents of enrolled children and the gender of the household head.
Water and sanitation	Water source	• Categorized as improved or unimproved [49]
	Toilet facility	• Categorized as improved or unimproved [49]
Socioeconomic status	Household Domestic Assets Index (HDAI)	• Weighted sum of livestock and non-livestock assets, according to their relative value using a system developed for use in sub-Saharan Africa [46] • *For dietary models:* Chickens and cattle were excluded from the HDAI, to test their association with dietary outcomes separately.
	Non-Livestock Asset Index (NLAI)	• Weighted sum of non-livestock assets only [46] • *For stunting and diarrhea models:* NLAI used rather than HDAI, to control for non-livestock wealth while testing a range of livestock variables separately as predictors of growth and diarrhea in children.
Livestock ownership	Livestock ownership	• Dichotomous variable (yes / no) for owning any form of livestock
	Cattle ownership	1. Dichotomous variable (yes / no) for owning cattle 2. Dichotomous variable for owning more or less than the median number of cattle in this population (i.e., > 7 vs. ≤ 7) 3. Number of cattle owned.
	Small ruminant ownership	1. Dichotomous variable (yes / no) for owning sheep or goats 2. Dichotomous variable for owning more or less than the median number of sheep or goats in this population (i.e., > 11 vs. ≤ 11) 3. Number of sheep or goats owned
	Chicken ownership	*For dietary models*, based on chicken ownership during the month of dietary assessment. *For stunting and diarrhea models*, based on ownership over the six-month periods preceding each round of anthropometry. In both cases: 1. Dichotomous variable (yes / no) for owning chickens 2. Dichotomous variable for owning more or less than the median number of sheep or goats in this population (i.e., >11 vs. ≤11) 3. Number of sheep or goats owned

Appendix B

Table A2. Univariable models [a] evaluating the significance of predictor variables for maternal and child dietary adequacy, dietary diversity and ASF consumption, showing p-values and the direction of associations (+/−). Grey shading indicates all suggestive associations ($p < 0.1$).

Predictor Variables	Dietary Adequacy	DD Score [b]	ASF Consumption			
			Any	Chicken	Egg	Milk
(a) Mothers						
Month of dietary assessment, May	<0.001 (+)	<0.001 (+)	<0.001(+)	0.694	0.343	<0.001 (+)
Maternal age	0.393	0.299	0.043 (−)	0.976	0.423	0.157
Maternal formal education, yes	0.090 (+)	0.095 (+)	0.939	0.465	0.959	0.239
Breastfeeding, yes	<0.001 (−)	< 0.001 (−)	0.022 (−)	0.887	0.018 (+)	0.377
Sex of household head, female	0.502	0.725	0.284	0.428	0.015 (+)	0.004 (−)
Number of household members	0.815	0.944	0.864	0.213	0.689	0.016 (+)
Language group, Sukuma	0.484	0.118	0.001 (+)	0.120	0.486	<0.001 (+)
Household domestic asset index [c,d]	<0.001 (+)	<0.001 (+)	<0.001 (+)	0.024 (+)	0.005 (+)	<0.001 (+)
Chickens owned, yes	0.004 (+)	0.003 (+)	0.003 (+)	0.036 (+)	0.685	0.011 (+)
Chickens, above median number	<0.001 (+)	0.009 (+)	0.011 (+)	0.463	0.148	0.003 (+)
Chickens, number owned [c]	<0.001 (+)	<0.001 (+)	<0.001 (+)	0.013 (+)	0.159	<0.001 (+)
Cattle owned, yes	0.003 (+)	0.002 (+)	<0.001 (+)	0.251	0.146	<0.001 (+)
Cattle, above median number	0.167	0.053 (+)	0.003 (+)	0.418	0.305	<0.001 (+)
Cattle, number owned [c]	0.003 (+)	0.001 (+)	<0.001 (+)	0.137	0.070 (+)	<0.001 (+)
(b) Breastfed children						
Month of dietary assessment, May	<0.001 (+)	<0.001 (+)	0.655	0.149	0.458	0.021
Child age	<0.001 (+)	<0.001 (+)	0.043 (+)	0.224	0.158	0.152
Sex of child, female	0.196	0.998	0.425	0.929	0.865	0.304
Child height-for-age Z-score	0.518	0.192	0.623	0.256	0.588	0.372
Maternal formal education, yes	0.673	0.517	0.460	0.134	0.326	0.680
Sex of household head, female	0.656	0.518	0.559	0.513	0.106	0.113
Number of household members	0.075 (+)	0.142	0.361	0.591	0.391	0.018 (+)
Language group, Sukuma	0.015 (+)	0.103	0.002 (+)	0.260	0.127	<0.001 (+)
Household domestic asset index [c,d]	<0.001 (+)	0.002 (+)	<0.001 (+)	0.162	0.214	<0.001 (+)
Chickens owned, yes	0.012 (+)	0.004 (+)	0.008 (+)	0.104	0.242	0.013 (+)
Chickens, above median number	0.005 (+)	<0.001 (+)	0.004 (+)	0.162	0.178	0.003 (+)
Chickens, number owned [c]	0.003 (+)	<0.001 (+)	<0.001 (+)	0.016 (+)	0.104	0.008 (+)
Cattle owned, yes	0.004 (+)	0.025 (+)	<0.001 (+)	0.181	N/A	<0.001 (+)
Cattle, above median number	<0.001 (+)	0.020 (+)	<0.001 (+)	0.289	0.704	<0.001 (+)
Cattle, number owned [c]	<0.001 (+)	0.004 (+)	<0.001 (+)	0.182	0.048 (+)	<0.001 (+)
(c) Non-breastfed children						
Month of dietary assessment, May	<0.001 (+)	<0.001 (+)	0.003 (+)	0.849	0.834	<0.001 (+)
Child age	0.138	0.023 (+)	0.884	0.163	0.045 (−)	0.950
Sex of child, female	0.123	0.180	0.015 (−)	0.799	0.328	0.288
Child height-for-age Z-score	0.044 (+)	0.060 (+)	0.568	0.434	0.976	0.323
Maternal formal education, yes	0.165	0.237	0.332	0.536	0.968	0.212
Sex of household head, female	0.307	0.892	0.565	0.482	0.266	0.082 (−)
Number of household members	0.789	0.709	0.924	0.080 (+)	0.185	0.116
Language group, Sukuma	0.289	0.063 (+)	0.003 (+)	0.231	0.751	<0.001 (+)
Household domestic asset index [c,d]	0.667	0.098 (+)	0.287	0.365	0.075 (+)	0.004 (+)
Chickens owned, yes	0.215	0.119	0.375	0.402	0.654	0.145
Chickens, above median number	0.725	0.097 (+)	0.169	0.998	0.432	0.021 (+)
Chickens, number owned [c]	0.361	0.025 (+)	0.056 (+)	0.521	0.103	0.007 (+)
Cattle owned, yes	0.491	0.111	0.090 (+)	0.600	0.629	<0.001 (+)
Cattle, above median number	0.768	0.531	0.051 (+)	N/A	0.554	<0.001 (+)
Cattle, number owned [c]	0.780	0.124	0.024 (+)	0.846	0.517	<0.001 (+)

[a] Generalized linear mixed models using binomial distribution, allowing for geographic clustering and longitudinal data; [b] Binomial totals of 10 for women (MDD-W) and 7 for children (IYCMDD); [c] log-transformed variables used to minimize excessive influence of large numbers; [d] Cattle and chickens excluded from HDAI, evaluated as separate predictor variables.

Table A3. Univariable models evaluating the significance of predictor variables for height-for-age Z-scores (HAZ) [a], probability of stunting (HAZ < −2) [b] and diarrhea frequency [b] in children, showing *p*-values and the direction of associations (+/−). Grey shading indicates all suggestive associations ($p < 0.1$).

Predictor Variables	HAZ	Stunting	Diarrhea
Child age	<0.001 (−)	<0.001 (+)	<0.001 (−)
Sex of child, female	0.006 (+)	0.003 (−)	0.681
Diarrhea frequency	0.004 (−)	0.558	N/A
Height-for-age Z-score	N/A	N/A	0.641
Month of data collection, May [c]	<0.001 (−)	0.011 (+)	0.031 (−)
Sex of household head, female	0.126	0.495	0.995
Number of household members	0.761	0.504	0.808
Maternal formal education, yes	0.794	0.305	0.351
Household language group, Sukuma	<0.001 (+)	0.001 (−)	0.512
Improved water source	0.312	0.627	0.298
Improved toilet facility	0.555	0.945	0.618
Household domestic asset index			
Livestock and non-livestock assets [d]	0.205	0.061 (−)	0.072 (−)
Non-livestock assets only [d]	0.076 (+)	<0.001 (−)	0.828
Non-livestock assets only, quintiles	<0.001 (+)	<0.001 (−)	0.558
Livestock			
Livestock owned, yes	0.086 (−)	0.368	0.327
"Livestock ladder" [e]	0.134	0.467	0.259
Chickens owned, yes	0.214	0.925	0.128
Chickens, above median	0.002 (−)	0.109	0.479
Chickens, number owned [d]	0.007 (−)	0.424	0.252
Chickens, location of overnight housing	0.651	0.692	0.101
Sheep or goats owned, yes	0.618	0.919	0.302
Sheep or goats, above median	0.121	0.035 (−)	0.398
Sheep or goats, number owned [d]	0.100 (+)	0.260	0.513
Cattle owned, yes	0.392	0.541	0.046 (−)
Cattle, above median	0.340	0.060 (−)	0.385
Cattle, number owned [d]	0.125	0.223	0.151
Children's diet, previous 24 h			
ASF consumption, yes	0.075 (−)	0.405	0.367
Chicken meat consumption, yes	0.181	0.324	0.050 (−)
Other meat or fish consumption, yes	0.001 (−)	0.531	0.473
Egg consumption, yes	0.587	0.814	0.584
Milk consumption, yes	0.084 (+)	0.554	0.042 (+)

[a] Linear mixed models, allowing for geographic clustering and longitudinal data; [b] Generalized linear mixed models using binomial distribution, allowing for geographic clustering and longitudinal data; [c] Two data collection months: May and November. Rainfall typically occurs between November and April in this area.; [d] log-transformed variables used to minimize excessive influence of large numbers; [e] Levels of livestock ownership (the "livestock ladder"): (1) none, (2) chickens only, (3) small ruminants +/− chickens, no cattle, (4) cattle +/− chickens and small ruminants.

References

1. Thornton, P.K.; Herrero, M. Adapting to climate change in the mixed crop and livestock farming systems in sub-Saharan Africa. *Nat. Clim. Chang.* **2015**, *5*, 830–836. [CrossRef]
2. Altieri, M.A.; Nicholls, C.I.; Henao, A.; Lana, M.A. Agroecology and the design of climate change-resilient farming systems. *Agron. Sustain. Dev.* **2015**, *35*, 869–890. [CrossRef]
3. Seo, S.N. Is an integrated farm more resilient against climate change? A micro-econometric analysis of portfolio diversification in African agriculture. *Food Policy* **2010**, *35*, 32–40. [CrossRef]
4. Murphy, S.P.; Allen, L.H. Nutritional importance of animal source foods. *J. Nutr.* **2003**, *133*, 3932S–3935S. [CrossRef] [PubMed]
5. Neumann, C.G.; Harris, D.M.; Rogers, L.M. Contribution of animal source foods in improving diet quality and function in children in the developing world. *Nutr. Res.* **2002**, *22*, 193–220. [CrossRef]

6. Randolph, T.F.; Ruel, M.; Schelling, E.; Grace, D.; Nicholson, C.F.; Leroy, J.L.; Cole, D.C.; Demment, M.W.; Omore, A.; Zinsstag, J. Invited review: Role of livestock in human nutrition and health for poverty reduction in developing countries. *J. Anim. Sci.* **2007**, *85*, 2788–2800. [CrossRef] [PubMed]
7. Penakalapati, G.; Swarthout, J.; Delahoy, M.J.; McAliley, L.; Wodnik, B.; Levy, K.; Freeman, M.C. Exposure to animal feces and human health: A systematic review and proposed research priorities. *Environ. Sci. Technol.* **2017**, *51*, 11537–11552. [CrossRef] [PubMed]
8. Zambrano, L.D.; Levy, K.; Menezes, N.P.; Freeman, M.C. Human diarrhea infections associated with domestic animal husbandry: A systematic review and meta-analysis. *Trans. R. Soc. Trop. Med. Hyg.* **2014**, *108*, 313–325. [CrossRef] [PubMed]
9. Crane, R.J.; Jones, K.D.; Berkley, J.A. Environmental enteric dysfunction: An overview. *Food Nutr. Bull.* **2015**, *36*, S76–S87. [CrossRef] [PubMed]
10. Mbuya, M.N.; Humphrey, J.H. Preventing environmental enteric dysfunction through improved water, sanitation and hygiene: An opportunity for stunting reduction in developing countries. *Matern. Child Nutr.* **2016**, *12*, 106–120. [CrossRef] [PubMed]
11. Ngure, F.M.; Reid, B.M.; Humphrey, J.H.; Mbuya, M.N.; Pelto, G.; Stoltzfus, R.J. Water, sanitation, and hygiene (WASH), environmental enteropathy, nutrition, and early child development: Making the links. *Ann. N. Y. Acad. Sci.* **2014**, *1308*, 118–128. [CrossRef] [PubMed]
12. Harper, K.M.; Mutasa, M.; Prendergast, A.J.; Humphrey, J.; Manges, A.R. Environmental enteric dysfunction pathways and child stunting: A systematic review. *PLoS Negl. Trop. Dis.* **2018**, *12*, e0006205. [CrossRef] [PubMed]
13. Fierstein, J.L.; Eliasziw, M.; Rogers, B.L.; Forrester, J.E. Nonnative cattle ownership, diet, and child height-for-age: Evidence from the 2011 Uganda Demographic and Health Survey. *Am. J. Trop. Med. Hyg.* **2017**, *96*, 74–82. [CrossRef] [PubMed]
14. Glatz, P.; Pym, R. Poultry housing and management in developing countries. In *Poultry Development Review*; FAO: Rome, Italy, 2013; pp. 24–28, ISBN 978-92-5-108067-2.
15. Guèye, E.F. Village egg and fowl meat production in Africa. *World's Poult. Sci. J.* **1998**, *54*, 73–86. [CrossRef]
16. Aini, I. Indigenous chicken production in South-East Asia. *World's Poult. Sci. J.* **1990**, *46*, 51–57. [CrossRef]
17. Sonaiya, E.B. Direct assessment of nutrient resources in free-range and scavenging systems. *World's Poult. Sci. J.* **2004**, *60*, 523–535. [CrossRef]
18. Bagnol, B. Gender issues in small-scale family poultry production: Experiences with Newcastle Disease and Highly Pathogenic Avian Influenza control. *World's Poult. Sci. J.* **2009**, *65*, 231–240. [CrossRef]
19. Guèye, E.F. Gender aspects in family poultry management systems in developing countries. *World's Poult. Sci. J.* **2005**, *61*, 39–46. [CrossRef]
20. Guèye, E.F. Women and family poultry production in rural Africa. *Dev. Pract.* **2000**, *10*, 98–102. [CrossRef] [PubMed]
21. Ruel, M.T.; Alderman, H. Nutrition-sensitive interventions and programmes: How can they help to accelerate progress in improving maternal and child nutrition? *Lancet* **2013**, *382*, 536–551. [CrossRef]
22. World Bank. *From Agriculture to Nutrition: Pathways, Synergies and Outcomes*; World Bank: Washington, DC, USA, 2007.
23. Headey, D.; Hirvonen, K. Is exposure to poultry harmful to child nutrition? An observational analysis for rural Ethiopia. *PLoS ONE* **2016**, *11*, e0160590. [CrossRef] [PubMed]
24. Headey, D.; Nguyen, P.; Kim, S.; Rawat, R.; Ruel, M.; Menon, P. Is exposure to animal feces harmful to child nutrition and health outcomes? A multicountry observational analysis. *Am. J. Trop. Med. Hyg.* **2017**, *96*, 961–969. [CrossRef] [PubMed]
25. Hetherington, J.B.; Wiethoelter, A.K.; Negin, J.; Mor, S.M. Livestock ownership, animal source foods and child nutritional outcomes in seven rural village clusters in Sub-Saharan Africa. *Agric. Food Secur.* **2017**, *6*, 9. [CrossRef]
26. Schmidt, W.P.; Boisson, S.; Routray, P.; Bell, M.; Cameron, M.; Torondel, B.; Clasen, T. Exposure to cows is not associated with diarrhoea or impaired child growth in rural Odisha, India: A cohort study. *Epidemiol. Infect.* **2016**, *144*, 53–63. [CrossRef] [PubMed]
27. Headey, D.; Hirvonen, K. Exploring Child Health Risks of Poultry Keeping in Ethiopia: Insights from the 2015 Feed the Future Survey. In *Essp ii Research Note 43*; International Food Policy Research Institute and Ethiopian Development Research Institute: Washington, DC, USA; Addis Ababa, Ethiopia, 2015.

28. Mosites, E.M.; Rabinowitz, P.M.; Thumbi, S.M.; Montgomery, J.M.; Palmer, G.H.; May, S.; Rowhani-Rahbar, A.; Neuhouser, M.L.; Walson, J.L. The relationship between livestock ownership and child stunting in three countries in Eastern Africa using national survey data. *PLoS ONE* **2015**, *10*, e0136686. [CrossRef] [PubMed]
29. Chilonda, P.; Otte, J. Indicators to monitor trends in livestock production at national, regional and international levels. *Livest. Res. Rural Dev.* **2006**, *18*, 117. Available online: http://www.lrrd.org/lrrd18/8/chil18117.htm (accessed on 1 August 2017).
30. Jahnke, H.E. *Livestock Production Systems and Livestock Development in Tropical Africa*; Kieler Wissenschaftsverlag Vauk: Kiel, Germany, 1982.
31. Dolberg, F. A livestock development approach that contributes to poverty alleviation and widespread improvement of nutrition among the poor. *Livestock Res. Rural Dev.* **2001**, *13*, 41. Available online: http://www.lrrd.org/lrrd13/5/dolb135.htm (accessed on 1 August 2017).
32. Maass, B.L.; Chiuri, W.L.; Zozo, R.; Katunga-Musale, D.; Metre, T.K.; Birachi, E. Using the 'livestock ladder' as a means for poor crop–livestock farmers to exit poverty in Sud Kivu province, eastern DR Congo. In *Agro-Ecological Intensification of Agricultural Systems in the African Highlands*; Vanlauwe, B., Asten, P.V., Blomme, G., Eds.; Earthscan, Routledge: London, UK, 2013; pp. 145–155, ISBN 978-0-415-53273-0.
33. Todd, H. Women climbing out of poverty through credit; or what do cows have to do with it? *Livest. Res. Rural Dev.* **1998**, *10*, 45–63.
34. Akinola, L.A.F.; Essien, A. Relevance of rural poultry production in developing countries with special reference to Africa. *World's Poult. Sci. J.* **2011**, *67*, 697–705. [CrossRef]
35. Alders, R.G.; Pym, R.A.E. Village poultry: Still important to millions, eight thousand years after domestication. *World's Poult. Sci. J.* **2009**, *65*, 181–190. [CrossRef]
36. Doran, M.H.; Low, A.R.C.; Kemp, R.L. Cattle as a store of wealth in Swaziland: Implications for livestock development and overgrazing in Eastern and Southern Africa. *Am. J. Agric. Econ.* **1979**, *61*, 41–47. [CrossRef]
37. Moll, H.A.J. Costs and benefits of livestock systems and the role of market and nonmarket relationships. *Agric. Econ.* **2005**, *32*, 181–193. [CrossRef]
38. Alders, R.; Aongola, A.; Bagnol, B.; de Bruyn, J.; Kimboka, S.; Kock, R.; Li, M.; Maulaga, W.; McConchie, R.; Mor, S.; et al. Using a one health approach to promote food and nutrition security in Tanzania and Zambia. *GRF Davos Planet@Risk* **2014**, *2*, 187–190.
39. Lema, M.; Majule, A. Impacts of climate change, variability and adaptation strategies on agriculture in semi arid areas of Tanzania: The case of Manyoni District in Singida Region, Tanzania. *Afr. J. Environ. Sci. Technol.* **2009**, *3*, 206–209.
40. FAO and FHI 360. *Minimum Dietary Diversity for Women: A Guide for Measurement*; FAO and FHI 360: Rome, Italy, 2016.
41. WHO. *Diarrhoeal Disease (Fact Sheet No. 330)*; WHO: Geneva, Switzerland, 2013.
42. WHO Multicentre Growth Reference Study Group. WHO Child Growth Standards based on length/height, weight and age. *Acta Pædiatr. Suppl.* **2006**, *450*, 76–85.
43. WHO. *WHO AnthroPlus for Personal Computers Manual: Software for Assessing Growth of the World's Children and Adolescents*; WHO: Geneva, Switzerland, 2009.
44. WHO. *Indicators for Assessing Infant and Young Child Feeding Practices. Part 1: Definitions*; WHO: Geneva, Switzerland, 2008.
45. Bandoh, D.A.; Kenu, E. Dietary diversity and nutritional adequacy of under-fives in a fishing community in the central region of Ghana. *BMC Nutr.* **2017**, *3*, 2. [CrossRef]
46. Alkire, S.; Meinzen-Dick, R.S.; Peterman, A.; Quisumbing, A.R.; Seymour, G.; Vaz, A. *The Women's Empowerment in Agriculture Index. Oxford Poverty and Human Development Initiative Working Paper No. 58*; University of Oxford: Oxford, UK, 2013.
47. Njuki, J.; Poole, J.; Johnson, N.; Baltenweck, I.; Pali, P.; Lokman, Z.; Mburu, S. *Gender, Livestock and Livelihood Indicators*; International Livestock Research Institute: Nairobi, Kenya, 2011.
48. Mabilia, M. Beliefs and practices in infant feeding among the Wagogo of Chigongwe (Dodoma Rural District), Tanzania: I. Breastfeeding. *Ecol. Food Nutr.* **1996**, *35*, 195–207. [CrossRef] [PubMed]
49. Selemani, I.S.; Eik, L.O.; Holand, Ø.; Ådnøy, T.; Mtengeti, E.; Mushi, D. The role of indigenous knowledge and perceptions of pastoral communities on traditional grazing management in north-western Tanzania. *Afr. J. Agric. Res.* **2012**, *7*, 5537–5547.

50. WHO; UNICEF. *Core Questions on Drinking-Water and Sanitation for Household Surveys*; WHO: Geneva, Switzerland, 2006.
51. Allegretti, A. 'Being Maasai' in markets and trade: The role of ethnicity-based institutions in the livestock market of northern Tanzania. *Nomadic Peoples* **2017**, *21*, 63–86. [CrossRef]
52. Savy, M.; Martin-Prevel, Y.; Traissac, P.; Eymard-Duvernay, S.; Delpeuch, F. Dietary diversity scores and nutritional status of women change during the seasonal food shortage in rural Burkina Faso. *J. Nutr.* **2006**, *136*, 2625–2632. [CrossRef] [PubMed]
53. Buza, J.J.; Mwamuhehe, H.A. Country report: Tanzania. In *Proceedings of SADC Planning Workshop on Newcastle Disease Control in Village Chickens, Maputo, Mozambique, 6–9 March 2000*; Alders, R.G., Spradbrow, P.B., Eds.; Australian Centre for International Agricultural Researc: Canberra, Australia, 2001; pp. 38–42.
54. Ministry of Health Community Development Gender Elderly and Children [Tanzania Mainland] (MoHCDGEC); Ministry of Health [Zanzibar] (MoH). *Tanzania Demographic and Health Survey and Malaria Indicator Survey 2015–16*; MoHCDGEC, MoH, NBS, OCGS and ICF: Dar es Salaam, Tanzania; Rockville, MD, USA, 2016.
55. Guèye, E.F. Employment and income generation through family poultry in low-income food-deficit countries. *World's Poult. Sci. J.* **2002**, *58*, 541–557. [CrossRef]
56. Pym, R.A.E.; Guerne Bleich, E.; Hoffman, I. *The Relative Contribution of Indigenous Chicken Breeds to Poultry Meat and Egg Production and Consumption in the Developing Countries of Africa and Asia. Presentation at XII European Poultry Conference, Verona, Italy, 10–14 September 2006*; CABI: Wallingford, UK, 2006.
57. de Bruyn, J.; Bagnol, B.; Darnton-Hill, I.; Maulaga, W.; Thomson, P.C.; Alders, R. Characterising infant and young child feeding practices and the consumption of poultry products in rural Tanzania: A mixed methods approach. *Matern. Child Nutr.* **2017**, *14*, e12550. [CrossRef] [PubMed]
58. Udo, H.M.J.; Aklilu, H.A.; Phong, L.T.; Bosma, R.H.; Budisatria, I.G.S.; Patil, B.R.; Samdup, D.; Bebe, B.O. Impact of intensification of different types of livestock production in smallholder crop-livestock systems. *Livest. Sci.* **2011**, *139*, 22–29. [CrossRef]
59. Neumann, C.G.; Murphy, S.P.; Gewa, C.; Grillenberger, M.; Bwibo, N.O. Meat supplementation improves growth, cognitive, and behavioral outcomes in Kenyan children. *J. Nutr.* **2007**, *137*, 1119–1123. [CrossRef] [PubMed]
60. Darwish, W.S.; Ikenaka, Y.; Nakayama, S.M.M.; Ishizuka, M. An overview on mycotoxin contamination of foods in Africa. *J. Vet. Med. Sci.* **2014**, *76*, 789–797. [CrossRef] [PubMed]
61. Gizachew, D.; Szonyi, B.; Tegegne, A.; Hanson, J.; Grace, D. Aflatoxin contamination of milk and dairy feeds in the Greater Addis Ababa milk shed, Ethiopia. *Food Control* **2016**, *59*, 773–779. [CrossRef]
62. Knight-Jones, T.; Hang'ombe, M.; Songe, M.; Sinkala, Y.; Grace, D. Microbial contamination and hygiene of fresh cow's milk produced by smallholders in Western Zambia. *Int. J. Environ. Res. Public Health* **2016**, *13*, 737. [CrossRef] [PubMed]
63. Budlender, D. The debate about household headship. *Soc. Dyn.* **2003**, *29*, 48–72. [CrossRef]
64. Rosenhouse Persson, S. *Identifying the Poor: Is "Headship" a Useful Concept? Living Standards Measurement Study Working Paper No. 58*; World Bank: Washington, DC, USA, 1989.
65. Kennedy, E.; Haddad, L. Are pre-schoolers from female-headed households less malnourished? A comparative analysis of results from Ghana and Kenya. *J. Dev. Stud.* **1994**, *30*, 680–695. [CrossRef]
66. Cronk, L. Preferential parental investment in daughters over sons. *Hum. Nat.* **1991**, *2*, 387–417. [CrossRef] [PubMed]
67. Miller, B.D. Social class, gender and intrahousehold food allocations to children in South Asia. *Soc. Sci. Med.* **1997**, *44*, 1685–1695. [CrossRef]
68. Espo, M.; Kulmala, T.; Maleta, K.; Cullinan, T.; Salin, M.L.; Ashorn, P. Determinants of linear growth and predictors of severe stunting during infancy in rural Malawi. *Acta Paediatr.* **2002**, *91*, 1364–1370. [CrossRef] [PubMed]
69. Ngare, D.K.; Muttunga, J.N. Prevalence of malnutrition in Kenya. *East Afr. Med. J.* **1999**, *76*, 376–380. [PubMed]
70. Wamani, H.; Åstrøm, N.; Peterson, S.; Tumwine, J.; Tylleskär, T. Boys are more stunted than girls in sub-Saharan Africa: A meta-analysis of 16 Demographic and Healthy Surveys. *BMC Pediatr.* **2007**, *7*, 17. [CrossRef] [PubMed]
71. Garenne, M. Sex differences in health indicators among children in African DHS surveys. *J. Biosoc. Sci.* **2003**, *35*, 601–614. [CrossRef] [PubMed]

72. Dumville, J.C.; Torgerson, D.J.; Hewitt, C.E. Reporting attrition in randomised controlled trials. *Br. Med. J.* **2006**, *332*, 969–971. [CrossRef] [PubMed]
73. Zafar, S.N.; Luby, S.P.; Mendoza, C. Recall errors in a weekly survey of diarrhoea in Guatemala: Determining the optimal length of recall. *Epidemiol. Infect.* **2009**, *138*, 264–269. [CrossRef] [PubMed]
74. Tomlinson, M.; Swartz, L.; Landman, M. Insiders and outsiders: Levels of collaboration in research partnerships across resource divides. *Infant Ment. Health J.* **2006**, *27*, 532–543. [CrossRef] [PubMed]
75. Webb, P.; Kennedy, E. Impacts of agriculture on nutrition: Nature of the evidence and research gaps. *Food Nutr. Bull.* **2014**, *35*, 126–132. [CrossRef] [PubMed]

nutrients

Article

Socio-Demographic Factors and Body Image Perception Are Associated with BMI-For-Age among Children Living in Welfare Homes in Selangor, Malaysia

Nur Nabilla A Rahim [1], Yit Siew Chin [1,2,*] and Norhasmah Sulaiman [1,2]

1 Department of Nutrition and Dietetics, Faculty of Medicine and Health Sciences, Universiti Putra Malaysia, Malaysia; nabilla022017@gmail.com (N.N.A.R.); norhasmah@upm.edu.my (N.S.)

2 Research Centre of Excellence, Nutrition and Non-Communicable Diseases, Faculty of Medicine and Health Sciences, Universiti Putra Malaysia, 43400 UPM Serdang, Selangor, Malaysia

* Correspondence: chinys@upm.edu.my; Tel.: +60-3-8947-2680

Received: 29 September 2018; Accepted: 25 December 2018; Published: 11 January 2019

Abstract: Considering the double burden of malnutrition in Malaysia, data on malnourished children living in welfare homes are limited. This study aimed to determine the body weight status of children living in welfare homes and its associated factors. A total of 307 children aged 7–17 years old living in 15 selected welfare homes completed a standardized questionnaire, and their body weight and height were measured by trained researchers. There were 54.4% orphans, 23.8% abandoned children, and 21.8% children from problematic families. There were 51.5% boys and 48.5% girls; 52.4% were Malays, followed by 31.3% Indians, 12.7% Chinese, and 3.6% from other ethnic groups. The prevalence of overweight and obesity (23.1%) was higher than the prevalence of thinness (8.5%). In bivariate analyses, socio-demographic factors of age ($p = 0.003$), sex ($p = 0.0001$), ethnicity ($p = 0.001$), and welfare home enrollment status ($p = 0.003$), and psychological factors of self-esteem ($p = 0.003$), body shape dissatisfaction ($p = 0.0001$), and underestimation of body weight status ($p = 0.002$), were significantly associated with body mass index (BMI)-for-age. In the multiple linear regression analysis, children who were either Malays ($\beta = 0.492$) or Chinese ($\beta = 0.678$), with a status of being abandoned ($\beta = 0.409$), with body shape dissatisfaction ($\beta = 0.457$), and underestimated body weight status ($\beta = 0.628$) significantly explained 39.7% of the variances in higher BMI-for-age ($F = 39.550$; $p < 0.05$). Besides socio-demographic background, the current findings emphasized the importance of incorporating body image perception in an obesity prevention intervention program in welfare homes.

Keywords: children; welfare home; body image; obesity; BMI-for-age

1. Introduction

While obesity has become a major nutritional problem worldwide, childhood obesity is a subject matter of priority as it determines obesity in adulthood and increases the risk of adult morbidity and mortality [1]. In a society where most adults, as well as children and adolescents, are attempting to lose weight, it is foreseeable that weight concerns and poor body image perception (body shape dissatisfaction and misperception of body weight status) are common.

Body image is a multidimensional construct encompassing how an individual perceive, think, feel, and act toward one's own body [2], and lies on a continuum from accurate and positive body perceptions to inaccurate and negative body perceptions [2,3]. With the growing concerns of body weight status among children, body dissatisfaction and body image misperception may affect their eating behaviors when they want to achieve an ideal body image and obtain a sense of control of their bodies, which can eventually cause clinical eating disorders and unhealthy body weight status [4,5]. Individuals who have poor body image perception have a low probability of taking part in healthy weight management behaviors; rather, they are more likely to adopt behaviors that could place them at risk of malnutrition and poor health status [6,7].

Body image perception as an associated factor with obesity has been widely discussed in the literature [8–11]. Previous local studies revealed that body shape dissatisfaction and misperception of body weight status were associated with unhealthy body weight status of Malaysian adolescents [12,13]. However, to the best of our knowledge, no prior studies in the related literature have assessed body shape dissatisfaction and misperception of body weight status among children living in welfare home setting. It is crucial to assess body image perception of these children in preventing unrealistic weight goals and unhealthy weight control behaviors, which may affect their growth and development.

A welfare home is considered to provide a foster family for children in need of care, such as orphans, abandoned children, and children from problematic families. In Malaysia, welfare homes are registered under the Social Welfare Department of Malaysia. The legal caregivers in welfare homes protect the children and provide them with basic necessities such as shelter, food, education, clothing, and school equipment. While a double burden of malnutrition is reported in Malaysia [14], data on malnourished children living in welfare homes are very limited. To the best of our knowledge, there are two local studies that reported about malnutrition among children living in welfare homes [15,16]. In 2008, Chee et al. [15] found that the prevalence of undernutrition (21.0%) was about five times higher than the prevalence of overnutrition (4.0%) among 73 children aged six to 17 years old in Kuala Lumpur. However, in 2015, Mohd Dzulkhairi et al. [16] reported that the prevalence of overnutrition (32.1%) was higher than that of undernutrition (6.2%) among 128 children below 18 years old in Selangor and Melaka. There is a shift in the malnutrition trend among children living in welfare homes from undernutrition to overnutrition within the last seven years. In the present study, malnutrition is determined based on body weight status of the children, assessed using z-score of body mass index (BMI)-for-age [14–16].

Children growing up in out-of-home care, such as those living in welfare homes, may have higher risks of adverse physical, emotional, and behavioral-related outcomes, which may further elevate risks of unstable life-course trajectories in later adulthood life [17–20]. As compared to children in the general population, children living in welfare homes have higher rates of chronic health conditions (CHCs) [21], including mental retardation and malnutrition. Similarly, children in the formal foster care were found to have high rates of health and mental health problems [22,23]. While depressive disorders refer to the presence of depression symptoms [24], Turney and Wilderman [22] reported that children placed in foster care have a greater likelihood of having depressive disorders than their counterparts. In addition, a previous study by Gürsoy et al. [25] has shown that children living in orphanages had low self-esteem scores, in which self-esteem reflects a person's overall evaluation or appraisal of one's own worth [26]. In spite of that, the potential association of self-esteem and depressive disorders with body weight status in the welfare home setting has not been explored further.

Previous reports by Chee et al. [15] and Mohd Dzulkhairi et al. [16] were limited to the study of dietary factors in relation to body weight status among girls [15], and knowledge, attitude, and practice with respect to nutritional status [16], respectively. Nevertheless, the inclusion of socio-demographic and psychological factors in the current study may facilitate the development of strategies for the prevention of disease related to nutritional status among children living in welfare homes. Therefore, this study aims to determine the body weight status among children living in welfare homes, and its association with socio-demographic and psychological factors.

2. Materials and Methods

2.1. Study Design and Respondents

This cross-sectional study was carried out in the Selangor state of Malaysia. Respondents of the present study were children living in welfare homes in Selangor, where there were three main categories of children, namely orphans, abandoned children, and children from problematic families. Children from problematic families included those with divorced parents, who lived in poverty, and were formerly abused by members of the family.

Based on the probability proportionate sampling, 524 children from 15 selected welfare homes were invited to participate in the current study. A total of 307 children who fulfilled the inclusion criteria of the study consented to participate in the study. The inclusion criteria of the children for this study were Malaysian, registered children in welfare homes and enrolled school-going children aged from 7 to 17 years old. Meanwhile, this study excluded children with disabilities and children who had physical and mental illnesses based on their health records.

The present study was conducted in accordance with the Declaration of Helsinki. Ethical approval was attained from the Ethics Committee for Research Involving Human Subjects, Universiti Putra Malaysia (UPM/TNCPI/RMC/1.4.18.1 (JKEUPM)/F2). Permissions to conduct this study were obtained from the Department of Social Welfare, Malaysia, and all selected welfare homes. Researchers explained about the study protocol to the children and their caregivers at the selected welfare homes, and informed consents were obtained from both the children and their caregivers. They were informed about their rights to voluntarily withdraw from the study. After getting informed consents from the caregivers and children, anthropometric measurements were taken by trained researchers. Respondents aged 10 years and above were requested to self-administer the questionnaire, whereas respondents aged below 10 years were interviewed by the researchers.

2.2. Study Measurements

2.2.1. Anthropometric Measurements

Body weight and height of respondents were measured with them in light clothing and barefooted using TANITA digital weighing scale Model HD-382 (TANITA Corporation, Japan) to the nearest 0.1 kg, and a portable SECA stadiometer Model 213 (SECA, Germany) to the nearest 0.1 cm, respectively. BMI-for-age (z-score) was determined by using the WHO Anthro- version 1.0.3 software [27]. Body weight status was classified using the WHO Growth Reference for 5-19 years [28].

2.2.2. Socio-Demographic Factors

Caregivers of the welfare homes were interviewed by using a socio-demographic questionnaire requesting information about the date of birth (age), sex, ethnicity, and enrollment status of the respondents.

2.2.3. Psychological Factors

Self-Esteem

Self-esteem was measured using the 10-item Rosenberg Self-Esteem Scale [26]. For items 1, 2, 4, 6 and 7, respondents had to give a score, with 1 = strongly agree, 2 = agree, 3 = disagree, and 4 = strongly disagree. Meanwhile, for items 3, 5, 8, 9 and 10, respondents had to give a score, with 1 = strongly disagree, 2 = disagree, 3 = agree, and 4 = strongly agree. The scores of all items were summed up to obtain the total self-esteem score, which ranged from 10 to 40. The categorization of the level of self-esteem was based on a previous research among children who lived in orphanages in Sharkia governorate [29], whereby a self-esteem score of below 15 signified low self-esteem. The internal consistency of the scale in this study was 0.53.

Depressive Disorders

The respondents' depressive disorders were assessed using the Children Depression Index [30], which is a standardized self-report developed for children and adolescents aged 6–17 years old. The questionnaire used in this study was an adapted version whereby a statement on "I want to kill myself" was removed, as it did not suit the Malaysian and welfare home context. There were 26 items, on a scale from zero (not a problem) to two (severe). The scores for all items were summed up to obtain a total score, which ranged from 0 to 52. A score of 19 and above indicated that the respondent had a higher likelihood of having depressive disorders [31]. The internal consistency of the scale in this study was 0.83.

Perception of Body Shape

A seven-figure Collins' body image silhouette [32] was used to assess the perception of body shape for children aged 7–12 years old, while a nine-figure Contour Drawing Rating Scale [33] was used to assess the perception of body shape for children aged 13–17 years old. Respondents were required to select the figure that resembled their actual body figure and the ideal body figure, respectively. Subtraction of the numeric values that corresponded to "actual" and "ideal" figures were used to calculate the body shape discrepancy score. The score indicated the degree of body shape dissatisfaction. A positive body shape discrepancy score signified the preference for a thinner body, while a negative score signified the preference for a bigger body.

Perception of Body Weight Status

Respondents were asked about their perception of body weight status [34]. The response options were "very thin" (1), "thin" (2), "normal" (3), "overweight" (4), and "obesity" (5). Then, the actual body weight status was compared with the perceived body weight status. Respondents were classified as correct estimators (perception equal to actual body weight status), under-estimators (perception is smaller than actual body weight status), and over-estimators (perception is bigger than actual body weight status).

2.3. Statistical Analyses

Statistical analyses were performed using IBM SPSS Statistics 21 software (version 21.0; SPSS Inc., Chicago, IL, USA), with a significance level set at $p < 0.05$. Frequency, percentage, mean, and standard deviation were used to describe the respondents' characteristics. The normality of the data was assessed by using the skewness test of normality. All continuous data of the present study were normally distributed, whereby a normal distribution was considered by the value of skewness within the range of $\pm$ 2.0 [35]. Statistical tests including the Pearson's product–moment correlation, independent samples t-test, one-way ANOVA, and chi-squared test were used in bivariate analyses, while a multiple linear regression (stepwise method) was performed to determine the factors associated with BMI-for-age.

3. Results

3.1. Body Weight Status of the Respondents

The mean body weight and height of the respondents were 43.1 $\pm$ 15.6 kg and 147.0 $\pm$ 14.0 cm, respectively. The mean BMI was 19.4 $\pm$ 4.7 kg/m^2 and the mean z-score of BMI-for-age was -0.06 ± 1.43. The present study found that about one-third of the respondents were facing malnutrition problems. Figure 1 shows that the prevalence of overweight and obesity were 15.0% and 8.1%, respectively, while the prevalence of severe thinness and thinness were 1.7% and 6.8%, respectively.

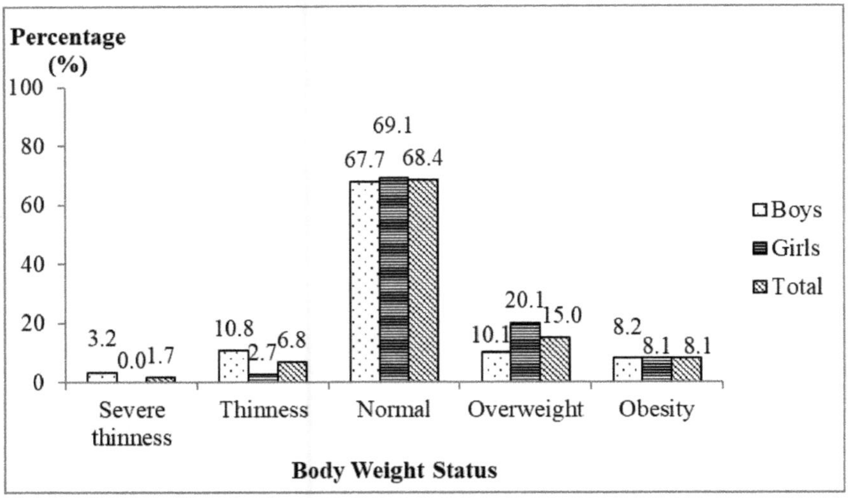

Figure 1. Distribution of respondents according to body weight status ($N = 307$).

3.2. Socio-Demographic Factors of the Respondents

The study consisted of a total of 307 respondents, with 51.5% boys and 48.5% girls (mean age of 13.0 $\pm$ 2.7 years old). About half of them (52.4%) were Malays, followed by 31.3% Indians, 12.7% Chinese, and 3.6% from other ethnic groups. More than half of the respondents living in the welfare homes were orphans (54.4%), followed by 23.8% abandoned children, and 21.8% children from problematic families (those with divorced parents, from poor families, or who had been abused).

3.3. Psychological Factors of the Respondents

Table 1 demonstrates the distribution of respondents according to psychological factors. The prevalence of low self-esteem was 16.3%, with a mean score of self-esteem was 18.2 $\pm$ 3.7. Meanwhile, the prevalence of high likelihood of depressive disorders was 38.4%, with a mean score of 16.5 $\pm$ 7.7. As for body image perception, the study found that the prevalence of body shape dissatisfaction was 73.0%, with a mean score of 0.1 $\pm$ 1.7. On the other hand, 37.8% of the respondents had reported to have underestimated their actual body weight status.

Table 1. Distribution of respondents according to psychological factors (N = 307).

Psychological Factors	Boys (n = 158)		Girl (n = 149)		Total (N = 307)		t/χ^2	p-Value
	Mean ± SD	n (%)	Mean ± SD	n (%)	Mean ± SD	n (%)		
Self-esteem	18.7 ± 3.9		17.6 ± 3.4		18.2 ± 3.7		2.565 [a]	0.011 *
Low		25 (15.8)		25 (16.8)		50 (16.3)		
Normal		133 (84.2)		124 (83.2)		257 (83.7)		
Depressive disorders	16.0 ± 7.7		16.9 ± 7.7		16.5 ± 7.7		−1.045 [a]	0.297
No likelihood of a depressive disorder		105 (66.5)		84 (56.4)		189 (61.6)		
High likelihood of a depressive disorder		53 (33.5)		65 (43.6)		118 (38.4)		
Perception of body shape	−0.5 ± 1.5		0.8 ± 1.7		0.1 ± 1.7		−7.185 [a]	0.0001 *
Satisfied		50 (31.6)		33 (22.1)		83 (27.0)		
Dissatisfied		108 (68.4)		116 (77.9)		224 (73.0)		
Perception of body weight status							2.242 [b]	0.326
Correct-estimator		79 (50.0)		86 (57.7)		165 (53.7)		
Over-estimator		13 (8.2)		13 (8.7)		26 (8.5)		
Under-estimator		66 (41.8)		50 (33.6)		116 (37.8)		

n, number of respondents; N, the sample size of this study; [a] refers to t, a statistic that compared whether sexes had different means through the independent samples t-test; [b] refers to χ^2, a statistic used for testing associations between categorical variables through chi-squared test; * Statistical significance at $p < 0.05$.

3.4. Associations between Socio-Demographic and Psychological Factors with BMI-for-Age

Table 2 shows the bivariate analyses of socio-demographic factors and BMI-for-age. Age was positively correlated with BMI-for-age of the respondents ($r = 0.169$; $p < 0.05$). Overall, girls had significantly higher BMI-for-age compared to boys ($t = -2.833$; $p < 0.05$). Across ethnicities, Malays and Chinese respondents had significantly higher mean BMI-for-age compared to Indians and other ethnic groups (F = 5.358; $p < 0.05$). By enrollment status, children being abandoned had the highest mean BMI-for-age compared to orphans and children from problematic families (F = 5.926; $p < 0.05$).

Table 2. Association between socio-demographic factors and BMI-for-age (z-score) (N = 307).

Socio-Demographic Factors	BMI-for-Age (*z*-Score)	*r*/*t*/F-Value	*p*-Value
	Mean ± SD		
Age of respondents		0.169 [b]	0.003 *
Sex			
Boys	−0.36 ± 1.54	−2.833 [c]	0.0001 *
Girls	0.26 ± 1.23		
Ethnicity		5.358 [d]	0.001 *
Malay	0.01 ± 1.37		
Chinese	0.60 ± 1.26		
Indian	−0.43 ± 1.47		
Others [a]	−0.19 ± 1.61		
Enrollment status		5.926 [d]	0.003 *
Orphan	−0.12 ± 1.51		
Abandoned	0.39 ± 1.25		
Problematic family	−0.41 ± 1.30		

N, sample size of this study was 307; [a] Others refer to aborigines and ethnics from Sabah and Sarawak; BMI, body mass index; SD, standard deviation; [b] refers to *r*, the correlation coefficient that measured the strength and direction of a linear relationship between two variables through Pearson's correlation analysis; [c] refers to *t*, a statistic that compared whether sexes had different means through the independent samples *t*-test; [d] refers to F, a statistic that compared differences between means of more than two groups through one-way ANOVA; *Statistical significance at $p < 0.05$.

Table 3 shows the bivariate analyses of psychological factors and BMI-for-age. Self-esteem score had inverse correlation with BMI-for-age ($r = -0.112$; $p < 0.05$). However, there was no correlation between the likelihood of depressive disorders and BMI-for-age ($r = 0.092$; $p > 0.05$). Body shape dissatisfaction was significantly correlated with BMI-for-age ($r = 0.551$; $p < 0.05$). In terms of perception of body weight status, respondents who underestimated their body weight status had the highest mean BMI-for-age compared to other categories (F = 6.523, $p < 0.05$).

Table 3. Association between psychological factors and BMI-for-age (z-score) (N = 307).

Psychological Factors	BMI-for-Age (*z*-Score)	*r*/F-Value	*p*-Value
	Mean ± SD		
Self-esteem		−0.112 [a]	0.003 *
Likelihood of depressive disorders		0.092 [a]	0.109
Body shape dissatisfaction		0.551 [a]	0.0001 *
Perception of body weight status			
Under-estimator	0.25 ± 1.60	6.523 [b]	0.002 *
Correct-estimator	−0.16 ± 1.22		
Over-estimator	−0.77 ± 1.56		

N, the sample size of this study, was 307; BMI, body mass index; SD, standard deviation; [a] refers to *r*, the correlation coefficient that measured the strength and direction of a linear relationship between two variables through Pearson's correlation analysis; [b] refers to F, statistic that compared differences between means of more than two groups through one-way ANOVA; *Statistical significance at $p < 0.05$.

Further, multiple linear stepwise regression was conducted to determine the factors contributing to BMI-for-age (z-score). As shown in Table 4, respondents who were abandoned, either Malay or Chinese, were dissatisfied with their body shape, and underestimated their body weight status had a higher BMI-for-age (z-score). The strongest factor of the BMI-for-age model was body shape dissatisfaction (ΔR^2 = 30.4%), followed by underestimation of body weight status (ΔR^2 = 4.8%), Malay (ΔR^2 = 1.7%) or Chinese (ΔR^2 = 1.6%) ethnic group, and abandoned status (ΔR^2 = 1.2%), which explained a total of 39.7% of the variances in BMI-for-age of the respondents (F = 39.550; $p < 0.05$).

Table 4. Multiple linear stepwise regression of BMI-for-age (z-score) (N = 307).

Variables	Unstandardized Coefficients		Standardized Coefficients	t	ΔR^2	p-Value
	β	Standard Error	Beta			
(Constant)	−0.796	0.131		−6.063		0.0001 *
Body shape dissatisfaction	0.457	0.038	0.549	12.126	0.304	0.0001 *
Underestimation of body weight status	0.628	0.134	0.213	4.691	0.048	0.0001 *
Malay	0.492	0.145	0.172	3.396	0.017	0.001 *
Chinese	0.678	0.214	0.158	3.162	0.016	0.002 *
Abandoned status	0.409	0.164	0.122	2.489	0.012	0.013 *

N, the sample size of this study, was 307; R, the multiple correlation coefficient, was 0.630; R^2, the coefficient of determination was 0.397; F, the ratio of the model mean square to the error mean square was 39.550; β, values for the regression equation for predicting the dependent variable from the independent variables, Beta was the standardized coefficient; t, a statistic used to check the significance of individual regression coefficients in the regression model; ΔR^2, incremental increase in the model R^2 resulting from the addition of a predictor to the regression equation; *Statistical significance at $p < 0.05$.

4. Discussion

The body weight status of children living in welfare homes in Selangor was unsatisfactory. Dual forms of malnutrition existed among children living in welfare homes, whereby the prevalence of overweight and obesity (23.1%) was about three times higher than the prevalence of thinness and severe thinness (8.5%). When compared to the recent report of the Adolescent Health Survey 2017 among school students aged 10 to 17 years old by Malaysia country and Selangor state [36], children living in the welfare homes generally had a lower overweight and obesity prevalence. The prevalence of overweight and obesity was 30.4% according to the national prevalence and 33.0% according to the Selangor state report, respectively [36]. On the other hand, more respondents were found thin in the welfare homes compared to the national survey. There were 6.6% and 6.7% of them were thin based on the national prevalence and the Selangor state prevalence, respectively [36].

In contrast to the current findings, previous studies of welfare homes in other countries such as Bangladesh, Nigeria, Ghana, and Sri Lanka reported that the prevalence of underweight was higher than that of overweight [37–40]. Nonetheless, the current findings are in agreement with a study among children living in welfare homes in Southeast Nigeria, wherein the prevalence of overweight (30.0%) was higher than the prevalence of underweight (2.2%) [41]. Our findings did not correspond to a local study by Chee et al. [15] in 2008, whereby they found that the undernutrition issue was more prevalent than overnutrition. However, a direct comparison of findings cannot be made as the present results used the WHO Growth Reference for those aged 5–19 years [28], while Chee et al. [15] classified children based on the Centers for Disease Control and Prevention (CDC) BMI-for-age Growth Chart [42]. As reported by Mohd Dzulkhairi et al. [16] in 2015, the trend of malnutrition among children living in welfare homes has changed over the last decade since Chee et al. [15] conducted the study in 2008. Our findings supported the findings of Mohd Dzulkhairi et al. [16] who reported that the prevalence of overweight and obesity (32.1%) was higher than that of thinness (6.2%), using the WHO (2007) classification. Based on our observation and informal communication with the caregivers, the current overweight and obesity problems among children living in the welfare homes may be due to the surplus of energy-dense foods such as pizza, fried chicken, hamburgers, fries, carbonated drinks, and ice-cream received from donors, which might lead to overeating. Possibly, children might be afraid of being hungry, and thus overeat whatever foods are given by their caregivers. Furthermore, children living in the welfare homes have always been given the opportunity to eat out, especially on weekends, and they usually go to western fast food outlets. An in-depth study about the eating behaviors and dietary intakes of children living in the welfare homes is needed.

The present study found that self-esteem was inversely associated with BMI-for-age in the bivariate analysis. Consistent with previous studies [43,44], low self-esteem was associated with the risk of overweight and obesity. The plausible explanation that low self-esteem is linked to overweight and obesity among the respondents was because children who have low self-esteem manifest their loneliness through disturbed eating habits and negative emotions related to eating during their stay in welfare homes. Nonetheless, there was no further significant association found between self-esteem and BMI-for-age in the multivariate analysis of the current findings. While about one-third of the children living in welfare homes had a high likelihood of having depressive disorders, there was no significant association between depressive disorders and BMI-for-age in the present study. Contradictory to a study by Luppino et al. [45], there was a reciprocal relationship between mental health and body weight status in which they reported that depression may be both a factor and an impact of obesity. On the other hand, the current findings are aligned with previous studies that focused on children in the general population, which reported no association between depression and body weight status [46]. In addition, a meta-analysis study revealed no significant association between body weight status and depression in the general population [47]. Although self-esteem and depressive disorders did not significantly contribute towards BMI-for-age of the children living in the welfare homes, both factors are still crucial to be addressed among children living in the welfare homes in promoting psychological stability and positive social activity in their later years of life.

Furthermore, the current study found that respondents with high BMI-for-age were those who were dissatisfied with their body shape, underestimated their body weight status, were Malays or Chinese, and had been abandoned. These factors explained about 40% of the variances in the BMI-for-age model. The current regression model was compared with other models on BMI-for-age in the Selangor state of Malaysia. It should be noted that our model was compared to the general population of Malaysia due to limited studies targeting respondents living in the welfare homes as their study respondents. For instance, a previous study in the Kajang district, Selangor, indicated that physical activity, body image, and energy intake explained 36.9% of the variances in BMI-for-age of adolescents aged 13 to 15 years old [48]. Physical activity was not included in the present study, yet our body image indicators, namely body shape dissatisfaction and body weight status underestimation, were consistent with the factors of negative body image found in their model [40]. Another BMI-for-age model of early adolescents aged 10 to 11 years old in Selangor showed that energy expenditure per kilogram body weight, being male, and the BMI of the mothers explained 66.7% of the variances in high BMI-for-age model [49]. In contrast to the model, our study found that sex did not contribute towards the high prevalence of overweight and obesity, while energy expenditure and maternal BMI were not assessed.

The present study also showed that Malay or Chinese respondents had higher BMI-for-age compared to other ethnicities. A previous study among Malaysian primary school children reported that the prevalence of overweight was higher among Chinese students (23.0%) compared to Indians (16.0%) and Malays (14.8%) [50]. Additionally, the prevalence of obesity was higher in Malays (7.6%), followed by Indians (5.1%) and Chinese (1.6%) [49]. Further studies may need to explore the underlying differences in ethnic groups that relate to the development of overweight and obesity in children. For instance, Zhang and Wang [51] suggested that Chinese people perceived having a large body size or being overweight and obese as a sign of wealth and success in their culture in China.

By enrollment status of the welfare homes, respondents with the enrollment by abandoned status had the highest BMI-for-age, followed by orphans, and children from problematic families. The possible explanation for these findings may be due to the immediate environment experienced by children who were abandoned from a young age (for example as newborns) when entering the welfare homes compared to other children. The immediate environment here refers to the welfare home as the first home of children being abandoned, which may be an obesogenic environment that encourages children to become overweight and obese from a very young age. On the other hand, most of the orphans and children from problematic families lived in their parents' home as their first home, which may indicate different early environment exposures as compared to abandoned children. Future research may need to consider the environment exposure prior to the enrollment when focusing on children living in welfare homes.

To the best of the authors' knowledge, no previous study in the related literature has assessed the perception of body image in the welfare home setting. However, the present findings support a study among children of general population from Nazrat et al. [52], in which girls desired for a smaller body size than boys. Likewise, Ozmen et al. [53] indicated that boys desired a larger body size. Furthermore, the association between body shape dissatisfaction and obesity was found in several studies in Malaysia [48,54,55]. Meanwhile, the present findings showed that there was an association between respondents under-estimating their body weight status and overweight and obese status. This is consistent with a study among adolescents of the general population aged 10 to 17 years in Malaysia, where the authors found that 12.2% of the overweight and obese respondents had under-estimated their actual body weight status [13]. Neumark-Sztainer et al. [56] highlighted that the association between poor body image (body shape dissatisfaction and underestimation of body weight status) and obesity was due to unhealthy weight control behaviors that put them at risk of weight gain. Further studies may focus on determining the types of unhealthy weight control behaviors among children.

There were several limitations in the current study. This cross-sectional study does not yield the evidence on the cause and effect of socio-demographic and psychological factors on BMI-for-age. However, the present study adds important information to the literature regarding the association of socio-demographic and psychological factors with body weight status among children living in welfare homes. Immediate action must be initiated to prevent excess weight gain and to treat those children who are already in the high BMI-for-age category.

5. Conclusions

The present study found that dual forms of malnutrition existed among children living in welfare homes. About one in four of the children were facing overweight and obesity problems, whereas about one in ten of them were thin and severely thin. Poor body image perception, being Malays or Chinese, and having been abandoned were associated with higher BMI-for-age among children living in welfare homes in Selangor. These findings suggest the need to have a regular assessment of body weight status among children, and preventive actions should be taken by the welfare homes' related agencies and donors. Additionally, an obesity intervention program that incorporates body image perception may improve the children's body weight status in future.

Author Contributions: Conceptualization, N.N.A.R., Y.S.C. and N.S.; Data curation, N.N.A.R.; Formal analysis, N.N.A.R.; Funding acquisition, Y.S.C.; Supervision, Y.S.C. and N.S.; Writing—original draft, N.N.A.R.; Writing—review and editing, Y.S.C. and N.S.

Funding: This research was funded by Universiti Putra Malaysia (Putra Grant (GP-IPS)) grant number GP-IPS/2014/9438732 for this research.

Acknowledgments: The authors acknowledge the support of Universiti Putra Malaysia. We thank all the caregivers and children who participated in this study. The authors appreciated trained researchers who assisted in data collection process for this study.

Conflicts of Interest: The authors declare that there is no conflict of interest about the publication of this article.

References

1. Sahoo, K.; Sahoo, B.; Choudhury, A.K.; Sofi, N.Y.; Kumar, R.; Bhadoria, A.S. Childhood obesity: Causes and consequences. *J. Fam. Med. Prim. Care* **2015**, *4*, 187–192.
2. Cash, T.F. Body image: Past, present, and future. *Body Image* **2004**, *1*, 1–5. [CrossRef]
3. Grogan, S. Promoting positive body image in males and females: Contemporary issues and future directions. *Sex Roles* **2010**, *63*, 757–765. [CrossRef]
4. Voelker, D.K.; Reel, J.J.; Greenleaf, C. Weight status and body image perceptions in adolescents: Current perspectives. *Adolesc. Health Med. Ther.* **2015**, *6*, 149–158. [PubMed]
5. Harriger, J.A.; Thompson, J.K. Psychological consequences of obesity: Weight bias and body image in overweight and obese youth. *Int. Rev. Psychiatry* **2012**, *24*, 247–253. [CrossRef] [PubMed]
6. Bibiloni Mdel, M.; Pich, J.; Pons, A.; Tur, J.A. Body image and eating patterns among adolescents. *BMC Public Health* **2013**, *13*, 1104. [CrossRef] [PubMed]
7. Rodgers, R.F.; McLean, S.A.; Marques, M.; Dunstan, C.J.; Paxton, S.J. Trajectories of body dissatisfaction and dietary restriction in early adolescent girls: A latent class growth analysis. *J. Youth Adolesc.* **2016**, *45*, 1664–1677. [CrossRef] [PubMed]
8. Malete, L.; Motlhoiwa, K.; Shaibu, S.; Wrotniak, B.H.; Maruapula, S.D.; Jackson, J.; Compher, C.W. Body image dissatisfaction is increased in male and overweight/obese adolescents in Botswana. *J. Obes.* **2013**, *2013*, 763624. [CrossRef]
9. Alipour, B.; Abbasalizad Farhangi, M.; Dehghan, P.; Alipour, M. Body image perception and its association with body mass index and nutrient intakes among female college students aged 18–35 years from Tabriz, Iran. *Eat. Weight Disord.* **2015**, *20*, 465–471. [CrossRef]
10. Kopcakova, J.; Veselska, Z.D.; Geckova, A.M.; van Dijk, J.P.; Reijneveld, S.A. Is being a boy and feeling fat a barrier for physical activity? The association between body image, gender and physical activity among adolescents. *Int. J. Environ. Res. Public Health* **2014**, *11*, 11167–11176. [CrossRef]
11. Slater, A.; Tiggemann, M. Gender differences in adolescent sport participation, teasing, self-objectification and body image concerns. *J. Adolesc.* **2011**, *34*, 455–463. [CrossRef]
12. Khor, G.L.; Zalilah, M.S.; Phan, Y.Y.; Maznah, B.; Norimah, A.K. Perception of body image among Malaysian male and female adolescents. *Singap. Med. J.* **2009**, *50*, 303–311.
13. Zainuddin, A.A.; Manickam, M.A.; Baharudin, A.; Omar, A.; Cheong, S.M.; Ambak, R.; Ahmad, M.H.; Ghaffar, S.A. Self-Perception of Body Weight Status and Weight Control Practices among Adolescents in Malaysia. *Asia Pac. J. Public Health* **2014**, *26*, 18S–26S. [CrossRef] [PubMed]
14. Institute for Public Health (IPH). National Health and Morbidity Survey 2015 (NHMS 2015). Volume II: Non-Communicable Diseases, Risk Factors & Other Health Problems. 2015. Available online: http://iku.moh.gov.my/images/IKU/Document/REPORT/nhmsreport2015vol2.pdf (accessed on 26 July 2015).
15. Chee, Y.F.; Roseline Yap, W.K.; Siti, S.B. Weight Status and Dietary Intake among Female Children and Adolescents Aged 6–17 Years in a Welfare Home, Kuala Lumpur. *Malays. J. Nutr.* **2008**, *14*, 79–89. [PubMed]
16. Mohd Dzulkhairi, M.R.; Syimir, S.; Zairina, A.R.; Wan Noraini, W.S.; Khairun Nain, N.; Nazefah, A.H. Nutritional status, knowledge, attitude, and practice among orphans living in institutions in Selangor and Melaka. *Med. J. Malays.* **2015**, *70*, 1.
17. Côté, S.M.; Orri, M.; Marttila, M.; Ristikari, T. Out-of-home placement in early childhood and psychiatric diagnoses and criminal convictions in young adulthood: A population-based propensity score-matched study. *Lancet Child Adolesc. Health* **2018**, *2*, 647–653. [CrossRef]
18. Brännström, L.; Vinnerljung, B.; Forsman, H.; Almquist, Y.B. Children Placed in Out-of-Home Care as Midlife Adults: Are They Still Disadvantaged or Have They Caught up with Their Peers? *Child Maltreat.* **2017**, *22*, 205–214. [CrossRef]
19. Forsman, H.; Brännström, L.; Vinnerljung, B.; Hjern, A. Does poor school performance cause later psychosocial problems among children in foster care? Evidence from national longitudinal registry data. *Child Abuse Negl.* **2016**, *57*, 61–71. [CrossRef]
20. Fallesen, P. Identifying divergent foster care careers for Danish children. *Child Abuse Negl.* **2014**, *38*, 1860–1871. [CrossRef]
21. Stein, R.E.K.; Hurlburt, M.S.; Heneghan, A. Chronic conditions among children investigated by child welfare. *Pediatrics* **2013**, *131*, 455–462. [CrossRef]

22. Turney, K.; Wildeman, C. Mental and Physical Health of Children in Foster Care. *Pediatrics* **2016**, *138*, e20161118. [CrossRef]
23. Horwitz, S.M.; Hurlburt, M.S.; Cohen, S.D.; Zhang, J.; Landsverk, J. Predictors of placement for children who initially remained in their homes after an investigation for abuse and neglect. *Child Abuse Negl.* **2011**, *35*, 188–198. [CrossRef]
24. Thompson, A.H. Childhood depression revisited: Indicators, normative tests and clinical course. *J. Can. Acad. Child Adolesc. Psychiatry* **2012**, *21*, 5–8.
25. Gürsoy, F.; Biçakçi, M.Y.; Orhan, E.; Bakırcı, S.; Çatak, S.; Yerebakan, Ö. Study on Self-Concept Levels of Adolescents in the Age Group of 13–18 who Live in Orphanage and those who do not Live in Orphanage. *Int. J. Soc. Sci. Educ.* **2012**, *2*, 56–66.
26. Rosenberg, M. *Society and the Adolescent Self-Image*; Princeton University Press: Princeton, NJ, USA, 1965.
27. WHO AnthroPlus for Personal Computers Manual. Software for Assessing the Growth of the World's Children and Adolescents. Geneva: World Health Organization. 2009. Available online: http://www.who.int/growthref/tools/en/ (accessed on 10 March 2014).
28. De Onis, M.; Onyango, A.W.; Borghi, E.; Siyam, A.; Nishida, C.; Siekmann, J. Development of a WHO growth reference for school-aged children and adolescents. *Bull. World Health Organ.* **2007**, *85*, 660–667. [CrossRef]
29. Fawzy, N.; Fouad, A. Psychosocial and Developmental Status of Orphanage Children: Epidemiological Study. *Curr. Psychiatry* **2010**, *17*, 41–48.
30. Kovacs, M. The Children's Depression Inventory (CDI). *Psychopharmacol. Bull.* **1985**, *21*, 995–998.
31. Kovacs, M. *The Children's Depression Inventory (CDI) Manual*; Multi-Health Systems: Toronto, ON, USA, 1992; pp. 15–25.
32. Collins, M.E. Body figure perceptions and preferences among preadolescent children. *Int. J. Eat. Disord.* **1991**, *10*, 199–208. [CrossRef]
33. Thompson, M.A.; Gray, J.J. Development and validation of a new body image assessment tool. *J. Pers. Assess.* **1995**, *64*, 258–269. [CrossRef]
34. Simko, M.D.; Cowell, C.; Hreha, M. *Practical Nutrition: A Quick Reference for the Health Care Practitioner*; Aspen Publishers: Rockville, MD, USA, 1989; pp. 282–286.
35. Reimann, C.; Filzmoser, P.; Garret, R.G.; Dutter, R. *Statistical Data Analysis Explained: Applied Environmental Statistics with R*; John Wiley & Sons: Hoboken, NJ, USA, 2008.
36. Institute for Public Health (IPH) 2017. National Health and Morbidity Survey (NHMS) 2017: Adolescent Nutrition Survey 2017, Malaysia. Available online: http://iku.moh.gov.my/images/IKU/Document/REPORT/NHMS2017/NutritionSurveyNHMS2017.pdf (accessed on 18 August 2018).
37. Obidual Hug, A.K.; Chowdhury, T.; Roy, P.; Formuzul Haque, K.M.; Bellal Hossain, M. Healthcare facilities and nutritional status of orphans residing in selected orphanage in capital city of Bangladesh. *Int. J. Curr. Microbiol. Appl. Sci.* **2013**, *2*, 118–125.
38. Nwaeri, D.U.; Omuemu, V.O. Intestinal helminthiasis and nutritional status of children living in orphanages in Benin-City, Nigeria. *Int. J. Clin. Pract.* **2013**, *16*, 243–248.
39. Sadik, A. Orphanage children in Ghana: Are their dietary needs met? *Pak. J. Nutr.* **2010**, *9*, 844–852. [CrossRef]
40. Jayasekera, C.R. Nutritional status of children under five in three State foster care institutions in Sri Lanka. *Ceylon Med. J.* **2006**, *51*, 63–65. [CrossRef]
41. Bismarck, E.C.; Onyeka, E.B.; Mildred, U.O.; Nnaemeka, I.A. Nutritional status of children living in motherless babies' homes in Enugu State Southeast Nigeria. *Indian J. Appl. Res.* **2014**, *4*, 478–482. [CrossRef]
42. CDC. About Child & Teen BMI: Centers for Disease Control and Prevention. Available online: https://www.cdc.gov/healthyweight/assessing/bmi/childrens_bmi/about_childrens_bmi.html (accessed on 20 September 2015).
43. Goldfield, G.S.; Moore, C.; Henderson, K.; Buchholz, A.; Obeid, N.; Flament, M.F. Body dissatisfaction, dietary restraint, depression, and weight status in adolescents. *J. Sch. Health* **2010**, *80*, 186–192. [CrossRef]
44. Yen, C.F.; Hsiao, R.C.; Ko, C.H.; Yen, J.Y. The relationship between overweight/obesity and self-esteem in adolescents: The moderating effects of socio-demographic characteristics, family support, academic achievement and peer interaction. *Taiwan J. Psychiatry* **2010**, *24*, 210–221.

45. Luppino, F.S.; de Wit, L.M.; Bouvy, P.F.; Stijnen, T.; Cuijpers, P.; Penninx, B.W.; Zitman, F.G. Overweight, obesity, and depression: A systematic review and meta-analysis of longitudinal studies. *Arch. Gen. Psychiatry* **2010**, *67*, 220–229. [CrossRef]
46. Wardle, J.; Williamson, S.; Johnson, F.; Edwards, C. Depression in adolescent obesity: Cultural moderators of the association between obesity and depressive symptoms. *Int. J. Obes.* **2006**, *30*, 634–643. [CrossRef]
47. Faith, M.S.; Matz, P.E.; Jorge, M.A. Obesity-depression associations in the population. *J. Psychosom. Res.* **2002**, *53*, 935–942. [CrossRef]
48. Fara Wahida, R.; Chin, Y.S.; Barakatun Nisak, M.Y. Obesity-related behaviors of Malaysian adolescents: A sample from Kajang district of Selangor state. *Nutr. Res. Pract.* **2012**, *6*, 458–465.
49. Woon, F.C.; Chin, Y.S.; Mohd Nasir, M.T. Association between behavioural factors and BMI-for-age among early adolescents in Hulu Langat district, Selangor, Malaysia. *Obes. Res. Clin. Pract.* **2015**, *9*, 346–356. [CrossRef]
50. Anuar Zaini, M.Z.; Lim, C.T.; Low, W.Y.; Harun, F. Factors affecting nutritional status of Malaysian primary school children. *Asia Pac. J. Public Health* **2005**, *17*, 71–80. [CrossRef]
51. Zhang, Y.; Wang, S. Prevalent change in overweight and obesity in children and adolescents from 1995 to 2005 in Shandong, China. *Asia Pac. J. Public Health* **2005**, *23*, 904–916. [CrossRef]
52. Nazrat, M.M.; Dawnavan Davis, M.S.; Yanovski, J.A. Body dissatisfaction, self-esteem, and overweight among innercity Hispanic children and adolescents. *J. Adolesc. Health* **2005**, *36*, 267.e16-20.
53. Ozmen, D.; Ozmen, E.; Ergin, D.; Cetinkaya, A.C.; Sen, N.; Dundar, P.E.; Taskin, E.O. The association of self-esteem, depression and body satisfaction with obesity among Turkish adolescents. *BMC Public Health* **2007**, *7*, 80. [CrossRef]
54. Chin, Y.S.; Taib, M.N.; Shariff, Z.M.; Khor, G.L. Development of Multidimensional Body Image Scale for Malaysian female adolescents. *Nutr. Res. Pract.* **2008**, *2*, 85–92. [CrossRef]
55. Nur Syuhada Zofiran, M.J.; Kartini, I.; Siti Sabariah, B.; Ajau, D. The relationship between eating behaviours, body image, and BMI status among adolescents age 13 to 17 years in Meru, Klang, Malaysia. *Am. J. Food Nutr.* **2011**, *1*, 185–192. [CrossRef]
56. Neumark-Sztainer, D.; Wall, M.; Story, M.; Standish, A.R. Dieting and unhealthy weight control behaviors during adolescence: Associations with 10-year changes in body mass index. *J. Adolesc. Health* **2012**, *50*, 80–86. [CrossRef]

nutrients

MDPI

Article

Canadian Children from Food Insecure Households Experience Low Self-Esteem and Self-Efficacy for Healthy Lifestyle Choices

Stephanie L. Godrich [1,*], Olivia K. Loewen [2], Rosanne Blanchet [3], Noreen Willows [3] and Paul Veugelers [2,*]

1 School of Medical and Health Science, Edith Cowan University, Bunbury, Western Australia 6230, Australia
2 School of Public Health, University of Alberta, Edmonton, AB T6G 2P5, Canada; oloewen@ualberta.ca
3 Department of Agricultural, Food & Nutritional Science, University of Alberta, Edmonton, AB T6G 2P5, Canada; rosanne.blanchet@ualberta.ca (R.B.); nwillows@ualberta.ca (N.W.)
* Correspondence: s.godrich@ecu.edu.au (S.L.G.); paul.veugelers@ualberta.ca (P.V.)

Received: 14 February 2019; Accepted: 17 March 2019; Published: 21 March 2019

Abstract: The objectives of this cross-sectional study were to: (i) determine whether there are differences in self-esteem and self-efficacy for healthy lifestyle choices between children living in food secure and food insecure households; and (ii) determine whether the association between household food insecurity (HFI), self-esteem and self-efficacy differs by gender. Survey responses of 5281 fifth-grade students (10 and 11 years of age) participating in the Canadian Children's Lifestyle and School Performance Study II were analyzed using logistic and linear regression. HFI status was determined by the six-item short-form Household Food Security Survey Module (HFSSM). Students from food insecure households had significantly higher odds of low self-esteem, and significantly lower scores for global self-efficacy to make healthy choices, compared to students from food secure households. These associations were stronger for girls than for boys and appeared independent of parental educational attainment. Household income appeared to be the essential underlying determinant of the associations of food insecurity with self-esteem and self-efficacy. Upstream social policies such as improving the household income of low-income residents will reduce food insecurity and potentially improve self-esteem and self-efficacy for healthy choices among children. This may improve health and learning, and in the long term, job opportunities and household earnings.

Keywords: food security; self-esteem; self-efficacy

1. Introduction

In Canada and the United States, household food insecurity (HFI) as measured on national surveys refers to self-reports of uncertain or insufficient food access, due to limited financial resources. Recent national prevalence data of HFI in Canada and the United States were reported as 12% [1] and 11.8% [2], respectively. These two countries use a validated tool, the 18-question Household Food Security Survey Module (HFSSM), to capture a gradient of deprivation within households. This ranges from anxiety about running out of food, to impacts on diet quality and quantity [2,3], which can have cognitive and physical health consequences [4].

Such consequences resulting from HFI include multiple poor health outcomes, higher health care utilization and costs [5,6], higher mortality rates [7] and adverse mental health outcomes such as behavioural issues, distress, anxiety, depression and suicidal thoughts [6,8–10]. Furthermore, HFI has a graded negative effect on a variety of physical and mental health outcomes, in which more severe food insecurity (FI) is associated with increased risk of adverse outcomes [10]. Among children, HFI has been associated with impaired mental health [11], reduced academic performance [12], absenteeism [13], and poorer behavioural outcomes [12,14]. HFI may affect girls and boys differently and associations between HFI, children's academic performance, social skills and feelings of fear have been shown to differ between gender, with the effect more pronounced for girls [15,16]. HFI seems to influence children's development through its effects as a component of overall family stress and poor functioning [12,17,18]. The evidence thus indicates that HFI is a critical public health issue that merits attention, given its importance in determining short and long-term health outcomes among children and adults [19,20].

As HFI experienced in childhood is a stressor and precursor to unfavourable cognitive outcomes in childhood and adulthood [12], it is important to build self-confidence early in life. Self-esteem can be described as the attitude towards oneself [21], which can be positive or negative [22]. Self-efficacy is an individual's belief in their ability to achieve goals [23], such as healthy eating (HE) or physical activity (PA) goals. People with high self-efficacy have higher confidence in their ability to translate intentions into behaviours [24]. With frequent practice, self-efficacy relating to healthy behaviour goals, such as meal preparation in the home environment, can be increased [25]. High self-efficacy has been shown in adult populations to increase diet quality [26]. The limited existing literature also suggests an association between FI and self-efficacy [27]. Self-efficacy seems to be impaired by FI [28] and improvements in food security (FS)—regular and reliable access to sufficient nutritious food [29]—have been shown to increase self-efficacy [30]. This may in turn enhance academic achievement and "economic productivity" [12]. Given that low self-esteem and self-efficacy in childhood may be an "enduring vulnerability" for mental health issues in adulthood [31,32], it is important to ensure positive self-esteem and self-efficacy are fostered in childhood [33]. This is particularly important among girls, who will become mothers, given HFI risk is increased by maternal depression [34] and food insecure mothers are more likely to report their own experiences of childhood deprivation [35]. Therefore, addressing FI during childhood could reduce the likelihood of intergenerational FI [35].

In order to prevent mental health issues, greater understanding of how FI influences self-esteem and self-efficacy among children is required. Further, the limited evidence of the association between household FS status and a child's perceived self-efficacy to make healthy lifestyle choices, such as PA and HE needs to be extended. Therefore, the aim of this paper is to examine the relationship between household FS and self-esteem and self-efficacy for healthy lifestyle choices among grade five children living in Nova Scotia, Canada, where 22.8% of children lived in FI households in 2015–16 [36]. The relationship is examined by classifying HFI using the six-item short form HFSSM into three levels (marginal, moderate and severe). The objectives included: (i) to determine whether there are differences in self-esteem and self-efficacy for healthy lifestyle choices between students living in households with FS and FI; and (ii) to determine whether there are gender differences within the association between FI, self-esteem and self-efficacy among children. We hypothesized that students from households experiencing FI would have lower self-esteem and lower self-efficacy for HE and participating in PA, and that this association would differ between genders.

2. Materials and Methods

2.1. Sampling and Recruitment

In this cross-sectional study, we used data from the Children's Lifestyle and School Performance Study II (CLASS II) conducted in 2011 in Nova Scotia, Canada. Nova Scotia is a province on the eastern coast of Canada, consisting of a peninsula and offshore islands with a population just under 1 million people [37]. CLASS II was a population-based survey that examined diet, physical activity, well-being, and school performance among fifth-grade students (10–11 years old). All grade five students in the province, their parent(s)/guardian(s), and school administrators were invited to participate in the study. Of all 286 provincial public schools with grade five students, 269 schools (94.1%) participated in the study. Once a school agreed to participate, parents or guardians received a home package containing a consent form and survey to complete. Parental consent to participate in the survey was given for 6591 of the 8736 students (75.4% consent rate). Of these, 1310 (19.9%) students did not complete the survey, were absent the day of the survey, or had returned an incomplete parent survey and were excluded from analysis, leaving 5281 eligible students. Of these, 5093 (96.4%) and 5113 (96.8%) had complete data for measures of self-esteem and self-efficacy items, respectively.

2.2. Instrument

The student survey consisted of questions on eating behaviours at school and home, physical activity, mental wellbeing, self-esteem, and self-efficacy. Parent(s)/guardian(s)' survey contained questions about the home environment, household FI experience, and sociodemographic factors. Specifically, the home survey contained the US Department of Agriculture 6-item short-form Household Food Security Survey Module (HFSSM), a tool that has been validated in the US and is recommended when there is the need to reduce respondent burden or when asking questions about children' FI is deemed too sensitive [3]. A score was calculated from the number of affirmative responses to the six questions about FI. Based on overall score, households were classified as food secure (score 0), marginal FI (score 1), moderate FI (score 2–4) or severe FI (5–6) [14]. FI status constituted the exposure of interest.

Outcomes included global self-esteem, assessed using a series of ten questions with a 3-point Likert scale response options similar to the Emotional Functioning and Social Functioning items on the PedsQL [38]. The following items were included (i) My future looks good to me; (ii) I like the way I look; (iii) I like myself; (iv) I feel like I do not have any friends; (v) I feel unhappy or sad; (vi) I worry a lot; (vii) I am in trouble with my teacher(s); (viii) I have trouble paying attention; (ix) I have trouble enjoying myself; (x) If I have problems there is someone I trust to go to for advice. Response choices for each of these items included 'never or almost never', 'sometimes', to 'often or almost always'. The responses were scored as 1, 2, 3, with the highest score representing good self-esteem. Scores were subsequently totaled. The inter-item reliability (Cronbach's alpha) of the 10 items was 0.70.

Outcomes also included self-efficacy for healthy lifestyle choices, assessed using 9 items, 4 for physical activity and 5 for healthy eating. Students were asked "If you wanted to, how confident are you that you could (i) be physically active no matter how tired you may be?; (ii) be physically active even if you have a lot of homework?; (iii) ask your parent or other adult to play a physical activity or sport with you?; (iv) be physically active for at least 60 min on 5 or more days per week?; (v) eat healthy food at school?; (vi) choose a healthy snack between school and dinner time?; (vii) eat healthy food if you are alone at home?; (viii) choose a healthy snack when you are bored?; (ix) choose a healthy snack when you are sad?" Response choices included 'not at all confident', 'a little bit confident', 'quite confident', and 'very confident'. The responses were scored as 1, 2, 3, 4, with the highest score representing higher self-efficacy. The scores were summed for global self-efficacy (all nine items), physical activity, and healthy eating. These scores were then transformed to a scale of 1 to 100 to make them comparable across the three measures on self-efficacy. The items for self-efficacy have each demonstrated good internal consistency [39]. The inter-item reliability (Cronbach's alpha) of the physical activity, healthy eating self-efficacy, and global self-efficacy items were 0.69, 0.83, and 0.83 respectively.

Covariates used in analyses included gender, region of residence (urban or rural; based on postal code), parental educational attainment, household income, and bodyweight status [40] (normal weight, overweight, or obese using age and gender specific cut-offs). Further information about the CLASS study can be found at www.nsclass.ca.

2.3. Data Collection

The student survey was pilot tested for ease of understanding and reliability. Trained CLASS research assistants travelled to participating schools and administered surveys to students who had returned a signed consent to participate. Research assistants measured students' height to the nearest 0.1 cm and weight to the nearest 0.1 kg on calibrated digital scales. Additional data collection information has been detailed elsewhere [41].

2.4. Data Entry and Analysis

We conducted descriptive analysis of associations between FI status, gender, region of residence, parent education, household income, and bodyweight status with self-esteem and self-efficacy using Chi^2 tests. For the descriptive analyses, self-efficacy scores were split into tertiles.

For self-esteem items, the responses were ordinal and the sum scores were not normally distributed. Self-esteem was therefore dichotomized whereby sum scores lower than the 15th percentile were defined as low self-esteem, which is similar to the parametric concept of one standard deviation below the mean, an approach commonly applied in self-esteem research [42]. Univariate logistic regression was used to examine the association of FI status and confounders with the dichotomized self-esteem scores. A multivariable mixed-effects logistic regression with robust standard errors was used to account for clustering of students within schools and the confounding potential of gender, region of residence, and bodyweight status. Later multivariable models were sequentially further adjusted for parent education and household income. In addition, these models were tested for gender-HFI interaction and found to be significant ($p = 0.006$). As such, gender-stratified multivariable models, adjusted for the same covariates (except gender), were used to examine whether the associations were distinct for girls and boys.

For the associations of self-efficacy with FI status, univariate linear regression models were conducted for global, PA, and HE self-efficacy scores. A multivariable linear regression model with robust standard errors was used to account for clustering of students and adjusted for gender, region of residence, and bodyweight status. This model was further adjusted for parental education and household income. Models were tested for gender-HFI interaction, but it was not found to be significant ($p = 0.251$). For consistency with self-esteem models, gender-stratified analyses was conducted using a multivariable model, adjusting for the same covariates (except gender).

All analyses were weighted to represent provincial estimates of the grade 5 student population in Nova Scotia. Responses rates in residential areas with lower household income were slightly lower than average and weights were calculated to account for this disproportionate non-response [43]. Missing values for potential confounders were considered as separate covariate categories, but their estimates are not presented. Normality and homoscedasticity were tested and found to be acceptable for all linear regression models. All analyses were conducted using the statistical software package Stata/IC 14 and $p < 0.05$ were considered significant.

The Health Sciences and Human Research Ethics Board of Dalhousie University approved the original study, including the informed consent procedure. The Health Research Ethics Board at the University of Alberta approved the data analysis of the present study. Edith Cowan University Human Research Ethics Committee provided multicentre research project approval.

3. Results

3.1. Participant Demographics

Table 1 presents characteristics of grade five students in Nova Scotia and shows that 52.2% were girls, 35.2% resided in rural regions, and 54.3%, 22.7%, and 17.8% had normal weight, overweight, or obesity, respectively.

Table 1. Characteristics of grade 5 students (aged 10–11 years) in Nova Scotia, Canada by self-esteem and self-efficacy. Children's Lifestyle and School performance Study (CLASS) 2011.

	Total Sample (n = 5281)	Self-Esteem (n = 5093)		Self-Efficacy (n = 5113)		
		Low	Normal	Lowest Tertile	Middle Tertile	Highest Tertile
Household Food Security Status						
Food secure	74.8%	66.8%	76.2%	72.2%	75.2%	77.5%
Marginal FI [1]	8.1%	10.1%	7.7%	7.9%	8.3%	8.2%
Moderate FI [1]	10.0%	13.7%	9.5%	11.6%	9.5%	8.6%
Severe FI [1]	7.1%	9.4%	6.6%	8.3%	7.0%	5.7%
Girls (%)	52.2%	47.8%	52.9%	49.5%	54.2%	52.9%
Bodyweight status (%)						
Normal weight	54.3%	43.3%	56.0%	50.5%	53.5%	59.9%
Overweight	21.7%	22.3%	21.7%	21.5%	22.7%	21.2%
Obesity	17.8%	28.2%	16.3%	20.9%	18.1%	14.1%
Missing	6.1%	6.3%	6.0%	7.1%	5.8%	4.9%
Rural Residence (%)	35.2%	41.6%	34.4%	37.3%	36.1%	32.9%
Household Income (%)						
<$20,000	20.7%	31.9%	18.8%	23.9%	19.4%	17.5%
$20,001–40,000	14.1%	14.5%	14.0%	15.0%	14.2%	12.6%
$40,001–60,000	25.4%	21.8%	26.0%	24.3%	26.6%	26.3%
>$60,000	20.6%	12.9%	21.8%	16.3%	21.5%	24.7%
Missing/prefer not to answer	19.2%	18.8%	19.4%	20.5%	18.3%	18.9%
Parent education (%)						
Secondary school or less	18.0%	23.0%	17.2%	20.8%	16.5%	16.2%
College	40.6%	44.5%	39.9%	41.7%	43.3%	36.0%
University	37.5%	27.0%	39.3%	32.5%	37.2%	42.3%
Missing	4.0%	5.6%	3.7%	5.1%	3.0%	3.5%

[1] Food insecurity.

3.2. Household Food Security Status

As shown in Table 1, 74.8% of students were from households classified as food secure, 8.1% from households with marginal FI, 10.0% from households with moderate FI, and 7.1% from households with severe FI, for a combined prevalence of 25.2% HFI.

3.3. Global Self-Esteem and Self-Efficacy for Healthy Lifestyle Choices

Of students with low self-esteem, 9.4% were from households experiencing severe FI whereas among students with normal self-esteem only 6.6% came from FI households. Likewise, among students in the lowest self-efficacy tertile, a higher percentage (8.3%) were from severe FI households relative to students in the highest self-efficacy tertile (5.7%). These differences were statistically significant (p's ≤ 0.001). Similar statistically significant gradients were observed for household income and parental education, with lower household income and parental education associated with lower self-esteem and self-efficacy (data not shown).

3.4. The Association between Household Food Security and Self-Esteem

Table 2 presents the univariate and multivariable associations between HFI status and low self-esteem for students. Students (girls and boys combined) from households with marginal, moderate, or severe FI had respectively 44%, 55%, and 54% higher odds of having low self-esteem compared to students from food secure households after adjusting for gender, region of residence and bodyweight. The interaction between FI and gender was found to be statistically significant ($p = 0.006$). In the gender-stratified Model 1, the association with lower self-esteem was only significant for girls from moderate FI households and boys from households with severe FI (girls: OR 2.19; boys: OR: 1.68, compared with their FS counterpart). This association was not significant among girls living in marginal or severe FI households or among boys living in marginal FI or moderate FI. When this model was further adjusted for parent educational attainment (Model 2), the association between HFI and low self-esteem remained significant only among students (girls and boys combined) and girls living in moderate FI households. They had respectively 40% and 2 times higher odds of low self-esteem when compared to their FS counterpart. Model 3 was further adjusted for household income. It showed that girls from moderate FI households had an associated 67% higher odds of low self-esteem when compared to their FS counterpart. This association was no longer significant for girls and boys combined.

Table 2. Relationship between food security and low self-esteem among grade 5 students (aged 10–11 years) in Nova Scotia, Canada.

Self-Esteem						
	All Students		**Girls**		**Boys**	
	OR (95%CI)	***p*-Value**	**OR (95%CI)**	***p*-Value**	**OR (95%CI)**	***p*-Value**
	Univariate					
Household Food Security Status						
Food secure	1		1	.	1	.
Marginal FI [1]	**1.49 (1.10, 2.03)**	**0.010**	**1.56 (1.05, 2.32)**	**0.028**	1.49 (0.93, 2.40)	0.095
Moderate FI [1]	**1.65 (1.25, 2.18)**	**<0.001**	**2.39 (1.71, 3.33)**	**<0.001**	1.07 (0.69, 1.68)	0.753
Severe FI [1]	**1.62 (1.19, 2.20)**	**0.002**	1.57 (0.97, 2.52)	0.066	**1.73 (1.16, 2.58)**	**0.007**
	Model 1					
Food secure	1		1	.	1	.
Marginal FI [1]	**1.44 (1.05, 1.97)**	**0.022**	1.47 (0.96, 2.23)	0.073	1.46 (0.91, 2.34)	0.120
Moderate FI [1]	**1.55 (1.18, 2.05)**	**0.002**	**2.19 (1.57, 3.07)**	**<0.001**	1.04 (0.66, 1.63)	0.869
Severe FI [1]	**1.54 (1.12, 2.12)**	**0.009**	1.42 (0.87, 2.31)	0.158	**1.68 (1.11, 2.53)**	**0.014**
	Model 2					
Food secure	1		1	.	1	.
Marginal FI [1]	1.35 (0.99, 1.85)	0.058	1.37 (0.90, 2.09)	0.146	1.38 (0.86, 2.20)	0.180
Moderate FI [1]	**1.40 (1.06, 1.85)**	**0.020**	**2.00 (1.42, 2.81)**	**<0.001**	0.93 (0.59, 1.45)	0.740
Severe FI [1]	1.35 (0.99, 1.85)	0.062	1.27 (0.77, 2.09)	0.352	1.46 (0.97, 2.19)	0.069
	Model 3					
Food secure	1		1	.	1	.
Marginal FI [1]	1.17 (0.85, 1.60)	0.330	1.16 (0.75, 1.79)	0.503	1.19 (0.74, 1.91)	0.474
Moderate FI [1]	1.16 (0.87, 1.55)	0.317	**1.67 (1.16, 2.41)**	**0.006**	0.77 (0.49, 1.23)	0.275
Severe FI [1]	1.01 (0.73, 1.41)	0.930	0.99 (0.58, 1.68)	0.972	1.06 (0.68, 1.65)	0.788

OR: Odds Ratio; 95% CI; 95% confidence interval; Model 1 is adjusted for region of residence, body weight status, and gender (in non-gender-stratified models). Model 2 is further adjusted for parental education and Model 3 is further adjusted for household income. Estimates are weighted to represent grade five students in Nova Scotia. Results in bold are statistically significant ($p < 0.05$); [1] Food insecurity.

3.5. The Association between Household Food Security Status and Self-Efficacy

Table 3 presents the associations between FI and self-efficacy. Students from moderate and severe FI households had significantly lower scores for global self-efficacy to make healthy choices than students from food secure households. The interaction between FI and gender in their association with self-efficacy was not statistically significant ($p = 0.251$). The associations of FI with global self-efficacy score remained statistically significant after adjusting for gender, bodyweight status, and region of residence, while they remained statistically significant only for girls in the gender-stratified Model 1. When these models were further adjusted for parent educational attainment, associations remained significant only for students (girls and boys combined) and for girls from moderate FI households (Model 2). The association between FI and global self-efficacy was no longer significant after further adjusting for household income.

The individual associations of FI with self-efficacy for physical activity and healthy eating are presented in the Supplementary Table S1. With respect to self-efficacy for physical activity, students from households with moderate and severe FI had significantly lower scores compared to students from food secure households. No differences were observed when comparing children from households with marginal FI and with FS. Associations remained after adjusting for gender, bodyweight status, and region of residence. In the gender-stratified models, this association remained only for girls. With the exception of girls from moderately FI households having significantly lower associated self-efficacy for physical activity after adjusting for parental education, associations did not remain statistically significant after further adjusting for parent education and household income.

Table 3. Relationship between food insecurity and global self-efficacy to make healthy choices among grade 5 students (aged 10–11 years) in Nova Scotia, Canada.

Global Self-Efficacy	All Students		Girls		Boys	
	B (95%CI)	*p*-Value	B (95%CI)	*p*-Value	B (95%CI)	*p*-Value
	Univariate					
Household Food Security Status						
Food secure	0.00	-	0.00	-	0.00	-
Marginal FI [1]	−1.03 (−2.69, 0.62)	0.221	−0.98 (−3.20, 1.23)	0.383	−1.32 (−3.55, 0.91)	0.244
Moderate FI [1]	**−2.73 (−4.19, −1.27)**	**<0.001**	**−3.16 (−4.92, −1.40)**	**<0.001**	−2.29 (−4.57, 0.00)	0.05
Severe FI [1]	**−2.27 (−4.04, −0.48)**	**0.013**	**−3.17 (−5.44, −0.90)**	**0.006**	−1.29 (−3.92, 1.33)	0.332
	Model 1					
Food secure	0.00	-	0.00	-	0.00	-
Marginal FI [1]	−0.82 (−2.48, 0.84)	0.331	−0.67 (−2.89, 1.56)	0.555	−1.14 (−3.32, 1.05)	0.305
Moderate FI [1]	**−2.41 (−3.83, −0.98)**	**0.001**	**−2.82 (−4.59, −1.04)**	**0.002**	−1.93 (−4.20, 0.33)	0.094
Severe FI [1]	**−2.02 (−3.78, −0.25)**	**0.025**	**−2.83 (−5.06, −0.60)**	**0.013**	−0.99 (−3.65, 1.66)	0.461
	Model 2					
Food secure	0.00		0.00	-	0.00	-
Marginal FI [1]	−0.31 (−1.97, 1.35)	0.710	−0.32 (−2.53, 1.89)	0.774	−0.51 (−2.71, 1.69)	0.646
Moderate FI [1]	**−1.58 (−3.01, −0.15)**	**0.030**	**−2.37 (−4.13, −0.62)**	**0.008**	−0.66 (−2.96, 1.63)	0.571
Severe FI [1]	−1.00 (−2.79, 0.79)	0.273	−2.24 (−4.48, 0.013)	0.051	0.52 (−2.12, 3.16)	0.699
	Model 3					
Food secure	0.00	-	0.00	-	0.00	
Marginal FI [1]	0.24 (−1.41, 1.90)	0.774	0.27 (−1.92, 2.47)	0.806	0.10 (−2.16, 2.36)	0.930
Moderate FI [1]	−0.90 (−2.38,0.58)	0.232	−1.80 (−3.61, 0.01)	0.052	0.084 (−2.33, 2.51)	0.946
Severe FI [1]	−0.081 (−2.03, 1.87)	−0.935	−1.56 (−4.04, 0.91)	0.215	1.64 (−1.17, 4.44)	0.249

B: regression coefficient; 95% CI; 95% confidence interval; Model 1 is adjusted for region of residence, body weight status, and gender (in non-gender-stratified models). Model 2 is further adjusted for parental education and Model 3 is further adjusted for household income. Estimates are weighted to represent grade five students in Nova Scotia. Results in bold are statistically significant ($p < 0.05$); [1] Food insecurity.

In terms of self-efficacy for healthy eating, students from moderately FI households had significantly lower scores than students from food secure households before and after adjusting for gender, bodyweight status, and region of residence. In gender-stratified models, this difference was significant for girls from moderate and severe FI households, but not for boys. The association with lower self-efficacy for healthy eating remained significant only among students (girls and boys combined) and girls living in moderate FI households after further considering parental education. When this model was further adjusted for household income, the association remained significant only for girls from moderately FI households (Supplementary Table S1).

4. Discussion

The objectives of this study were to: (i) to determine whether there are differences in self-esteem and self-efficacy for healthy lifestyle choices between students living in households with FS and FI; and (ii) to determine whether there are gender differences within the association between FI, self-esteem and self-efficacy among children. Our findings revealed that one quarter (25.2%) of children who participated in the CLASS II study were living in food insecure households. We demonstrated that these children living in households with FI were more likely to have low global self-esteem and low self-efficacy for healthy lifestyle choices. These associations were generally more pronounced for girls than for boys and independent of region of residence, bodyweight status and parental educational attainment. Household income appeared to be the essential underlying determinant of the associations of FI with self-esteem and self-efficacy, to some extent lesser in the association in girls. Although 7.1% of children lived in households with severe FI, we did not observe a gradient of severity of HFI with likelihood of low self-esteem and self-efficacy for physical activity and healthy eating.

Our observed FI prevalence (25.2%) was relatively consistent with provincial estimates of HFI for the same year (2011) in that 23% of Nova Scotian households with children were food insecure [19]. Findings from the present study relating to FI, self-esteem and self-efficacy are supported by previous literature [30,44]. However, as existing research that has measured the association between FI and self-esteem among children is limited, we have positioned our findings amongst studies of adults. Laraia et al. (2006) reported a negative association among self-esteem and FI among women [44]. A similar inverse relationship between self-efficacy and FI was observed among adults in the United States; FI was associated with low levels of self-efficacy [27]. Martin et al. (2016) investigated whether an association existed between self-efficacy and FS among adults. The authors found a significant inverse association between FI and self-efficacy [30]. Our findings corroborate these results.

4.1. Policy, Practice and Research Recommendations

Given we found self-esteem and self-efficacy were compromised among children from food insecure households, especially among girls, upstream policy actions targeting the structural determinants of HFI [45] should be prioritized. Our research is suggestive that such action would not only reduce FI prevalence but could also prevent resultant implications for children's mental health status and life chances, given that living in households with FI manifests in mental health issues in adolescence and adulthood [12,46,47]. As such, our recommendation to address HFI includes social policy interventions to increase the household income of low-income residents [48]. The relationship between income and HFI suggests increasing these residents' income, such as through a Basic Income Guarantee, could have a substantial impact on FI [49]. Other important implications of this research include incorporating strategies to increase self-esteem and self-efficacy, such as for example in school settings [27] because improved lifestyle behaviours have also been related to better school achievement and reduced prevalence of mental health issues [50,51]. Further, promoting childhood self-esteem and self-efficacy for healthy lifestyle choices may improve health and learning, and herewith future job opportunities and earnings. Population groups that require targeted support include girls, given the current study suggests they are more vulnerable to low self-esteem and self-efficacy if they are living in food insecure households [47,52]. Additionally, there is a relationship between positive self-efficacy and mental wellbeing [32]. Therefore, strategies must be implemented to ensure the lasting trajectory towards both FI and negative psychological outcomes is mitigated during childhood [46].

Further research demonstrating the relationship between HFI and low self-esteem and self-efficacy is warranted, given that low self-esteem contributes to depression in youth [32,53]. This research should also be undertaken in other similar countries, for comparison purposes.

4.2. Strengths and Limitations

Strengths of this study include the large population-based sample, increasing the study's representativeness. Sampling accounted for urban and rural residents, with all public schools in the province invited to participate. The relative high participation rate was another strength. To our knowledge, no other studies have investigated the gender differences in children between HFI modelled as three levels of severity and self-esteem and self-efficacy, reinforcing the importance of our contribution to the scarce evidence base. However, there were limitations associated with this study. This research was cross-sectional in nature, and therefore we could not establish causation. A review of longitudinal studies investigating associations between FI and mental health in adults suggested a bidirectional relationship existed (for example FI increasing depression and depression increasing FI) [54]. Therefore, low self-esteem may contribute to increasing FI over time in adults. However, research among children is insufficient to understand this relationship. A previous study has suggested that the cost of treating children's mental health care may negatively impact household finances, thus resulting in HFI [55]. However, further research in the field is required and the cross-sectional nature of the present study precludes further investigation into the temporality of the association among our sample. Although responses rates were lower than average among residential areas with lower household income, weights were calculated to correct for this disproportionate non-response. The use of the 6-item HFSSM does not capture the most severe range of FI, nor does it capture anxiety or concerns with regards to accessing food [3]. In addition, it does not inquire about FI among children within the household, and thus, limits our ability to directly associate findings with child FI. However, evidence suggests that HFI independently predicts individuals' health [56] and that living in an adult food insecure household is sufficient for children to suffer from consequences of FI [3]. Further, the six-item short-form is slightly less reliable and sensitive than the full 18-item questionnaire [3,57], and as such, the prevalence reported in our research may be underestimated. This shortcoming also has the potential to diminish the strength of association between HFI and self-esteem and self-efficacy. Lastly, though having demonstrated good internal reliability, the lack of standardized self-esteem and self-efficacy tools is a limitation of this research.

5. Conclusions

Various studies examined the association between HFI and poor mental health in high-income countries such as Canada. These studies generally concluded that HFI is associated with poor mental health outcomes. In this study, we examined in children if self-esteem and self-efficacy were associated with HFI at three increasing levels of severity. Given there is a hypothetical cyclical relationship between FI and self-esteem and self-efficacy, interventions that address both child poverty, low-self-esteem and low self-efficacy are required to break the cycle of intergenerational HFI. Such actions could improve physical and cognitive health among children now and throughout their entire lifespan. This is critically important, given the link between mental health problems in childhood and in later life [11].

Supplementary Materials: The following are available online at http://www.mdpi.com/2072-6643/11/3/675/s1, Table S1: Relationship between food insecurity and self-efficacy for physical activity and healthy eating among grade 5 students (aged 10–11 years) in Nova Scotia, Canada.

Author Contributions: Conceptualization, S.L.G., O.K.L., R.B., N.W. and P.V.; Data curation, O.K.L. and P.V.; Formal analysis, O.K.L.; Funding acquisition, S.L.G. and P.V.; Investigation, P.V.; Methodology, S.L.G., O.K.L., R.B., N.W. and P.V.; Resources, P.V.; Software, O.K.L.; Validation, O.K.L.; Writing–original draft, S.L.G., O.K.L. and R.B.; Writing–review & editing, S.L.G., O.K.L., R.B., N.W. and P.V.

Funding: This research was funded by the Collaborative Research and Innovation Opportunities (CRIO) Team program from Alberta Innovates (AI grant number 201300671) to Veugelers. Godrich was funded through an Edith Cowan University School of Medical and Health Sciences Research Collaboration Travel Grant. Blanchet is funded by a Banting Postdoctoral Fellowship.

Acknowledgments: The authors would like to sincerely thank the participants of this study.

Conflicts of Interest: The authors declare no conflicts of interest. The funders had no role in the design of the study; in the collection, analyses, or interpretation of data; in the writing of the manuscript, or in the decision to publish the results.

References

1. Tarasuk, V.; Mitchell, A.; Dachner, N. *Household Food Insecurity in Canada, 2014*; Research to Identify Policy Options to Reduce Food Insecurity (PROOF): Toronto, ON, Canada, 2016.
2. Coleman-Jensen, A.; Rabbitt, M.P.; Gregory, C.A.; Singh, A. *Household Food Security in the United States in 2015*; United States Department of Agriculture Economic Research Service: Washington, DC, USA, 2016.
3. Bickel, G.; Nord, M.; Price, C.; Hamilton, W.; Cook, J. *Guide to Measuring Household Food Security, Revised 2000*; U.S. Depatment of Agriculture, Food and Nutrition Service: Alexandria, Egypt, 2000.
4. Ke, J.; Ford-Jones, E.L. Food insecurity and hunger: A review of the effects on children's health and behaviour. *Paediatr. Child Health* **2015**, *20*, 89–91. [CrossRef] [PubMed]
5. Tarasuk, V.; Cheng, J.; de Oliveira, C.; Dachner, N.; Gundersen, C.; Kurdyak, P. Association between household food insecurity and annual health care costs. *Can. Med. Assoc. J.* **2015**, *187*, E429–E436. [CrossRef] [PubMed]
6. Tarasuk, V.; Cheng, J.; Gundersen, C.; de Oliveira, C.; Kurdyak, P. The Relation between Food Insecurity and Mental Health Care Service Utilization in Ontario. *Can. J. Psychiatry* **2018**, *63*, 557–569. [CrossRef] [PubMed]
7. Gundersen, C.; Tarasuk, V.; Cheng, J.; de Oliveira, C.; Kurdyak, P. Food insecurity status and mortality among adults in Ontario, Canada. *PLoS ONE* **2018**, *13*, e0202642. [CrossRef] [PubMed]
8. Che, J.; Chen, J. Food insecurity in Canadian households. *Health Rep.* **2001**, *12*, 11–22. [PubMed]

9. Muldoon, K.A.; Duff, P.K.; Fielden, S.; Anema, A. Food insufficiency is associated with psychiatric morbidity in a nationally representative study of mental illness among food insecure Canadians. *Soc. Psychiatry Psychiatr. Epidemiol.* **2013**, *48*, 795–803. [CrossRef] [PubMed]
10. Jessiman-Perreault, G.; McIntyre, L. The household food insecurity gradient and potential reductions in adverse population mental health outcomes in Canadian adults. *SSM Popul. Health* **2017**, *3*, 1–9. [CrossRef] [PubMed]
11. Althoff, R.R.; Ametti, M.; Bertmann, F. The role of food insecurity in developmental psychopathology. *Prev. Med.* **2016**, *92*, 106–109. [CrossRef] [PubMed]
12. Ashiabi, G.S.; O'Neal, K.K. A Framework for Understanding the Association Between Food Insecurity and Children's Developmental Outcomes. *Child Dev. Perspect.* **2008**, *2*, 71–77. [CrossRef]
13. Cook, J. Impacts of child food insecurity and hunger on health and development in children. In Proceedings of the Workshop on Research Gaps and Opportunities on the Causes and Consequences of Child Hunger, Washington, DC, USA, 8–9 April 2013.
14. Kirk, S.F.; Kuhle, S.; McIsaac, J.L.; Williams, P.L.; Rossiter, M.; Ohinmaa, A.; Veugelers, P.J. Food security status among grade 5 students in Nova Scotia, Canada and its association with health outcomes. *Public Health Nutr.* **2015**, *18*, 2943–2951. [CrossRef]
15. Jyoti, D.F.; Frongillo, E.A.; Jones, S.J. Food Insecurity Affects School Children's Academic Performance, Weight Gain, and Social Skills. *J. Nutr.* **2005**, *135*, 2831–2839. [CrossRef] [PubMed]
16. Molcho, M.; Gabhainn, S.; Kelly, C.; Friel, S.; Kelleher, C. Food poverty and health among schoolchildren in Ireland: Findings from the Health Behaviour in School-aged Children (HBSC) study. *Public Health Nutr.* **2007**, *10*, 364–370. [CrossRef]
17. Cook, J.T.; Frank, D.A. Food Security, Poverty and Human Development in the United States. *Ann. New York Acad. Sci.* **2008**, *1136*, 193–209. [CrossRef]
18. Fram, M.; Frongillo, E.; Jones, S.; Williams, R.; Burke, M. Children Are Aware of Food Insecurity and Take Responsibility for Managing Food. *J. Nutr.* **2011**, *141*, 1114–1119. [CrossRef] [PubMed]
19. Tarasuk, V.; Mitchell, A.; Dachner, N. *Household Food Insecurity in Canada, 2011. Research to Identify Policy Options to Reduce Food Insecurity*; PROOF: Toronto, ON, Canada, 2013.
20. Bhattacharya, J.; Currie, J.; Haider, S. Poverty, food insecurity, and nutritional outcomes in children and adults. *J. Health Econ.* **2004**, *23*, 839–862. [CrossRef] [PubMed]
21. Merriam-Webster. Self-Esteem. Available online: https://www.merriam-webster.com/dictionary/self-esteem (accessed on 13 February 2019).
22. Rosenberg, M.; Schooler, C.; Schoenbach, C.; Rosenberg, F. Global self-esteem and specific self-esteem: Different concepts, different outcomes. *Am. Sociol. Rev.* **1995**, *60*, 141–156. [CrossRef]
23. Bandura, A. *Self-Efficacy: The Exercise of Control*; W.H. Freeman and Company: New York, NY, USA, 1997.
24. Richert, J.; Reuter, T.; Wiedemann, A.U.; Lippke, S.; Ziegelmann, J.; Schwarzer, R. Differential effects of planning and self-efficacy on fruit and vegetable consumption. *Appetite* **2010**, *54*, 611–614. [CrossRef] [PubMed]
25. Chu, Y.L.; Fung, C.; Kuhle, S.; Storey, K.E.; Veugelers, P.J.; Farmer, A. Involvement in home meal preparation is associated with food preference and self-efficacy among Canadian children. *Public Health Nutr.* **2014**, *16*, 108–112. [CrossRef]
26. Bartfield, J.K.; Ojehomon, N.; Huskey, K.W.; Davis, R.B.; Wee, C.C. Preferences and self-efficacy for diet modification among primary care patients. *Obesity* **2010**, *18*, 430–432. [CrossRef]
27. Kamimura, A.; Jess, A.; Trinh, H.N.; Aguilera, G.; Nourian, M.M.; Assasnik, N.; Ashby, J. Food Insecurity Associated with Self-Efficacy and Acculturation. *Popul. Health Manag.* **2017**, *20*, 66–73. [CrossRef]
28. Vijayaraghavan, M.; Jacobs, E.A.; Seligman, H.; Fernandez, A. The association between housing instability, food insecurity, and diabetes self-efficacy in low-income adults. *J. Health Care Poor Underserved* **2011**, *22*, 1279–1291. [CrossRef]
29. Committee on World Food Security. Coming to terms with terminology: Food security, nutrition security, food security and nutrition, food and nutrition security. In Proceedings of the Thirty-Ninth Session of the EuFMD Commission, Rome, Italy, 27–28 April 2011.
30. Martin, K.S.; Colantonio, A.G.; Picho, K.; Boyle, K.E. Self-efficacy is associated with increased food security in novel food pantry program. *SSM Popul. Health* **2016**, *2*, 62–67. [CrossRef] [PubMed]

31. Masselink, M.; Van Roekel, E.; Oldehinkel, A.J. Self-esteem in Early Adolescence as Predictor of Depressive Symptoms in Late Adolescence and Early Adulthood: The Mediating Role of Motivational and Social Factors. *J. Youth Adolesc.* **2018**, *47*, 932–946. [CrossRef] [PubMed]
32. Mulligan, A. The Relationship between Self-Esteem and Mental Health Outcomes in Children and Youth. Available online: file:///D:/sgodric0/Downloads/eis_self_esteem_mh.pdf (accessed on 13 February 2019).
33. Bandura, A.; Pastorelli, C.; Barbaranelli, C.; Caprara, G.V. Self-Efficacy Pathways to Childhood Depression. *J. Personal. Soc. Psychol.* **1999**, *76*, 258–269. [CrossRef]
34. Hromi-Fiedler, A.; Bermúdez-Millán, A.; Segura-Pérez, S.; Pérez-Escamilla, R. Household food insecurity is associated with depressive symptoms among low-income pregnant Latinas. *Matern. Child Nutr.* **2011**, *7*, 421–430. [CrossRef] [PubMed]
35. Chilton, M.; Knowles, M.; Bloom, S.L. The Intergenerational Circumstances of Household Food Insecurity and Adversity. *J. Hunger Environ. Nutr.* **2017**, *12*, 269–297. [CrossRef]
36. PROOF. Latest Household Food Insecurity Data Now. Available online: https://proof.utoronto.ca/new-data-available/ (accessed on 13 February 2019).
37. Finance and Treasury Board. Economics and Statistics. Available online: https://www.novascotia.ca/finance/statistics/archive_news.asp?id=13441&dg=&df=&dto=0&dti=3 (accessed on 13 February 2019).
38. Varni, J.; Seid, M.; Rode, C.A. The PedsQL: Measurement model for the pediatric quality of life inventory. *Med. Care* **1999**, *37*, 126–139. [CrossRef]
39. Maximova, K.; Khan, M.K.; Austin, S.B.; Kirk, S.F.; Veugelers, P.J. The role of underestimating body size for self-esteem and self-efficacy among grade five children in Canada. *Ann. Epidemiol.* **2015**, *25*, 753–759. [CrossRef]
40. BMI-for-Age (5–19 Years). Available online: https://www.who.int/growthref/who2007_bmi_for_age/en/ (accessed on 22 March 2018).
41. Fung, C.; McIsaac, J.D.; Kuhle, S.; Kirk, S.F.L.; Veugelers, P.J. The impact of a population-level school food and nutrition policy on dietary intake and body weights of Canadian children. *Prev. Med.* **2013**, *57*, 934–940. [CrossRef]
42. Hesketh, K.; Wake, M.; Waters, E. Body mass and parent-reported self-esteem in elementary school children: Evidence for a causal relationship. *Int. J. Obes.* **2004**, *28*, 1233–1237. [CrossRef]
43. Veugelers, P.; Fitzgerald, A. Effectiveness of School Programs in Preventing Childhood Obesity: A Mulltilevel Comparison. *Am. J. Public Health* **2005**, *95*, 432–435. [CrossRef]
44. Laraia, B.A.; Siega-Riz, A.M.; Gundersen, C.; Dole, N. Psychosocial factors and socioeconomic indicators are associated with household food insecurity among pregnant women. *J. Nutr.* **2006**, *136*, 177–182. [CrossRef]
45. Rychetnik, L.; Webb, K.; Story, L.; Katz, T. *Food Security Options Paper: A Planning Framework and Menu of Options for Policy and Practice Interventions*; NSW Centre for Public Health Nutrition: Sydney, Australia, 2003.
46. Vozoris, N.T.; Tarasuk, V.S. Household Food Insufficiency is Associated with Poorer Health. *J. Nutr.* **2003**, *133*, 120–126. [CrossRef]
47. Melchior, M.; Caspi, A.; Howard, L.M.; Ambler, A.P.; Bolton, H.; Mountain, N.; Moffitt, T.E. Mental Health Context of Food Insecurity: A Representative Cohort of Families With Young Children. *Pediatrics* **2009**, *124*, E564–E572. [CrossRef]
48. Emery, J.C.H.; Fleisch, V.C.; McIntyre, L. How a Guaranteed Annual Income Could Put Food Banks Out of Business. In *SPP Research Paper*; The School of Public Policy: Calgary, AB, Canada, 2013; pp. 6–37.
49. Tarasuk, V. *Implications of a Basic Income Guarantee for Household Food Insecurity*; Northern Policy Institute: Thunder Bay, ON, Canada, 2017.
50. Faught, E.L.; Ekwaru, J.P.; Gleddie, D.; Storey, K.E.; Asbridge, M.; Veugelers, P.J. The combined impact of diet, physical activity, sleep and screen time on academic achievement: A prospective study of elementary school students in Nova Scotia, Canada. *Int. J. Behav. Nutr. Phys. Act.* **2017**, *14*, 29. [CrossRef]
51. Loewen, O.K.; Ekwaru, J.P.; Faught, E.L.; Maximova, K.; Ohinmaa, A.; Veugelers, P. Adherence to recommendations for lifestyle behaviours in childhood and mental health in subsequent years: A prospective study of Canadian children. In Proceedings of the International Society for Behavioural Nutrition and Physical Activity Conference 2018, Hong Kong, China, 4–6 June 2018.
52. Garg, A.; Toy, S.; Tripodis, Y.; Cook, J.; Cordella, N. Influence of Maternal Depression on Household Food Insecurity for Low-Income Families. *Acad. Pediatr.* **2015**, *15*, 305–310. [CrossRef]

53. Orth, U.; Robins, R.W. Understanding the Link Between Low Self-Esteem and Depression. *Assoc. Psychol. Sci.* **2013**, *22*, 455–460. [CrossRef]
54. Maynard, M.; Andrade, L.; Packull-McCormick, S.; Perlman, C.M.; Leos-Toro, C.; Kirkpatrick, S.I. Food Insecurity and Mental Health among Females in High-Income Countries. *Int. J. Environ. Res. Public Health* **2018**, *15*, 1424. [CrossRef] [PubMed]
55. Burke, M.; Martini, L.H.; Cayir, E.; Hartline-Grafton, H.L.; Meade, R.L. Severity of household food insecurity is positively associated with mental disorders among children and adolescents in the United States. *J. Nutr.* **2016**, *146*, 2019–2026. [CrossRef] [PubMed]
56. PROOF. Household Food Insecurity in Canada: A Guide to Measurement and Interpretation. Available online: https://proof.utoronto.ca/wp-content/uploads/2018/11/Household-Food-Insecurity-in-Canada-A-Guide-to-Measurement-and-Interpretation.pdf (accessed on 30 January 2019).
57. Blumberg, S.J.; Bialostosky, K.; Hamilton, W.L.; Briefel, R.R. The effectiveness of a short form of the Household Food Security Scale. *Am. J. Public Health* **1999**, *89*, 1231–1234. [CrossRef] [PubMed]

nutrients

MDPI

Article

South West Food Community: A Place-Based Pilot Study to Understand the Food Security System

Stephanie Louise Godrich [1,*], Jennifer Payet [1], Deborah Brealey [1], Melinda Edmunds [2], Melissa Stoneham [2] and Amanda Devine [3]

1 School of Medical and Health Sciences, Edith Cowan University, Bunbury, WA 6230, Australia; j.payet@ecu.edu.au (J.P.); d.brealey@ecu.edu.au (D.B.)
2 Public Health Advocacy Institute of Western Australia, Curtin University, Bentley, WA 6102, Australia; melinda.edmunds@curtin.edu.au (M.E.); M.Stoneham@curtin.edu.au (M.S.)
3 School of Medical and Health Sciences, Edith Cowan University, Joondalup, WA 6027, Australia; a.devine@ecu.edu.au
* Correspondence: s.godrich@ecu.edu.au; Tel.: +61-(08)-6304-2032

Received: 29 January 2019; Accepted: 26 March 2019; Published: 29 March 2019

Abstract: The objectives of this study were to: (i) Identify initiatives supporting healthy food availability, access and utilisation in the South West region of Western Australia (WA); and (ii) understand how they were functioning as a system to enhance community-level food security (FS). This study used a novel approach; a Systemic Innovation Lab, to interview initiative leaders/stakeholders about their FS initiative. Initiative characteristics measured included those which were associated with creating the effective conditions for FS systems change. Information was uploaded to an innovative online tool, creating a 'transition card' (matrix) of initiatives and partnering organisations. Fifty-one participants reported on 52 initiatives. Initiatives were most likely to possess characteristics relating to reinforcing changes towards an enhanced way of working to address FS and creating disruption to the old way of working. The initiative characteristic that initiatives were least likely to possess related to identifying the different causal factors of FS, and working with other stakeholders on specific components of FS. The South West Food Community pilot project used a comprehensive yet defined approach to demonstrate the value of a place-based, co-design project. Participants and stakeholders could strengthen specific initiative characteristics to facilitate enhanced community-level FS.

Keywords: food security; public health; place-based; co-design

---

1. Introduction

Food security (FS) refers to sufficient physical, economic and social access to safe and nutritious food at all times [1]. At a community level, this extends to all community residents obtaining adequate food through a sustainable food system that maximizes self-reliance [2]. Suboptimal or inadequate food access results in food insecurity (FI) [3], which is known as a complex 'wicked' problem [4]. The unique issue is not well understood, nor resolved by any particular individual solution [5]. To facilitate understanding of the issue's components, four pillars of FS are typically defined: Food availability, access, utilisation, and stability of the first three pillars [6–8]. Within these pillars, a range of determinants are described. Food availability drivers include well-located retail options selling affordable, nutritious food of sufficient quantity [9–12]. Determinants of food access include adequate resources to access food, private, public and active transport opportunities [9,10,12,13]. Within the food utilisation pillar, determinants include adequate food preparation, cooking and storage facilities, cultural considerations, nutrition knowledge and cooking skills to achieve physiological needs [9,10,12].

The stability of the first three pillars refers to the ability of all individuals, households and communities to have sustained access to nutritious food at all times [12], thus being food secure.

By and large, most Australians are thought to be food secure [10], with the reported household FI prevalence at 4% [14] nationally. However, other Australian research suggests this is an underestimate, with the prevalence reported to be as high as 36% [15]. FS can be particularly challenging to ensure, especially in rural and remote locations, given the poorer food availability, quality and higher cost [9,16,17]. Additional challenges associated with financial and physical access to food or nutrition knowledge and food preparation skills can hamper efforts to achieve FS [9,10,13,16]. Recommendations to enhance FS across food availability, access, utilisation and stability pillars have included local, sustainable food supply options, enhanced social support and increasing the number and duration of food literacy programs [9]. However, given the complexity of this issue, the need to move beyond viewing FS through pillars alone, and thus adopting a systemic approach, is necessary [18].

Approaches to increase FS systemically include the use of 'lab' approaches. These experimental methods identify societal issues, develop and test impactful ideas to solve such issues [19]. Labs use varying methods, focus areas, processes and typically possess one or more features identified in the literature to address wicked issues [19]. However, given the varied scope, their efficacy is limited. To more effectively address complex issues, a novel lab type coined a 'Systemic Innovation Lab' [20], can be used. This new, holistic lab type includes all elements recommended to address complex concepts, such as FS [20]. The process is based on a series of principles that create enabling conditions for adopting a more effective way of addressing complex problems [20]. Features include addressing the unpredictability of complex problems that have interconnected determinants [20,21], a place-based focus engaging a variety of stakeholders [18,19,22] transitioning to a new, more effective way of working [20,23], and self-organisation [20,24]. When these elements are collectively used, this approach facilitates place-based data collection and identifies governments' enabling influences for change [20]. It also involves a range of stakeholders from various levels of government and community throughout the process [20]. Community participation or citizen engagement in health promotion projects ensures research meets community needs, increases public awareness, improves research translation and decision-making [25]. It also results in more effective solution generation, increases trust, empowers participants and increases the potential for proposed strategies or outcomes to be accepted by the wider community [26].

A critical component of the new Systemic Innovation Lab approach is the nine embedded Focus Areas, which align with the aforementioned principles to create enabling conditions for change. Specific Focus Areas include: (1) Create a disequilibrium state (shaking up the current way of working); (2) Amplify action (transitioning towards a new and better way of working); (3) Encourage self-organisation (organisations working in new ways); (4) Stabilise feedback (locking in the new way of working); (5) Enable information flows (disseminating information throughout the system); (6) Unplanned exploration at the interface between a government bureaucracy and the community (aligning community organisations' work with government priorities); (7) Unplanned exploration at the interface between the elected members of a government and the community (community organisations shaping government policies); (8) Planned exploitation at the interface between the community and a government bureaucracy (government using community knowledge and ideas); and (9) Planned exploitation at the interface between the community and the elected members of a government (government sharing information about community initiatives). Further detail about these Focus Areas and their characteristics has been previously published [18,27].

Whilst previous research has investigated the determinants and the prevalence of household FI in Western Australia (WA) [9,13,16,17,28], a systemic examination of FS at a community level has yet to be conducted. We currently lack a broad understanding of the initiatives being used to improve FS in WA. We also lack a comprehensive map of these initiatives across regions, local government areas and communities. Further, existing partnerships that support these initiatives are yet to be identified. This highlights a clear gap in evidence and practice, and hampers potential action to enhance FS in WA.

The resultant piece-meal approach impedes the understanding and improvement of FS, particularly in rural and remote areas where food system challenges are heightened. The objectives of this pilot project were therefore to: (i) Identify the initiatives supporting healthy food availability, access and utilisation in South West WA; and (ii) understand how they are functioning as a system to enhance FS.

2. Materials and Methods

2.1. Sampling and Recruitment

This pilot study took place in the South West region of WA, south of Perth and covers 23,970 km^2 [29] and includes inner regional and outer regional towns [30]. The project utilised a Systemic Innovation Lab [18] approach, which was based on appropriate features for addressing complex issues such as FS [20]. This process, developed by the organisation Wicked Lab (www.wickedlab.com.au), aligned with systemic design and was underpinned by complex systems leadership theories and complex adaptive systems [18,27]. The methodology used, including the steps of Form, Explore, Map, Learn, Address and Share (FEMLAS) [20], is explained in detail elsewhere [20] and thus a summary is presented in this paper. A cross-institutional core team and reference group provided guidance, feedback and oversight of project processes. Structured individual or group interviews were deemed the most appropriate data collection method, for FS initiatives and their characteristics. This approach facilitated assessment of alignment between initiatives' characteristics and those associated with transitioning to a more effective way of increasing FS [18].

A Microsoft Excel database was compiled by the project team via an Internet (Google) search of programs and projects (initiatives) operating in the selected geographical boundary; the South West region of WA. To be included in the database, initiatives had to focus on one or more FS pillars in the South West region of WA. Within these pillars, initiatives were required to address one or more of the determinants of FS, for example healthy food promotion, social support, nutrition knowledge and cooking skills [6,10]. Example search terms included a broad scope such as 'food security programs in South West Western Australia'. Search terms also related to FS pillars, such as 'food availability in South West Western Australia', and FS determinants such as 'social support programs South West Western Australia' and 'nutrition education programs South West Western Australia'. The initiative database included the initiative name, a description, start and finish date (if ceased), initiative owner/stakeholder name, email address, website URL and partnering organisations involved with the initiative. Interview participants were identified as project coordinators, staff, volunteers or committee members working on one or more initiatives. In addition, database contacts were added from existing stakeholder network databases. An organisation database included the administering organisation's name, a description of the organisation, sector (i.e., business, not-for-profit organisation) and website URL.

To increase stakeholder buy-in, recruitment and to identify additional initiatives, stakeholders from state and local government, community organisations and community members were invited to a project launch. During this launch, the proposed process was outlined and participants were engaged in a scoping activity to outline the current South West region initiatives focusing on the FS pillars. The purpose of this activity was to familiarise attendees with the local FS system and identify further potential initiatives for inclusion. Identified stakeholders from the Internet search and project launch (n = 79) were invited by email to participate in an interviewer-administered survey and sent an information letter and consent form. A minimum of three follow up contacts were made to recruit participants. Of these, 51 stakeholders consented to participate in an interview (65% response rate).

2.2. Instrument

A 45-item survey tool was developed by the project team and was linked to Wicked Lab's Tool for Systemic Change [31], a digital tool designed specifically to address wicked problems. The Tool for Systemic Change was based on a model focusing on 36 initiative characteristics embedded within the nine aforementioned Focus Areas. These Focus Areas and their characteristics were associated with creating desirable conditions for systems change; transitioning to a more effective way of enhancing FS [18,20]. Each Focus Area characteristic was linked to a survey question. The survey was cross-checked by Wicked Lab consultants to ensure the questions retained the intent of the Focus Area characteristics. An example of a Focus Area 1 characteristic included 'cultivate a passion for action.' [18]. The related interview question was "Does your initiative create a passion for the community to take action around food security? (i.e. encouraging/influencing the system to a new way of working, such as community getting involved with creating a local edible garden)". See Supplementary Table S1 for a complete list of Focus Areas, their associated characteristics and survey interview questions. Response options to questions included 'Yes' or 'No'. Participants were asked to provide a comment on why they believed that their initiative did or did not contain this characteristic. Additional survey items included demographic questions such as worker type, years working in the field, a description of their initiative/s and partner organisations with whom they were working.

2.3. Data Collection

Interviews

Qualitative interviews were the chosen data collection method, and are deemed appropriate for the investigation of novel concepts or issues [32]. Interviews afford a greater understanding of such issues [33]. Data collection occurred between July–October 2018 by two interviewers. Individual or group interviews using the survey tool were conducted in person (n = 3) or via telephone (n = 38) with a total of 51 participants. To ensure rigour and consistency, both interviewers co-conducted the first interview, which commenced with a verbal preamble about the study purpose, format and number of questions. Interviewees were advised there were no correct or incorrect answers; the responses were based on their perception of their initiative. Interviewers proceeded to ask all questions to respondents, taking notes during each interview and digitally entering responses into a Microsoft Excel spreadsheet thereafter.

2.4. Data Entry and Analysis

Microsoft Excel was used to manage interview data before being uploaded to Wicked Lab's Tool for Systemic Change [18,31]. The Tool for Systemic Change captured information about the organisation that owned the initiative, contact details, any partnering organisations working on the initiative and details about the length of time the initiative had been operating. The Tool for Systemic Change also included a series of tick boxes relating to each Focus Area and their characteristics, which were ticked where the initiative met the characteristics [20]. In addition, text boxes captured open-ended responses explaining how the initiative did or did not possess the characteristic. This enabled the creation of a visual 'transition card' (matrix) displaying the initiatives and the characteristics they possessed, within the nine Focus Areas (Figure 1) [18]. If the initiative possessed the characteristic within the Focus Area, the cell on the transition card corresponding to the tick box response was filled. This provided a visual representation of each initiative's contribution to systemic change [20]. In addition, it displayed how the 'solution ecosystem' of initiatives and their partner organisations collectively contributed towards systemic change in the South West WA region. The transition card was subsequently analysed initiative by initiative and as a whole, to highlight gaps in opportunity that could be harnessed to improve FS across the region. Reports generated in Microsoft Excel format by the Wicked Lab tool included descriptive statistics of: The total number of initiatives; total number of partnering organisations; number of organisations by sector (i.e., business, not for profit); the number of partner organisations per initiative; and number of initiative per organisation [18]. A report also provided the number and proportion (%) of initiatives that met each Focus Area's characteristics. Initiatives were then summed by FS pillar in an additional report; categorised into 'food availability', 'food access' or 'food utilisation' pillars. Food availability initiatives were categorised where they aligned with the definition of "sufficient quantities of food of appropriate quality, supplied through domestic production, imports" [34]. This included food sourced through formal or informal means, such as through community gardens. It incorporated initiatives that aligned with one or more of the food availability pillar determinants of food availability, food price, location of outlets, food quality, promotion, or food variety [6,9,10]. An example includes a health and wellbeing plan supporting local agricultural development, with the purpose of increasing healthy food availability. Food access was defined as "the resources and ability that communities, households and individuals have in order to acquire and consume a healthy diet" [34]. Initiatives were categorised within this pillar if they aligned with one or more of its determinants of social support, household finances, transport, distance to outlets and mobility [6,9,10]. An example initiative included a fresh produce swapping group open to any community member. The food utilisation definition included "utilisation of food through adequate diet, clean water, sanitation to reach a state of nutritional wellbeing, where all physiological needs are met [34]." Initiatives were categorised within this pillar if they aligned with one or more of its determinants of nutrition knowledge and cooking skills, food preferences, storage or cooking facilities or time to purchase and prepare food [6,9,10]. An example initiative is a community strategy that supports nutrition education.

After results were reviewed by the project team, participants were invited together in a results-sharing and action planning forum. Forum participants (n = 20) were provided with a second briefing paper which outlined the process taken and a copy of the overall transition card. In addition, each participant was provided with an individual summary report for their initiative/s, to facilitate understanding of strengths and 'windows of opportunity' to strengthen. A facilitated action-planning session with provision of examples allowed participants to develop initiative action plans, which outlined strategies to fill identified gaps and enhance their initiative/s functioning to address FS. Participants also discussed potential new FS initiatives, which could be explored to fill identified gaps in the system. A workshop video recording and Microsoft Power Point slides were sent along with individual action plans to participants not able to attend the workshop.

All participants gave their informed consent for inclusion before they participated in the study. The study was conducted in accordance with the Declaration of Helsinki of 1975, revised in 2013, and the protocol was approved by the Edith Cowan University Human Research Ethics Committee (project 20508).

3. Results

3.1. Participant Demographics

A total of 41 individual or group interviews were conducted, with 51 participants. Interviewees were most often volunteers, volunteer leaders or committee members (n = 13), followed by directors, managers or coordinators (n = 11). Participants had worked, on average, three years in their field. Table 1 presents a demographic profile of study participants' worker type.

3.2. Partnering Organisations

There were 83 partnering organisations working on identified initiatives. The majority of interviewees reported partnering with not-for-profit groups (37%), businesses (24%) and state government organisations (19%) to deliver their initiative/s. Table 1 outlines the frequency of partnering organisation type.

Table 1. Participant Demographics.

Worker type	*n* (%)
Education professional	1 (2)
Food producer/farmer	6 (11)
Environmental health officer	1 (2)
Community development officer, services worker or support officer	7 (13)
Director, manager or coordinator	11 (21)
Volunteer, volunteer leader or committee member	13 (24)
Health professional (i.e., health promotion officer, nutritionist, dietitian, nurse)	9 (17)
CEO or President	2 (4)
Social enterprise manager	1 (2)
Sustainability or recycling officer	2 (4)
Total	**53 * (100)**
Partner organisation	***n* (%)**
Local government	9 (11)
State Government	16 (19)
Education	1 (1)
Not-for-profit	31 (37)
Business	20 (24)
Formal community group	3 (4)
Informal community group	3 (4)
Total	**83 (100)**

* Some participants performed more than one role in their initiative/s.

3.3. Initiative Characteristics

A total of 52 initiatives were captured in the mapping process. Initiatives were categorised by FS pillar, with 32 initiatives relating to the 'food availability' pillar. Example initiatives within this pillar included farmers' markets, food trails, local government plans and agritourism initiatives. Thirty initiatives related to the 'food access' pillar and included produce swapping groups, community gardens and community plans outlining objectives or strategies to increase community food access. A total of 31 initiatives were categorised within the 'food utilisation' pillar and were provided by way of community nutrition education initiatives, educational farm stays and other examples including fundraising activities through FS awareness-raising events. No initiatives were categorised in the 'stability' pillar. Most initiatives focused on a combination of food availability, access and/or utilisation dimensions.

3.4. Focus Areas and Initiative Characteristics

Overall, initiatives were most likely to possess characteristics within Focus Area 4, 'stabilise feedback', which related to reinforcing progression to an enhanced way of working (Table 2). This was followed by Focus Area 1, 'create a disequilibrium state', which related to disrupting the old/previous way of working. The initiative characteristic met by the majority of initiatives (92%) included the Focus Area 1 characteristic 'highlight the need to organise communities differently'. This characteristic related to the initiative encouraging communities to address FS in a new or innovative way. Equally, 92% of initiatives reportedly possessed the Focus Area 5 characteristic 'assist in the connection, dissemination and processing of information'. This was achieved either through a newsletter, website or through social media.

The initiative characteristic that was least likely to be met included the Focus Area 2 characteristic of 'partition the system' (*n*= 10, 19%). This could include identifying the different causal factors (parts) of FS and working with other stakeholders on specific parts of FS. An example provided to participants that exemplified this characteristic included a working group made up of members of various sectors, collectively working towards a strategy. This was followed by only 14% of initiatives addressing the characteristic of 'assist elected members to frame policies in a manner which enables community adaptation of policies'. An example provided to participants included a local government putting a call out for community ideas supporting healthy food access through social media.

Table 2 depicts the frequency and proportion of initiatives that met Focus Area characteristics. Results were determined by interviewee responses to the survey questions that linked to each characteristic. A detailed explanation of these characteristics has been published elsewhere [27].

Table 2. Frequency of initiatives meeting Focus Areas and characteristics.

Focus Areas and Characteristics Met by Initiatives	n (%)
Focus Area 1: Create a disequilibrium state (Shaking up the current way of working)	
Highlight the need to organise communities differently	48 (92)
Cultivate a passion for action	39 (75)
Manage initial starting conditions	46 (88)
Specify goals in advance	43 (83)
Establish appropriate boundaries	46 (88)
Embrace uncertainty	34 (65)
Surface conflict	34 (65)
Create controversy	25 (48)
Focus Area 2: Amplify action (moving to a new and better way of working)	
Enable safe fail experimentation	41 (79)
Enable rich interactions in relational spaces	42 (81)
Support collective action	38 (73)
Partition the system	10 (19)
Establish network linkages	40 (77)
Frame issues to match diverse perspectives	21 (40)
Focus Area 3: Encourage self-organisation (organisations working in new and more effective ways with each other)	
Create correlation through language and symbols	40 (77)
Encourage individuals to accept positions as role models for the change effort	27 (52)
Enable periodic information exchanges between partitioned subsystems	40 (77)
Enable resources and capabilities to recombine	31 (60)
Focus Area 4: Stabilise feedback (the new way of working becomes the dominant way of working among the organisations in the system).	
Integrate local constraints	42 (81)
Provide a multiple perspective context and system structure	39 (75)
Enable problem representations to anchor in the community	47 (90)
Enable emergent outcomes to be monitored	42 (81)
Focus Area 5: Enable information flows (helping to get information spread throughout the system)	
Assist system members to keep informed and knowledgeable of forces influencing their community system	34 (65)
Assist in the connection, dissemination and processing of information	48 (92)
Enable connectivity between people who have different perspectives on community issues	40 (77)
Retain and reuse knowledge and ideas generated through interactions	34 (65)
Focus Area 6: Public administration–adaptive community interface (Helping the work undertaken by community organisations to align with government priorities)	
Assist public administrators to frame policies in a manner which enables community adaptation of policies	21 (40)
Remove information differences to enable the ideas and views of citizens to align to the challenges being addressed by governments	22 (42)
Encourage and assist street level workers to take into account the ideas and views of citizens	28 (54)
Focus Area 7: Elected government–adaptive community interface (Creating government policies that are shaped by community organisations)	
Assist elected members to frame policies in a manner which enables community adaptation of policies	14 (27)
Assist elected members to take into account the ideas and views of citizens	21 (40)
Focus Area 8: Community innovation–public administration interface (Government using community knowledge and ideas)	
Encourage and assist street level workers to exploit the knowledge, ideas and innovations of citizens	20 (38)
Bridge community-led activities and projects to the strategic plans of governments	23 (44)
Gather, retain and reuse community knowledge and ideas in other contexts	21 (40)
Focus Area 9: Community innovation–elected government interface (The government sharing information about community initiatives operating in their area)	
Encourage and assist elected members to exploit the knowledge, ideas and innovations of citizens	20 (38)
Collect, analyse, synthesise, reconfigure, manage and represent community information that is relevant to the electorate or area of portfolio responsibility of elected members	24 (46)

Figure 1 provides a visual representation of the 'transition card' of initiatives (y-axis) and their associated Focus Area characteristics (x-axis). The visual representation identifies gaps and opportunities from a set of unlinked community-based initiatives. As seen by the uncoloured cells, and as presented in Table 2, initiatives were least likely to possess characteristics within Focus Areas 6–9, which focused on the community–government interface. Example characteristics included government staff working with community groups through a committee, or investigating how the government could support initiatives that were addressing the objectives in the government Strategic Plan. Each initiative owner received an individual summary report highlighting their associated row within Figure 1.

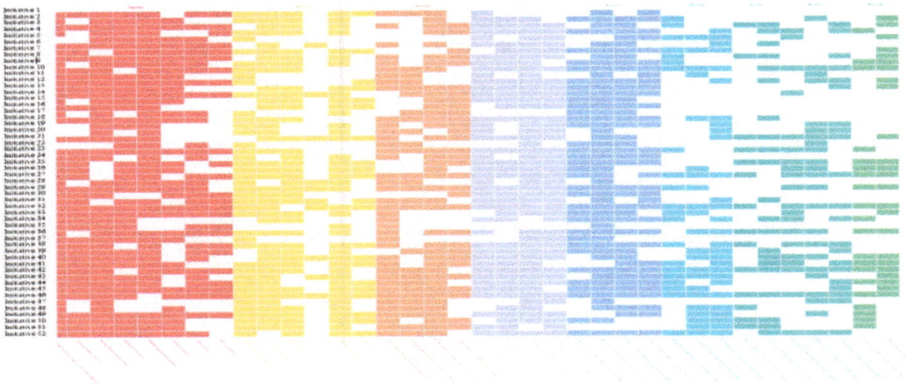

Figure 1. South West WA Food Community 'transition card' at baseline mapping.

4. Discussion

The objectives of this project were to: (i) Identify the initiatives supporting healthy food availability, access and utilisation in South West WA; and (ii) understand how they were functioning as a system to enhance FS. This pilot project resulted in the identification of 52 initiatives in the South West solution ecosystem. Of these, 32 initiatives related to healthy food availability, 30 focused on food access and 31 initiatives focused on food utilisation. Most initiatives focused on a combination of availability, access and/or utilisation dimensions. To deliver their initiatives, organisations partnered with state and local government, as well as the not-for-profit and business sectors. Initiatives were investigated to determine presence of characteristics associated with addressing complex problems, and encouragingly, many communities addressed FS in a new or different way. Information dissemination about FS was also a common attribute, and the majority of initiatives possessed this characteristic. Initiatives were least likely to partition the FS system, for example working with cross-sector stakeholders to address components of FS, or achieve the Focus Areas of 8 and 9—the interface with public administration and elected members.

Previous literature has demonstrated the value of encouraging communities to take a new approach to address complex problems [23,27], to disrupt the system; a characteristic that the majority of initiatives in this project possessed. Similarly, the importance of ensuring information flows throughout the system, whilst it is transitioning from old to new approaches has been reinforced [23,27]. Most of the initiatives captured in this project shared information through the FS system via newsletters or electronic means. Previous evidence has reported the value of stakeholder engagement opportunities afforded by social networking sites, such as awareness raising, sharing program success, or support fundraising efforts [35]. Although less than half of the initiatives possessed the characteristic 'partition the system', previous evidence has acknowledged this characteristic is imperative to support stakeholders to be co-creators of initiatives [20,36]. The value of co-creation lies in its facilitation of needs-based research design, effective decision-making and solution generation, community empowerment and resultant action [25,26].

This project has answered the call of previous research, contributing to a greater understanding of how FI can be addressed as a wicked problem through the use of a Systemic Innovation Lab approach [18]. The approach utilised in this project has supported the South West FS system of organisations and initiatives to identify where their initiatives are functioning effectively to address FS. It also assisted participants to identify where changes were required within their initiatives, to incorporate characteristics within specific areas to leverage change. For example, an outcome of participating in the action-planning forum could include a Local Government Authority hosting a community consultation to review their proposed Public Health Plan, to ensure it meets their needs associated with healthy food availability, access and use. This change would result in the initiative possessing characteristics associated with creating policies that the community shape. Another example could include a community group providing their local government staff with a solution template about FS, explaining how their initiative supports it. This action would result in the community initiative possessing a characteristic associated with sharing information about community initiatives. If multiple initiatives changed their practice and incorporated strategies that linked to associated characteristics they were previously lacking, the system of initiatives would have transitioned to a new and more effective way of supporting FS. Thus, resulting in systemic change and enhancing community-level FS in the region [20]. In addition, the project has used steering strategies to create opportunities for government and community stakeholders to interact, resulting in the collaborative design of adaptations to existing and potential new FS initiatives. For example, cross-pollination of ideas and advice between such stakeholders at the action-planning forum. Therefore, supporting enhanced FS governance [18]. However, further research is now required to evaluate changes to initiatives that occur as a result of the Systemic Innovation Lab approach [20]. This work will involve interviewing initiative leaders to ascertain changes to initiative characteristics and then recreating the transition card to measure impact on the food security system. In addition, conducting further research on a larger scale would likely ensure initiatives addressing the 'stability' FS pillar are captured and would facilitate region-to-region comparisons.

This project possessed a number of strengths, such as a more rigorous evaluation of initiatives' capacity to transition towards enhancing FS. A known limitation of FS initiatives to date has been limited assessment of this impact [37]. Another strength was the innovative Systemic Innovation Lab [20] approach used to support multiple initiatives to transition to a more effective way of enhancing FS [20]. By taking a solution ecosystem approach, the complexity associated with FS was considered [20]. The place-based nature of the project also enabled the identification of synergies within the local context and across social, economic, environmental and cultural dimensions [20]. The use of a common platform to connect the various stakeholders participating in the project was another strength [20,38], which increased stakeholder awareness of the characteristics their initiative/s possessed, as well as the opportunities for improvement. The engagement of these stakeholders as co-creators [20] was another strength. However, the pilot project is not without limitations. This project included a small sample of stakeholders (n = 51), limiting its generalisability and also limiting the capture of all existing initiatives in the South West region of WA. Secondly, given the variability in respondents' roles, varying levels of details about initiatives were captured. In addition, this project did not involve verification of respondents' comments about initiative characteristics with document analysis or collection of any other program information. Thirdly, the transitioning to a more effective way of working may not have been the intention of the organisations, and the possession of the desired characteristics may have been by chance. This project required translation from complex academic language associated with theories that underpinned the constructs, to plain English. Two team members had participated in a six-month Complex Systems Leadership Program [39], delivered by Wicked Lab and focusing on the constructs that underpinned the project model. Therefore, these team members led the development of the survey tool used in interviews as well as crosschecking the tool with Wicked Lab's consultants, to ensure language used was appropriate for all participants whilst retaining the integrity of the model. However, the other project team members had not participated in the training. Full team member training would likely facilitate enhanced understanding of project concepts among participating stakeholders. Finally, as this project was a pilot, a limited number of initiatives were uncovered in the discrete project timeframe. This resulted in no identification of initiatives addressing the 'stability' pillar of FS. Though it remains unknown whether such initiatives exist in the region.

5. Conclusions

FS focuses on ensuring physical, social and economic access to food. While FS in rural and remote locations can be challenging to sustain, the South West region provided numerous opportunities to increase community-level FS. This pilot project investigated FS strategies being implemented across the South West region of WA. It mapped their initiative characteristics to desirable characteristics using an online tool. This comprehensive but defined approach demonstrated the value of a place-based co-design approach to addressing FS.

Supplementary Materials: The following are available online at http://www.mdpi.com/2072-6643/11/4/738/s1, Table S1: Focus Areas, embedded characteristics, and associated survey interview questions.

Author Contributions: Conceptualization, S.L.G., J.P., D.B., M.E., M.S. and A.D.; Data curation, J.P. and D.B.; Formal analysis, S.L.G.; Funding acquisition, S.L.G.; Investigation, S.L.G.; Methodology, S.L.G., J.P., D.B., M.E., M.S. and A.D.; Project administration, S.L.G.; Software, S.L.G.; Writing—original draft, S.L.G., J.P., D.B., M.E., M.S. and A.D.; Writing—review & editing, S.L.G., J.P., D.B., M.E., M.S. and A.D.

Funding: This research was funded by an Edith Cowan University School of Medical and Health Sciences Research Grant Scheme.

Acknowledgments: The authors would like to sincerely thank the participants of this project and Wicked Lab consultants Emily Humphreys and Dr Sharon Zivkovic.

Conflicts of Interest: The authors declare no conflict of interest. The funders had no role in the design of the study; in the collection, analyses, or interpretation of data; in the writing of the manuscript, or in the decision to publish the results.

References

1. Food and Agriculture Organization. Rome Declaration on World Food Security and World Food Summit Plan of Action. Available online: http://www.fao.org/docrep/003/w3613e/w3613e00.HTM (accessed on 4 December 2018).
2. Hamm, M.W.; Bellows, A.C. Community food security: background and future directions. *J. Nutr. Educ. Behav.* **2003**, *35*, 37–43. [CrossRef]
3. Household Food Insecurity in Canada, 2011. Research to Identify Policy Options to Reduce Food Insecurity (PROOF). Available online: https://proof.utoronto.ca/resources/proof-annual-reports/annual-report/ (accessed on 4 December 2018).
4. Grochowska, R. Specificity of food security concept as a wicked problem. *JAST* **2014**, *4*, 823–831.
5. Conklin, J. *Dialogue Mapping: Building Shared Understanding of Wicked Problems*; Wiley: Hoboken, NJ, USA, 2006.
6. Food Security: The What, How, Why and Where to of Food Security in NSW: Discussion Paper. Available online: https://ses.library.usyd.edu.au/handle/2123/9082 (accessed on 19 December 2018).
7. An Introduction to the Basic Concepts of Food Security. Available online: www.fao.org/docrep/013/al936e/al936e00.pdf (accessed on 19 December 2018).
8. Bach, C.; Aborisade, B. Assessing the Pillars of Sustainable Food Security. *Eur. Int. J. Sci.Technol.* **2014**, *3*, 117–125.
9. Godrich, S.L.; Davies, C.R.; Darby, J.; Devine, A. What are the determinants of food security among regional and remote Western Australian children? *Aust. N. Z. J. Public Health* **2017**, *41*, 172–177. [CrossRef] [PubMed]
10. Food Security Options Paper: A Planning Framework and Menu of Options for Policy and Practice Interventions. Available online: https://www.health.nsw.gov.au/heal/Publications/food-security.pdf (accessed on 19 December 2018).

11. Lawlis, T.; Islam, W.; Upton, P. Achieving the four dimensions of food security for resettled refugees in Australia: A. systematic review. *Nutr. Diet.* **2018**, *75*, 182–192. [CrossRef] [PubMed]
12. Food Security. Available online: http://www.fao.org/fileadmin/templates/faoitaly/documents/pdf/pdf_Food_Security_Cocept_Note.pdf (accessed on 19 December 2018).
13. Pollard, C.; Nyaradi, A.; Lester, M.; Sauer, K. Understanding food security issues in remote Western Australian Indigenous communities. *Health Promot. J. Aust.* **2014**, *25*, 83–89. [CrossRef] [PubMed]
14. 4364.0.55.009-Australian Health Survey: Nutrition-State and Territory results, 2011-12. Available online: http://www.abs.gov.au/ausstats/abs@.nsf/Lookup/4364.0.55.009main+features12011-12 (accessed on 19 December 2018).
15. Butcher, L.M.; O'Sullivan, T.A.; Ryan, M.M.; Lo, J.; Devine, A. Utilising a multi-item questionnaire to assess household food security in Australia. *Health Prom. J. Aust.* **2018**, *30*, 9–17. [CrossRef] [PubMed]
16. Pollard, C.; Landrigan, T.; Ellies, P.; Kerr, D.; Lester, M.; Goodchild, S. Geographic Factors as Determinants of Food Security: A Western Australian Food Pricing and Quality Study. *Asia Pac. J. Clin. Nutr.* **2014**, *23*, 703–713. [PubMed]
17. Pollard, C.; Savage, V.; Landrigan, T.; Hanbury, A.; Kerr, D. *Food Access and Cost Survey*; Department of Health: Perth, Australia, 2015.
18. Zivkovic, S. Addressing food insecurity: A systemic innovation approach. *Soc. Enterprise J.* **2017**, *13*, 234–350. [CrossRef]
19. Innovation Teams and Labs, a Practice Guide. Available online: https://media.nesta.org.uk/documents/innovation_teams_and_labs_a_practice_guide.pdf (accessed on 22 December 2018).
20. Zivkovic, S. Systemic Innovation Labs: A lab for wicked problems. *Soc. Enterprise J.* **2018**, *14*, 348–366. [CrossRef]
21. Snowden, D.J.; Boone, M.E. A leader's framework for decision making. *Harv. Bus. Rev.* **2007**, *85*, 69–76.
22. The Evaluation of Place-Based Approaches. Available online: https://www.horizons.gc.ca (accessed on 22 December 2018).
23. Goldstein, J.; Hazy, J.; Lichtenstein, B. *Complexity and the Nexus of Leadership*; Palgrave MacMillan: Basingstoke, UK, 2010.
24. Sorensen, E.; Torfing, J. Metagoverning collaborative innovation in governance networks. *Am. Rev. Public Adm.* **2017**, *47*, 826–839. [CrossRef]
25. Consumers Health Forum of Australia. Statement on Consumer and Community Involvement in Health and Medical Research. Available online: https://www.nhmrc.gov.au/sites/default/files/documents/reports/consumer-community-involvement.pdf (accessed on 22 December 2018).
26. Developing Effective Citizen Engagement: A How-to Guide for Community Leaders. Available online: http://www.rural.palegislature.us/effective_citizen_engagement.pdf (accessed on 22 December 2018).
27. Zivkovic, S. A complexity based diagnostic tool for tackling wicked problems. *Emerg. Complex. Organ.* **2015**. [CrossRef]
28. Godrich, S.L.; Lo, J.; Davies, C.R.; Darby, J.; Devine, A. Prevalence and socio-demographic predictors of food insecurity among regional and remote Western Australian children. *Aust. N. Z. J. Public Health.* **2017**, *41*, 585–590. [CrossRef] [PubMed]
29. Our WA Regions. Available online: http://www.drd.wa.gov.au/regions/Pages/default.aspx (accessed on 22 December 2018).
30. Australian Statistical Geography Standard (ASGS). Available online: http://www.abs.gov.au/websitedbs/d3310114.nsf/home/australian+statistical+geography+standard+(asgs) (accessed on 22 December 2018).
31. A Tool for Systemic Change. Available online: http://www.wickedlab.com.au/tool-for-systemic-change.html (accessed on 22 December 2018).
32. Corbin, J.; Strauss, A. *Basics of Qualitative Research: Techniques and Procedures for Developing Grounded Theory*, 3rd ed.; SAGE Publications Inc.: Thousand Oaks, CA, USA, 2009.
33. Jamshed, S. Qualitative research method-interviewing and observation. *J.Basic Clin. Pharm.* **2014**, *5*, 87–88. [CrossRef] [PubMed]
34. Agriculture and Development Economics Division. Available online: http://www.fao.org/economic/agricultural-development-economics/en/ (accessed on 20 December 2018).
35. Waters, R.D.; Burnett, E.; Lamm, A.; Lucas, J. Engaging stakeholders through social networking: How nonprofit organizations are using Facebook. *Public Relat. Review.* **2009**, *35*, 102–106.

36. Surie, G.; Hazy, J.K. Generative leadership: Nurturing innovation in complex systems. *Emerg. Complex. Organ.* **2006**, *8*, 13–26.
37. Collins, P.A.; Power, E.M.; Little, M.H. Municipal-level responses to household food insecurity in Canada: A call for critical, evaluative research. *Can. J. Public Health* **2014**, *105*, e138–e141. [CrossRef] [PubMed]
38. State of the Future. Available online: http://www.millennium-project.org/publications-2-3/ (accessed on 22 December 2018).
39. Zivkovic, S. Determining and increasing the performance of a Complex Systems Leadership Program. In Proceedings of the 9th International Social Innovation Research Conference, Melbourne, Australia, 12–14 December 2017.

nutrients

MDPI

Article

Food-Insecure Household's Self-Reported Perceptions of Food Labels, Product Attributes and Consumption Behaviours

Lucy M. Butcher [1,2,*], Maria M. Ryan [3], Therese A. O'Sullivan [1], Johnny Lo [4] and Amanda Devine [1]

1 School of Medical and Health Sciences, Edith Cowan University, Joondalup, WA 6027, Australia; t.osullivan@ecu.edu.au (T.A.O.); a.devine@ecu.edu.au (A.D.)
2 Foodbank Western Australia, Perth Airport, WA 6105, Australia
3 School of Business and Law, Edith Cowan University, Joondalup, WA 6027, Australia; m.ryan@ecu.edu.au
4 School of Science, Edith Cowan University, Joondalup, WA 6027, Australia; j.lo@ecu.edu.au
* Correspondence: lucy.butcher@foodbankwa.org.au; Tel.: +61-08-9463-3215

Received: 4 March 2019; Accepted: 9 April 2019; Published: 12 April 2019

Abstract: Dietary compromises related to food insecurity profoundly undermine health and constitute a serious public health issue, even in developed nations. The aim of this study was to explore the impact of food labelling and product attributes on the purchasing choices of food-insecure households in Australia. An online survey containing 19 food choice and 28 purchasing behaviours questions was completed by 1056 adults responsible for household grocery shopping. The short form of the US Household Food Security Survey Module was used as the food security indicator. Multinomial logistic regression modelling was employed to analyse the survey data. Respondents were classified as having either high-marginal (63.4%, $n = 670$), low (19.8%, $n = 209$) or very low (16.8%, $n = 177$) food security. Respondents with low or very low food security status were less likely to self-report understanding the information on the back of packaging ($p < 0.001$), find information on food labels useful ($p = 0.002$) or be influenced by product nutrition information ($p = 0.002$). Convenience ($p < 0.001$), organic ($p = 0.027$) and supermarket-branded products ($p < 0.001$) were more likely to be rated as important by food-insecure respondents when compared to their food-secure counterparts. When asked to rate "how healthy" their diet was, high–marginal FS respondents were twice as likely describe their diet as healthy than very low FS respondents ($p = 0.001$).

Keywords: vulnerable groups; food poverty; food insecurity; food literacy; public health

---

1. Introduction

A nutritionally adequate diet is increasingly viewed as the leading modifiable factor in the prevention of chronic disease [1]. Regardless of this, the majority of Australians have suboptimal intakes of nutrient dense foods, such as fruit and vegetables, and compliance to the national dietary guidelines is low [2]. Food-insecure households are thought to be a particularly vulnerable subpopulation and are more likely exhibit a poorer diet quality than the general Australian population [3–6]. Food insecurity exists "whenever the availability of nutritionally adequate and safe foods, or the ability to acquire acceptable food in socially acceptable ways, is limited or uncertain" [7]. The current reported national prevalence of food insecurity is 3.7% [2]. However, other Australian researchers have found the rate of food insecurity to be as high as 25% [8] to 36% [9] when a more sensitive food insecurity measure has been applied.

Food insecurity occurs on a continuum of severity which may exist with or without hunger depending on the scarcity of nutritious food. Individuals experiencing mild or "low" food security may try to avoid hunger by reducing portion sizes, skipping meals, choosing cheaper foods or reducing diet variety [10]. Reduced intake of fruit and vegetables, overconsumption of high energy, nutrient-poor foods and decreased diet diversity, are frequently viewed as characterising features of mild forms of food insecurity in developed nations [11–13]. However, when food is simply not available, coping strategies prove ineffective and hunger is inevitable. Food insecurity with hunger is synonymous with severe food insecurity or "very low" food security (FS) [10]. The dietary compromises related to even mild forms of food insecurity have been cited as significant, profoundly undermining health [8,14]. When prevalence is considered, food insecurity constitutes a serious public health issue, even in developed nations such as Australia [15].

Recently, as a strategy to improve purchasing behaviours and address poor dietary intakes of Australians, there has been conscious effort to improve and simplify food labelling (particularly front of pack information including nutrition claims) [16]. In other developed nations, the majority of consumers report using food labels to assist in food choices [17,18]. While interest in food labels may be high, Sharf, et al. [19] suggests the public's actual understanding of the topic is low.

The nutritionally inferior dietary patterns of food-insecure people are generally regarded as a symptom of economic constraints [11]. There is limited research about other factors (such as food labels and product attributes) influencing food choices and the flow-on effect to consumption behaviours in this subpopulation. To the authors' knowledge, no Australian research has been conducted into food-insecure households' self-reported use or understanding food labels. In addition, only one study outside Australia has investigated this, specifically how food-insecure people residing in America interpret food labels [20]. This research forms one component of a multidisciplinary study investigating food shopping and consumption behaviours. The purpose of this article is to explore the impact of food labelling and product attributes on the food choices of food-insecure individuals.

2. Materials and Methods

The aims of this study were to: (1) Assess the extent to which food-insecure people find food labels useful when making food choices, (2) determine if other product attributes, such as cost and quality, affect purchasing choices and (3) consider how these factors may translate into consumption behaviours.

An online survey investigating food choices and purchasing behaviours was conducted between November 2014 and February 2015. All participants were recruited through a commercial research company, and survey administration was through Qualtrics (Provo, Utah, USA). Respondents were required to be over 18 years of age, the main household grocery purchaser and located in one of five Australian states (New South Wales, Victoria, Western Australia, South Australia and Queensland). As the survey was disseminated online, internet access was necessary for participation. No further inclusion or exclusion criteria were applied. In Australia, approximately a third of primary household grocery shoppers are thought to be male [21]. Therefore, an adequate quota for male representation was set at a minimum proportion of 30% in an effort to make the sample population comparable to the Australian general population. Quotas were also established for age and location, in order to align with the general Australian population [22].

2.1. Survey Content

The survey comprised: Twelve sociodemographic questions (including age, gender, immigration, occupation, education, household income, household structure and marital status), the six-item US Household Food Security Survey Module (HFSSM), twenty-eight food purchasing and nineteen consumption questions.

The six-item HFSSM was included as a food security indicator. The short form was selected due to the comparable accuracy with the longer 18 item form (correctly identified 97.7% of households), while simultaneously having the added benefit of reduced respondent burden [23]. Food security (FS) status was categorised and named in accordance with the HFSSM user notes [24], and the authors' previous research outlines a more detailed methodology [9]. The three levels of household FS referred to in this study are: High-marginal FS (no anxiety about accessing adequate food), low FS (reduced quality, variety and desirability of diet, but no reduction in quantity of food) and very low FS (intermittent disruption of eating patterns and reduced food intake of one or more household members) [10]. For the purpose of this research, food insecurity is considered a broader term encompassing households reporting both low and very low FS [24].

The food purchasing behaviour indicators consisted of a total of 28 questions: Eleven on product attributes, nine on food label reading and an additional eight on nutrition claims. The selection of product attributes questions was influenced by an extensive literature review, not included in this paper, of the associated factors of food insecurity. Food label reading questions were developed to demonstrate how useful consumers found nutrition information on packaging. Questions relate to both the front of pack nutrition claims and the back of pack information (including the nutrition information panel and the ingredient list). In Australia, nutrition claims are statements about the content of particular substances or nutrients in a food product, for example "low fat" or "high protein" [25]. Nutrition claims reflected eight commonly used terms on food packages at the time of survey administration: Low glycaemic index, kilojoules, sugar, preservatives, carbohydrates, saturated fats, sodium and high protein [26].

Food and beverage consumption questions were based on the standard serve or serving sizes outlined in the 2013 Australian Dietary Guidelines [27]. Respondents were asked to estimate the number of standard serves consumed for each food grouping on a typical day. Foods and drinks were classified into 18 distinct groupings for analysis. In conjunction with the dietary intake questions, respondents were also asked to rate the perceived healthiness of their diet.

2.2. Statistics

Response categories for the food purchasing questions were collapsed from a five-point scale (strongly agree to strongly disagree) to a three-point scale (agree, neither agree nor disagree and disagree), due to low cell counts in some categories. The response categories for the 18 food consumption indicators are defined by a five-point scale (0, 1, 2, 3, 4 or more serves) and were collapsed, if necessary, when low counts were observed.

All food purchasing and consumption behaviour indicators were entered into a multinomial logistic regression model to formally examine their relationship with FS status. Age, household income, marital status and education were established as significant sociodemographic predictors of FS status in the authors' previous research [9]. These variables were controlled for in all models. Statistical Package for Social Sciences (SPSS) (IBM Corp. Version 20, Armonk, NY, USA) was employed to analyse the survey data. Statistical significance was set at $p \leq 0.05$.

2.3. Ethics Approval

Ethics approval was granted by Edith Cowan University's Human Research Ethics Committee (# 11118). All participants involved in this study provided informed written consent upon agreeing to complete the survey. All survey data were non-identifiable, with no individual identifier labels ever utilised.

3. Results

3.1. Sample Demographics

The survey was completed by 1056 Australian participants (5442 invited, response rate: 19.4%). Table 1 describes the respondent group using characteristics, with the exception of gender, previously established to be associated with FS. The majority of respondents were classified as having high–marginal FS status (63.4%, n = 670), followed by low (19.8%, n = 209) and then very low (16.8%, n = 177). In relation to household income, respondents were most likely to indicate an income in the low (31.6 %, n = 334), followed by the middle (24.3 %, n = 257) and high (24.1%, n = 255) brackets (Table 1). Approximately two thirds (62.4 %, n = 659) of respondents were in a de facto relationship or married. Over 73% (n = 771) of respondents had attained some form of post-secondary education.

Table 1. Characteristics of survey respondents compared by food security status.

Independent Variable	Category	Overall Significance [b]	Total n (% of n = 1056)	High–Marginal Food Security n = 670 (63.4%)	Low Food Security n = 209 (19.8%)	Very Low Food Security n = 177 (16.8%)
Gender		0.256				
	Male		329 (31.2%)	225 (33.6%)	56 (26.8%)	48 (27.1%)
	Female		727 (68.8%)	445 (66.4%)	153 (73.2%)	129 (72.9%)
Age (years)		<0.001 **				
	19–24		81 (7.7%)	53 (7.9%)	14 (6.7%)	14 (7.9%)
	25–34		195 (18.5%)	102 (15.3%)	52 (24.9%)	41 (23.2%)
	35–44		212 (20.1%)	128 (19.1%)	44 (21.1%)	40 (22.6%)
	45–54		219 (20.7%)	141 (21.0%)	42 (20.1%)	36 (20.3%)
	55–64		181 (17.1%)	120 (17.9%)	30 (14.4%)	31 (17.5%)
	65–84		168 (15.9%)	126 (18.8%)	27 (12.8%)	15 (8.5%)
Marital status		0.006 **				
	Widowed		37 (3.5%)	27 (4.0%)	5 (2.4%)	5 (2.8%)
	Divorced/Separated		108 (10.2%)	56 (8.4%)	21 (10.0%)	31 (17.5%)
	Married/De facto		659 (62.4%)	440 (65.7%)	127 (60.8%)	92 (52.0%)
	Single		252 (23.9%)	147 (21.9%)	56 (26.8%)	49 (27.7%)
Household income ($AUD)		<0.001 **				
	Very low (<$18,000)		35 (3.3%)	16 (2.4%)	6 (2.9%)	13 (7.3%)
	Low ($18,001–37,000)		334 (31.6%)	181 (27.0%)	78 (37.3%)	75 (42.4%)
	Middle ($37,001–87,000)		257 (24.3%)	166 (24.8%)	45 (21.5%)	46 (26.0%)
	High ($87,001–180,000)		255 (24.1%)	180 (26.9%)	51 (24.5%)	24 (13.6%)
	Very high (>$180,000)		75 (7.1%)	64 (9.5%)	8 (3.8%)	3 (1.7 %)
	Did not answer		100 (9.6%)	63 (9.4%)	21 (10.0%)	16 (9.0%)
Education completed		<0.001 **				
	Secondary or less		285 (27.0%)	161 (24.1%)	66 (31.6%)	58 (32.7%)
	Vocational [a]		401 (38.0%)	240 (35.8%)	89 (42.6%)	72 (40.7%)
	University		370 (35.0%)	269 (40.1%)	54 (25.8%)	47 (26.6%)

[a] Vocational considered to be post-secondary; [b] Multinomial logistic regression was used to establish significance; ** p-value < 0.01.

3.2. Food Purchasing Behaviours and Food Security Status

From the 28 food purchasing indicators assessed, just under half ($n = 11$) were significantly associated with FS status (refer to Tables 2 and 3). Of the significant indicators, five were related to "food labels" (Table 2) and six were "food product attributes" (Table 3). None of the nutrition claims were found to be significant. All models were adjusted for education, household income, marital status and age. The response rates (Tables S1–S3) and analysis of all indicators (Tables S4–S6) can be found in the Supplementary Materials.

3.2.1. Food Label Indicators

Respondents with high–marginal FS status were more likely to agree that they understood the information on the back of packaging ($p < 0.001$) and that food label information was useful ($p = 0.002$), in comparison to those with low or very low FS status (Table 2). In contrast to the high–marginal FS group, low or very low FS respondents were less likely to read food labels ($p < 0.001$), be influenced by product nutrition information ($p = 0.002$) and were more likely to think there was too much information on a food packages ($p < 0.001$) (Table 2).

3.2.2. Food Product Characteristics

No significant relationships were reported between FS status and cost ($p = 0.117$), Australian grown products ($p = 0.889$), those in season ($p = 0.614$), local ($p = 0.205$) or unprocessed products ($p = 0.521$). High–marginal FS respondents were more likely to rate quality ($p = 0.010$) and nutrition ($p = 0.021$) as important when compared to low or very low FS respondents (Table 3). Conversely, convenience ($p < 0.001$), organic ($p = 0.027$) and supermarket-branded products ($p < 0.001$) were more likely to be rated as important by low FS respondents than those with high–marginal FS (Table 3).

3.3. Food Consumption

When adjusted for sociodemographic variables, eight food groupings (bread, fruit juice, salad and vegetables, potato (not including chips), pasta, rice or noodles, poultry, nuts and seeds and water) were significantly associated with FS status (Table 4). High–marginal FS respondents were more likely to report higher consumption of salad and vegetables ($p = 0.003$), pasta, rice or noodles ($p = 0.007$) and nuts and seeds ($p < 0.001$) compared to food-insecure respondents. Very low FS respondents cited the lowest consumption of bread ($p = 0.014$), potato ($p < 0.001$) and poultry ($p = 0.020$). Food-insecure respondents reported the highest fruit juice ($p = 0.043$) intake and, conversely, the lowest water ($p < 0.001$) intake. Refer to Table S7 in the Supplementary Materials for consumption indicator response rates. When asked to rate "how healthy" their diet was, high–marginal FS respondents were twice as likely to describe their diet as healthy than very low FS respondents ($p = 0.001$).

Table 2. Significant food label and single consumption indicators. [a]

Outcome	Category	Overall Significance [a]	Post Hoc Analysis					
			High–Marginal vs. Very Low Food Security		High–Marginal vs. Low Food Security		Low Food Security Vs. Very Low Food Security	
			OR (95% CI)	*p*-Value	OR (95% CI)	*p*-Value	OR (95% CI)	*p*-Value
I understand the information provided on the back of food packages	Agree	<0.001 **	2.83 (1.72, 4.66)	<0.001 **	1.46 (0.86, 2.49)	0.146	1.93 (1.07, 3.51)	0.030 *
	Neither agree nor disagree		1.67 (0.98, 2.86)	0.062	0.73 (0.42, 1.27)	0.261	2.29 (1.23, 4.26)	0.009 **
	Disagree		1.00 (ref)		1.00 (ref)		1.00 (ref)	
The ingredients and nutritional information on the back of the package does not influence my purchasing decisions	Agree	0.002 **	0.82 (0.52, 1.30)	0.399	0.52 (0.35, 0.78)	0.001 **	1.58 (0.94, 2.65)	0.088
	Neither agree nor disagree		0.60 (0.40, 0.90)	0.013 *	0.58 (0.39, 0.86)	0.007 **	1.02 (0.63, 1.66)	0.929
	Disagree		1.00 (ref)		1.00 (ref)		1.00 (ref)	
The nutrition information offers useful information about the product	Agree	0.002 **	3.26 (1.67, 6.37)	0.001 **	1.59 (0.77, 3.27)	0.208	2.05 (0.95, 4.42)	0.066
	Neither agree nor disagree		2.04 (1.01, 4.11)	0.046	1.08 (0.51, 2.28)	0.843	1.89 (0.85, 4.12)	0.117
	Disagree		1.00 (ref)		1.00 (ref)		1.00 (ref)	
There is too much nutritional information on food packaging	Agree	<0.001 **	0.44 (0.28, 0.70)	<0.001 **	0.57 (0.36, 0.92)	0.020 *	0.77 (0.44, 1.34)	0.352
	Neither agree nor disagree		1.02 (0.68, 1.54)	0.924	0.52 (0.36, 0.75)	0.001 **	1.95 (1.21, 3.15)	0.007 **
	Disagree		1.00 (ref)		1.00 (ref)		1.00 (ref)	
I never read the nutritional information and ingredients on food packages	Agree	<0.001 **	0.48 (0.29, 0.79)	0.004 **	0.54 (0.34, 0.87)	0.011 *	0.86 (0.50, 1.58)	0.678
	Neither agree nor disagree		0.44 (0.29, 0.66)	<0.001 **	0.33 (0.23, 0.48)	0.001 **	1.32 (0.83, 2.09)	0.245
	Disagree		1.00 (ref)		1.00 (ref)		1.00 (ref)	
How healthy would you say your diet was?	Healthy	0.001 **	2.17 (1.44, 3.27)	<0.001	1.31 (0.87, 1.95)	0.195	1.66 (1.04, 2.67)	0.034 *
	Unhealthy		1.00 (ref)		1.00 (ref)		1.00 (ref)	

[a] Multinomial logistic regression model was adjusted for sociodemographic variables (age, household income, education and marital status). * p-value < 0.05; ** p-value < 0.01; OR = odds ratio; CI = confidence interval; 1.00 (ref) = reference level.

Table 3. Significant food product attributes. [a]

Outcome	Category	Overall Significance [a]	Post Hoc Analysis: High–Marginal vs. Very Low Food Security		High–Marginal vs. Low Food Security		Low Food Security vs. Very Low Food Security	
			OR (95% CI)	*p*-Value	OR (95% CI)	*p*-Value	OR (95% CI)	*p*-Value
Nutrition	Important	0.021 *	1.00 (ref)		1.00 (ref)		1.00 (ref)	
	Neither important nor unimportant		0.49 (0.30, 0.81)	0.005 **	0.53 (0.34, 0.84)	0.006 **	0.93 (0.54, 1.59)	0.790
	Unimportant		0.73 (0.28, 1.91)	0.531	0.82 (0.33, 2.05)	0.667	0.90 (0.30,2.69)	0.853
Quality	Important	0.010 *	1.00 (ref)		1.00 (ref)		1.00 (ref)	
	Neither important nor unimportant		0.40 (0.20, 0.81)	0.011 *	0.40 (0.21, 0.76)	0.005 **	1.00 (0.47, 2.11)	0.994
	Unimportant		0.36 (0.10, 1.28)	0.115	0.383 (0.12, 1.28)	0.119	0.94 (0.25, 3.53)	0.932
Organic	Important	0.027 *	0.65 (0.42, 1.01)	0.056	0.55 (0.36, 0.83)	0.005 **	1.19 (0.70, 2.00)	0.520
	Neither important nor unimportant		1.01 (0.66, 1.56)	0.963	0.73 (0.49, 1.08)	0.116	1.39 (0.83, 2.33)	0.205
	Unimportant		1.00 (ref)		1.00 (ref)		1.00 (ref)	
Raw food (natural state)	Important	0.024 *	1.119 (0.71, 1.77)	0.632	0.57 (0.35, 0.93)	0.023 *	1.96 (1.10, 3.47)	0.022 *
	Neither important nor unimportant		1.60 (0.98, 2.62)	0.059	0.77 (0.47, 1.273)	0.309	2.08 (1.13, 3.82)	0.018 *
	Unimportant		1.00 (ref)		1.00 (ref)		1.00 (ref)	
Convenience (pre-packaged to save time) e.g., pre-cut vegetables, pre-marinated meats, bottle sauces	Important	<0.001 **	0.53 (0.34, 0.83)	0.005 **	0.40 (0.27, 0.61)	<0.001 **	1.31 (0.77, 2.22)	0.325
	Neither important nor unimportant		0.55 (0.36, 0.85)	0.007 **	0.52 (0.35, 0.79)	0.002 **	1.06 (0.63, 1.78)	0.833
	Unimportant		1.00 (ref)		1.00 (ref)		1.00 (ref)	
Supermarket branded (home brand, Coles Select)	Important	<0.001 **	0.37 (0.23, 0.60)	<0.001 **	0.214 (0.13, 0.35)	<0.001 **	1.74 (0.97, 3.12)	0.066
	Neither important nor unimportant		0.83 (0.53, 1.28)	0.391	0.475 (0.30, 0.74)	0.001 **	1.74 (0.99, 3.05)	0.053
	Unimportant		1.00 (ref)		1.00 (ref)		1.00 (ref)	

[a] Multinomial logistic regression model was adjusted for sociodemographic variables (age, household income, education and marital status). * *p*-value < 0.05; ** *p*-value < 0.01; OR = odds ratio; CI = confidence interval; 1.00 (ref) = reference level.

Table 4. Consumption behaviours related to food and beverages (with example serve sizes [a] given) by food security status. [b]

	Question	Serves	*n* (%)	Overall Significance	Post-Hoc Analysis: High–Marginal vs. Very Low Food Security		High–Marginal vs. Low Food Security		Low Food Security vs. Very Low Food Security	
					OR (95% CI)	*p*-Value	OR (95% CI)	*p*-Value	OR (95% CI)	*p*-Value
On a Typical Day, How Many Serves of the Following Foods Would You Eat?										
Breakfast cereals	2/3 cup breakfast cereals, cooked oats	0	200 (19.5%)	0.525	1.00 (Ref)		1.00 (Ref)		1.00 (Ref)	
	2 wheat-biscuits	1	736 (71.7%)		1.41 (0.91, 2.19)	0.127	1.13 (0.74, 1.73)	0.566	1.25 (0.74, 2.09)	0.403
		2 or more	90 (8.8%)		1.49 (0.7, 3.17)	0.296	0.9 (0.47, 1.71)	0.739	1.67 (0.71, 3.89)	0.238
Milk, yoghurt, cheese and dairy alternatives	1 cup of milk or soy milk	0	76 (7.4%)	0.496	1.00 (Ref)		1.00 (Ref)		1.00 (Ref)	
	2 slices of cheese	1	568 (55.4%)		1.39 (0.71, 2.72)	0.332	1.24 (0.66, 2.32)	0.501	1.12 (0.52, 2.4)	0.766
	1 tub of yoghurt	2	288 (28.1%)		1.67 (0.81, 3.42)	0.163	1.66 (0.85, 3.27)	0.139	1 (0.44, 2.29)	0.998
		3 or more	94 (9.2%)		1.86 (0.77, 4.46)	0.166	1.16 (0.53, 2.53)	0.714	1.6 (0.6, 4.32)	0.350
Bread	1 slice of bread	0	71 (6.9%)	0.014 *	1.00 (Ref)		1.00 (Ref)		1.00 (Ref)	
	1 crumpet or English muffin	1	414 (40.4%)		1.85 (0.95, 3.6)	0.069	0.85 (0.41, 1.77)	0.669	2.17 (0.96, 4.93)	0.064
		2	428 (41.7%)		3.05 (1.55, 5.99)	0.001 **	1.17 (0.56, 2.44)	0.674	2.6 (1.13, 6.01)	0.025 *
		3 or more	113 (11%)		2.64 (1.15, 6.05)	0.022 *	0.79 (0.35, 1.81)	0.579	3.34 (1.25, 8.92)	0.016 *
Fruit (not including juice)	1 medium banana, apple or orange	0	56 (5.5%)	0.080	1.00 (Ref)		1.00 (Ref)		1.00 (Ref)	
	2 small kiwi fruit, apricots or plums	1	480 (46.8%)		2.52 (1.24, 5.09)	0.010 **	1.14 (0.53, 2.47)	0.735	2.2 (0.95, 5.13)	0.067
	1 cup canned fruit	2	327 (31.9%)		3.45 (1.65, 7.21)	0.001 **	1.39 (0.63, 3.06)	0.416	2.48 (1.03, 6.01)	0.043 *
	A handful of dried fruit (e.g., 4 apricot halves)	3 or more	163 (15.9%)		2.6 (1.17, 5.8)	0.020 **	1.32 (0.56, 3.1)	0.525	1.97 (0.75, 5.18)	0.169
Fruit juice	1 cup fruit juice	0	288 (28.1%)	0.043 *	1.00 (Ref)		1.00 (Ref)		1.00 (Ref)	
		1	598 (58.3%)		1.39 (0.92, 2.11)	0.117	0.87 (0.58, 1.28)	0.472	1.61 (0.98, 2.64)	0.060
		2 or more	140 (13.6%)		0.78 (0.44, 1.36)	0.374	0.54 (0.32, 0.93)	0.027 *	1.43 (0.75, 2.72)	0.281
Salad and vegetables (not including potato)		0	44 (4.3%)	0.003 **	1.00 (Ref)		1.00 (Ref)		1.00 (Ref)	
	1 cup salad vegetables (e.g., lettuce, cucumber, tomato) ½	1	463 (45.1%)		4.08 (1.74, 9.56)	0.001 **	3.13 (1.38, 7.11)	0.006 **	1.3 (0.55, 3.08)	0.547
	cup cooked or canned vegetables	2	292 (28.5%)		5.03 (2.09, 12.08)	<0.001 **	4.6 (1.97, 10.75)	<0.001 **	1.09 (0.44, 2.7)	0.847
		3	148 (14.4%)		3.81 (1.5, 9.69)	0.005 **	3.32 (1.36, 8.08)	0.008 **	1.15 (0.44, 3.03)	0.778
		4 or more	79 (7.7%)		4.58 (1.61, 13.04)	0.004 **	6.18 (2.17, 17.57)	0.001 **	0.74 (0.23, 2.4)	0.619
Potato (not including chips)	½ medium potato	0	80 (7.8%)	<0.001 **	1.00 (Ref)		1.00 (Ref)		1.00 (Ref)	
	½ cup mashed potato	1	763 (74.4%)		3.88 (2.09, 7.19)	<0.001 **	2.46 (1.35, 4.51)	0.003 **	1.57 (0.81, 3.07)	0.185
		2 or more	183 (17.8%)		2.78 (1.37, 5.66)	0.005 **	0.64 (0.33, 1.24)	0.185	1.63 (0.75, 3.54)	0.218
Pasta, rice, or noodles		0	74 (7.2%)	0.007 **	1.00 (Ref)		1.00 (Ref)		1.00 (Ref)	
	½ cup cooked pasta or rice, noodles	1	739 (72%)		2.89 (1.5, 5.59)	0.002 **	2.5 (1.35, 4.61)	0.003 **	1.16 (0.57, 2.35)	0.682
		2 or more	213 (20.8%)		2.63 (1.26, 5.5)	0.010 **	1.99 (1.01, 3.92)	0.046 *	1.32 (0.6, 2.93)	0.491
Meat alternatives	1 cup baked beans, cooked legumes or tofu	0	121 (11.8%)	0.151	1.00 (Ref)		1.00 (Ref)		1.00 (Ref)	
		1	764 (74.5%)		1.8 (1.06, 3.05)	0.031 *	1.65 (1.01, 2.71)	0.046 *	1.09 (0.6, 1.97)	0.786
	2 large eggs	2 or more	141 (13.7%)		1.53 (0.78, 2.99)	0.218	1.67 (0.88, 3.16)	0.119	0.92 (0.42, 1.99)	0.825

Table 4. *Cont.*

	Question	Serves	*n* (%)	Overall Significance	High–Marginal vs. Very Low Food Security		High–Marginal vs. Low Food Security		Low Food Security vs. Very Low Food Security	
					OR (95% CI)	*p*-Value	OR (95% CI)	*p*-Value	OR (95% CI)	*p*-Value
On a Typical Day, How Many Serves of the Following Foods Would You Eat?										
Fish	A cooked fish fillet about the size of an open hand (100 g)	0	141 (13.7%)	0.272	1.00 (Ref)		1.00 (Ref)		1.00 (Ref)	
		1	747 (72.8%)		1.47 (0.9, 2.41)	0.128	0.9 (0.54, 1.5)	0.694	1.63 (0.89, 2.96)	0.111
	One small can of fish (100 g)	2 or more	138 (13.5%)		1.25 (0.64, 2.45)	0.505	0.65 (0.35, 1.22)	0.179	1.93 (0.89, 4.19)	0.095
Poultry	Cooked lean poultry such as chicken or turkey, about the size of an open hand (80 g)	0	69 (6.7%)	0.020 *	1.00 (Ref)		1.00 (Ref)		1.00 (Ref)	
		1	758 (73.9%)		2.25 (1.19, 4.27)	0.013 *	1.1 (0.53, 2.28)	0.798	2.05 (0.91, 4.6)	0.084
		2 or more	199 (19.4%)		1.96 (0.95, 4.05)	0.069	0.68 (0.31, 1.48)	0.334	2.87 (1.18, 6.98)	0.020 *
Red meat	Cooked lean meat, about the size of a deck of playing cards (65 g)	0	95 (9.3%)	0.611	1.00 (Ref)		1.00 (Ref)		1.00 (Ref)	
		1	736 (71.7%)		1.42 (0.78, 2.58)	0.249	1.1 (0.61, 2)	0.745	1.29 (0.63, 2.63)	0.489
		2 or more	195 (19%)		1.6 (0.79, 3.21)	0.189	0.93 (0.48, 1.81)	0.837	1.71 (0.75, 3.89)	0.199
Nuts and seeds	A handful of nuts /seeds	0	174 (17%)	0.001 **	1.00 (Ref)		1.00 (Ref)		1.00 (Ref)	
		1	662 (64.5%)		2.3 (1.45, 3.64)	<0.001 **	1.23 (0.78, 1.95)	0.370	1.86 (1.08, 3.2)	0.025 *
		2 or more	190 (18.5%)		1.33 (0.76, 2.34)	0.322	0.73 (0.42, 1.27)	0.266	1.82 (0.95, 3.48)	0.071
Savoury snacks	2 slices of processed meat	0	157 (15.3%)	0.396	1.00 (Ref)		1.00 (Ref)		1.00 (Ref)	
	12 hot chips	1	676 (65.9%)		1.61 (0.99, 2.6)	0.054	1.02 (0.63, 1.65)	0.928	1.57 (0.88, 2.81)	0.127
	$\frac{1}{2}$ small packet of crisps (20 g)	2 or more	193 (18.8%)		1.29 (0.72, 2.33)	0.392	0.94 (0.53, 1.67)	0.835	1.37 (0.68, 2.76)	0.371
Sweet snacks	2 scoops ice cream	0	107 (10.4%)	0.165	1.00 (Ref)		1.00 (Ref)		1.00 (Ref)	
	1 doughnut, slice of cake, muffin	1	718 (70%)		1.97 (1.14, 3.4)	0.015 *	1.51 (0.89, 2.58)	0.130	1.3 (0.69, 2.44)	0.412
	$\frac{1}{2}$ regular bar of chocolate (25 g)	2 or more	201 (19.6%)		1.92 (1.01, 3.62)	0.045 *	1.49 (0.8, 2.77)	0.207	1.29 (0.62, 2.67)	0.500
	2–3 biscuits									
Water (including tea and coffee)	1 cup (250 mL)	0	38 (3.7%)	<0.001 **	1.00 (Ref)		1.00 (Ref)		1.00 (Ref)	
		1	185 (18%)		5.41 (2, 14.61)	0.001 **	2.8 (1.09, 7.18)	0.033 *	1.94 (0.74, 5.03)	0.175
		2	118 (11.5%)		5.83 (2.05, 16.59)	0.001 **	3.69 (1.36, 10.01)	0.010 **	1.58 (0.56, 4.45)	0.386
		3	140 (13.6%)		5.41 (1.95, 15.05)	0.001 **	4.19 (1.55, 11.36)	0.005 **	1.29 (0.47, 3.57)	0.623
		4 or more	545 (53.1%)		10.63 (4.12, 27.4)	<0.001 **	5.07 (2.05, 12.54)	<0.001 **	2.1 (0.85, 5.15)	0.107
Additional drinks (not including alcohol)	1 can of soft drink (375 mL)	0	255 (24.9%)	0.076	1.00 (Ref)		1.00 (Ref)		1.00 (Ref)	
	2 cups of cordial (500 mL)	1	564 (55%)		1.16 (0.75, 1.81)	0.505	0.87 (0.57, 1.32)	0.508	1.34 (0.79, 2.28)	0.282
	1 can energy drink (330 mL)	2	143 (13.9%)		0.79 (0.44, 1.43)	0.437	0.68 (0.39, 1.19)	0.174	1.16 (0.58, 2.32)	0.666
	2 cups of Sports drink (500 mL)	3 or more	64 (6.2%)		0.41 (0.2, 0.87)	0.019 *	0.47 (0.23, 0.97)	0.042 *	0.87 (0.38, 2)	0.750
Alcohol	30 mL spirits	0	270 (26.3%)	0.202	1.00 (Ref)		1.00 (Ref)		1.00 (Ref)	
	60 mL fortified wine	1	367 (35.8%)		1.33 (0.86, 2.08)	0.204	1.2 (0.79, 1.83)	0.390	1.11 (0.66, 1.86)	0.698
	100 mL wine	2	214 (20.9%)		1.4 (0.84, 2.35)	0.198	1.34 (0.82, 2.19)	0.239	1.05 (0.57, 1.92)	0.885
	425 mL light beer	3	81 (7.9%)		1.43 (0.68, 3.01)	0.341	1.12 (0.58, 2.18)	0.731	1.28 (0.54, 3.01)	0.575
	285 mL regular beer	4 or more	94 (9.2%)		3.56 (1.49, 8.51)	0.004 **	1.26 (0.69, 2.32)	0.455	2.82 (1.09, 7.34)	0.033
	Small bottle of premix drink or "alco-pop" (300 mL)									

[a] Serves as defined by the Australian Dietary Guidelines [b] Multinomial logistic regression model was adjusted for sociodemographic variables (age, household income, education and marital status). * *p*-value < 0.05; ** *p*-value < 0.01; OR = odds ratio; CI = confidence interval; 1.00 (ref) = reference level.

4. Discussion

This study contributes to the understanding of how food labels and other factors are associated with the purchasing decisions of a food-insecure population. These findings indicate those experiencing food insecurity are less likely to self-report understanding, using or being influenced by food labels. Similarly, Gittelsohn, Song, Anliker, Sharma and Mattingly [20] found food-insecure households in Baltimore City in the USA had the lowest label reading scores, and the procurement of healthy food was directly related to this nutrition knowledge. Interest in food labels is generally thought to be high, with approximately 70% individuals reporting taking notice of food labels in both Israel and the United Kingdom [17,18]. Similarly, the majority of our study's respondents (53% low and very low FS to 59%—high–marginal FS) indicated they read food labels. However, Sharf, Sela, Zentner, Shoob, Shai and Stein-Zamir [19] suggested consumer understanding of these labels is low. Self-reported understanding of food labels in our study was relatively low in general (59%) but was significantly lower in the food-insecure group (48%). This significance remained even when formal education was controlled for, implying that higher educational attainment may not necessarily translate into the demonstration of greater food literacy skills in food-insecure populations. This lack of knowledge or food literacy may result in an inability to decode or apply information and may be linked to a sense of being deliberately misled, which may ultimately impact healthy food choices [28].

Despite nutrition labels not being rated as important, our study revealed that convenience, organic status and supermarket-branded products were seen as important by food-insecure individuals. Cost or perceived cost of healthy food is frequently cited as a significant barrier for food-insecure households [8,29–33], yet cost was not found to be significantly related to food insecurity in our research. A possible explanation for this is that the vast majority of respondents, regardless of FS status, considered cost an important determining factor in their purchasing decision process. Food-insecure respondents did, however, look for supermarket "home" brands or "no name" brands more than their food-secure counterparts, and these tend to be a cheaper option. Previous research has identified purchasing supermarket-branded products as a cost-saving measure employed by food-insecure households [11]. Other coping strategies identified in the literature are reducing the quality and nutritional value of food as a means of maximising the household spending power [34]. These coping strategies are reflected in the present research, where quality and nutrition were rated as less important by food-insecure respondents.

Lack of time has been cited as a barrier to obtaining and preparing healthy foods in food-insecure households in several studies [29,33,35,36]. Indeed, food-insecure respondents in our research highly valued convenience, but it is unclear how these individuals make trade-offs between convenience and price. Another product attribute considered important by food-insecure respondents in this study was organic produce. This mirrored the results from our previous research, where food-insecure interviewees indicated that organic food equated to healthy food, and this was one of the reasons cited for the perceived higher cost of nutritious food [36]. It is plausible that increased provision of food literacy education, with an emphasis on understanding food labels, identification of cost-effective and convenient healthy food options, may assist those experiencing low food security in maximising their income and diet diversity [37]. More research is warranted in this area.

There is a growing body of evidence demonstrating food insecurity is associated with suboptimal nutritional status and poorer diet quality [38–40]. Certainly, food-insecure respondents in our study were more likely to perceive their diets to be "unhealthy" when compared to their food-secure counterparts. There is agreeance in the research that food insecurity is related to ongoing dietary compromise [4,6,20], but there is debate about the exact concessions made. Respondents classified as having low FS in this study reported greater or similar intakes to their high–marginal FS counterparts for many food groups. This implies, in line with the definition of low FS, that whilst these respondents may be reducing the quality or variety within the food groups, the overall volume of food consumed appears to be similar. Australian adults experiencing food insecurity in this study consumed significantly less pasta, noodles or rice, salad or other vegetables and water compared to those who were food-secure.

On the other hand, fruit juice intake was higher in food-insecure households. In agreeance with our findings, several other studies have indicated food-insecure households may displace water intake with sugar sweetened beverages [39,41]. Canadian and US studies have demonstrated greater consumption of fast food, sugary drinks, fruit juice and snack foods in food-insecure populations [11,42–44]. Nevertheless, findings from outside of North America are less consistent, perhaps highlighting differing eating patterns and behaviours based on geographical location and culture. For example, food-insecure Pacific Island families residing in New Zealand were more likely to favour nutritionally dense foods (bread, fruit and vegetables) instead of energy dense foods (sugary drinks, ice cream and alcohol) [45].

Approximately 90% of all respondent groups in our study cited vegetable intakes below the recommendation of five serves [27], results similar to Australian national survey findings [46]. Despite the overall low intake of vegetables by participants in our study, the food-insecure group still demonstrated a significantly lower consumption rate in comparison to those who were food-secure. Compared to the results of a New Zealand study, our findings also suggest food-insecure households may be prepared to reduce spending on vegetables or bread but not meat products, with the exception of poultry. Furthermore, poultry and nuts and seeds are perceived as 'luxury' or expensive items in Australia [38], and this may explain limited intake of these foods in food-insecure households.

Although this study utilised a large, representative sample size, there are several limitations that need to be considered when interpreting the results. Firstly, self-reported research is subject to various disadvantages, including social desirability bias [47]. This study only investigated the self-reported understanding and use of food labels. Observational research has found consumer interaction with food labels was considerably lower than self-reported usage and understanding [48]. Therefore, the actual food label behaviours of the respondents may be different from those cited in this study's survey. Secondly, the dietary consumption tool used in this study did allow for comparison to the Australian dietary guidelines; however, changes in food quality and variety over time [5,6], fast food intake [8] or cyclical eating patterns [49] were not captured. These are potentially important dietary considerations for food-insecure populations. Thirdly, aspects not considered in this study were the impact of Aboriginal and Torres Strait Islander status or geographical remoteness. This may be important as both the aforementioned aspects are considered noteworthy social determinants of FS in Australia [50–52], and therefore, generalising these results across all sub populations is cautioned.

5. Conclusions

This research indicates food-insecure respondents are less likely to self-report understanding, using or being influenced by food labels when making purchasing decisions. However, factors such as convenience, super-market-branded and organic status were viewed as important by this subpopulation. Food-insecure respondents in this study were more likely to consider their diet "unhealthy", and there were variances in reported dietary intake when compared to their food-secure counterparts. It is possible that factors other than the income or financial constraints outlined in this study may have an impact on the dietary intake of food-insecure people, but more research is needed to support this theory.

Supplementary Materials: The following are available online at http://www.mdpi.com/2072-6643/11/4/828/s1, Table S1: Response, by three categories of food security, frequencies and proportions for a single consumption and food label indicators, Table S2: Response, by three categories of food security, frequencies and proportions for nutrition claim indicators, Table S3: Response, by three categories of food security frequencies and proportions for product attribute indicators, Table S4: Response, by three categories of food security *p*-values and odds ratios of single consumption and food label indicators, Table S5: Response, by three categories of food security *p*-values and odds ratios of nutrition claim indicators, Table S6: Response, by three categories of food security *p*-values and odds ratios of product attribute indicators, Table S7: Response, by three categories of food security, frequencies and proportions for consumption behaviours.

Author Contributions: All authors were involved in the conceptualisation and design of the study. Manuscript draft preparation was conducted by L.M.B. Results were analysed by L.M.B., with assistance from A.D., M.M.R., T.A.O. and J.L. A.D., M.M.R., T.A.O. and J.L. provided review, editing and supervision.

Funding: This research received no external funding.

Conflicts of Interest: The authors declare no conflict of interest.

References

1. McCullough, M.; Feskanich, D.; Stampfer, E.; Giovannucci, E.; Rimm, E.; Hu, F.; Spiegelman, D.; Hunter, D.; Colditz, G.; Willett, W. Diet quality and major chronic disease risk in men and women: Moving towards improved dietary guidance. *Am. J. Clin. Nutr. Diet.* **2002**, *76*, 1261–1271. [CrossRef]
2. Australian Bureau of Statistics. *Australian Health Survey: Nutrition First Results—Foods and Nutrients, 2011–2012*; ABS: Canberra, Australia, 2014.
3. Howard, L. Food insecurity experiences predict children's fruit and vegetable consumption in the USA. *ISRN Nutr.* **2013**, *2013*, 426029. [CrossRef] [PubMed]
4. Robaina, K.A.; Martin, K.S. Food insecurity, poor diet quality, and obesity among food pantry participants in hartford, CT. *J. Nutr. Educ. Behav.* **2013**, *45*, 159–164. [CrossRef] [PubMed]
5. Ko, B.-J.; Park, K.H.; Shin, S.; Zaichenko, L.; Davis, C.R.; Crowell, J.A.; Joung, H.; Mantzoros, C.S. Diet quality and diet patterns in relation to circulating cardiometabolic biomarkers. *Clin. Nutr.* **2016**, *35*, 484–490. [CrossRef] [PubMed]
6. Bocquier, A.l.; Vieux, F.; Lioret, S.; Dubuisson, C.; Caillavet, F.; Darmon, N. Socio-economic characteristics, living conditions and diet quality are associated with food insecurity in france. *Public Health Nutr.* **2015**, *18*, 2952–2961. [CrossRef] [PubMed]
7. Radimer, K. Measurement of household food security in the USA and other industrialized countries. *Public Health Nutr.* **2002**, *5*, 859–864. [CrossRef] [PubMed]
8. Ramsay, R.; Giskes, K.; Turrell, G.; Gallegos, D. Food insecurity among adults residing in disadvantaged urban areas: Potential health and dietary consequences. *Public Health Nutr.* **2012**, *15*, 227–237. [CrossRef]
9. Butcher, L.M.; O'Sullivan, T.A.; Ryan, M.M.; Lo, J.; Devine, A. Utilising a multi-item questionnaire to assess household food security in australia. *Health Promot. J. Aust. Off. J. Aust. Assoc. Health Promot. Prof.* **2019**, *30*, 9–17. [CrossRef]
10. United States Department of Agriculture. Definitions of Food Security. Available online: https://www.ers.usda.gov/topics/food-nutrition-assistance/food-security-in-the-us/definitions-of-food-security.aspx (accessed on 8 February 2019).
11. Dachner, N.; Ricciuto, L.; Kirkpatrick, S.I.; Tarasuk, V. Food purchasing and food insecurity among low-income families in toronto. *Can. J. Diet. Pract. Res.* **2010**, *71*, e50–e56.
12. Lee, S.; Gundersen, C.; Cook, J.; Laraia, B.; Johnson, M. Food insecurity and health across the lifespan. *Adv. Nutr.* **2012**, *3*, 744–745. [CrossRef]
13. Mercille, G.; Receveur, O.; Potvin, L. Household food insecurity and canadian aboriginal women's self-efficacy in food preparation. *Can. J. Diet. Pract. Res.* **2012**, *73*, 134–140. [CrossRef]
14. Seligaman, H.K.; Laraia, B.A.; Kushel, M.B. Food insecurity is associated with chronic disease among low-income nhanes participants. *J. Nutr. Nutr. Dis.* **2010**, *140*, 304–310. [CrossRef]
15. Lindberg, R.; Lawrence, M.; Gold, L.; Friel, S.; Pegram, O. Food insecurity in australia: Implications for general practitioners. *Aust. Fam. Physician* **2015**, *44*, 859–862.
16. Food Regulation Secretariat. Review of Food Labelling Law and Policy. Available online: http://foodregulation.gov.au/internet/fr/publishing.nsf/Content/review-food-labelling (accessed on 23 March 2018).
17. Hall, C.; Osses, F. A review to inform understanding of the use of food safety messages on food labels. *Int. J. Consum. Stud.* **2013**, *37*, 422–432. [CrossRef]
18. Barreiro-Hurlé, J.; Gracia, A.; de-Magistris, T. Does nutrition information on food products lead to healthier food choices? *Food Policy* **2010**, *35*, 221–229. [CrossRef]
19. Sharf, M.; Sela, R.; Zentner, G.; Shoob, H.; Shai, I.; Stein-Zamir, C. Figuring out food labels. Young adults' understanding of nutritional information presented on food labels is inadequate. *Appetite* **2012**, *58*, 531–534.
20. Gittelsohn, J.; Song, H.-J.; Anliker, J.A.; Sharma, S.; Mattingly, M. Food insecurity is associated with food-related psychosocial factors and behaviors among low-income african american adults in baltimore city au—Suratkar, sonali. *J. Hunger Environ. Nutr.* **2010**, *5*, 100–119.

21. Watson, W.L.; Kelly, B.; Hector, D.; Hughes, C.; King, L.; Crawford, J.; Sergeant, J.; Chapman, K. Can front-of-pack labelling schemes guide healthier food choices? Australian shoppers' responses to seven labelling formats. *Appetite* **2014**, *72*, 90–97. [CrossRef]
22. Australian Bureau of Statistics (Ed.). *Australian Demographic Statistics*; Australian Bureau of Statistics: Canberra, Australia, 2016.
23. Blumberg, S.; Bialostosky, K.; Hamilton, W.; Briefel, R. The effectiveness of a short form of the household food security scale. *Am. J. Public Health* **1999**, *89*, 1231–1234. [CrossRef]
24. Economic Research Service. *U.S. Household Food Security Survey Module: Six-Item Short Form*; United States Department of Agriculture, Ed.; United States Department of Agriculture: Washington, DC, USA, 2012.
25. Zealand, F.S.A.N. Nutrition, health and related claims. In *Australia New Zealand Food Standards Code*; Food Standards Australia New Zealand: Canberra, Australia, 2016.
26. Williams, P.; Yeatman, H.; Ridges, L.; Houston, A.; Rafferty, J.; Roesler, A.; Sobierajski, M.; Spratt, B. Nutrition function, health and related claims on packaged australian food products—Prevalence and compliance with regulations. *Asia Pac. J. Clin. Nutr.* **2006**, *15*, 10–20.
27. National Health and Medical Research Council. *Australian Dietary Guidelines*; National Health and Medical Research Council: Canberra, Australia, 2013.
28. Lioutas, E.D. Food consumer information behavior: Need arousal, seeking behavior, and information use. *J. Agric. Food Inf.* **2014**, *15*, 81–108. [CrossRef]
29. Wright, L.; Epps, J. Evaluation of a nutrition education program to increase fruit and vegetable intake in children from food insecure households. *J. Community Nutr. Health* **2013**, *2*, 76–83.
30. Innes-Hughes, C.; Bowers, K.; King, L.; Chapman, K.; Eden, B. *Food Security: The What, How, Why and Where to of Food Security in NSW; Discussion Paper*; NSW Centre for Public Health Nutrition: Sydney, NSW, Austrilia, 2013.
31. Drewnowski, A. Obesity, diets, and social inequalities. *Nutr. Rev.* **2009**, *67*, 36–39. [CrossRef]
32. Scheier, L. What is the hunger-obesity paradox? *J. Am. Diet. Assoc.* **2005**, *105*, 883–886. [CrossRef]
33. Crawford, B.; Yamazaki, R.; Franke, E.; Amanatidis, S.; Ravulo, J.; Steinbeck, K.; Ritchie, J.; Torvaldsen, S. Sustaining dignity? Food insecurity in homeless young people in urban australia. *Health Promot. J. Aust.* **2014**, *25*, 71–78. [CrossRef]
34. Hanson, K.L.; Connor, L.M. Food insecurity and dietary quality in us adults and children: A systematic review. *Am. J. Clin. Nutr.* **2014**, *100*, 684–692. [CrossRef]
35. Dimitri, C.; Rogus, S. Food choices, food security, and food policy. *J. Int. Aff.* **2014**, *67*, 19–31.
36. Butcher, L.M.; Ryan, M.M.; O'Sullivan, T.A.; Lo, J.; Devine, A. What drives food insecurity in western australia? How the perceptions of people at risk differ to those of stakeholders. *Nutrients* **2018**, *10*, 1059. [CrossRef]
37. Begley, A.; Paynter, E.; Butcher, L.M.; Dhaliwal, S.S. Examining the association between food literacy and food insecurity. *Nutrients* **2019**, *11*, 445. [CrossRef]
38. Smith, C.; Parnell, W.R.; Brown, R.C.; Gray, A.R. Balancing the diet and the budget: Food purchasing practices of food-insecure familiesin new zealand. *Nutr. Diet.* **2013**, *70*, 278–285. [CrossRef]
39. Mark, S.; Lambert, M.; O'Loughlin, J.; Gray-Donald, K. Household income, food insecurity and nutrition in canadian youth. *Can. J. Public Health* **2012**, *103*, 94–99.
40. Araújo, M.L.D.; Mendonça, R.D.D.; Lopes Filho, J.D.; Lopes, A.C.S. Association between food insecurity and food intake. *Nutrition* **2018**, *54*, 54–59. [CrossRef]
41. Mello, J.; Gans, K.; Risica, P.; Kirtania, U.; Strolla, L.; Fournier, L. How is food insecurity associated with dietary behaviors? An analysis with low-income, ethnically diverse participants in a nutrition intervention study. *J. Am. Diet. Assoc.* **2010**, *110*, 1906–1911. [CrossRef]
42. Zizza, C.; Duffy, P.; Gerrior, S. Food insecurity is not associated with lower energy intakes. *Obesity* **2008**, *16*, 1908–1913. [CrossRef]
43. Cunningham, T.; Barradas, D.; Rosenberg, K.; May, A.; Kroelinger, C.; Ahluwalia, I. Is maternal food security a predictor of food and drink intake among toddlers in oregon? *Matern. Child Health J.* **2012**, *16*, 339–346. [CrossRef]
44. Sharkey, J.; Nalty, C.; Johnson, C.; Dean, W. Children's very low food security is associated with increased dietary intakes in energy, fat, and added sugar among mexican-origin children (6–11 y) in texas border colonias. *BMC Pediatr.* **2012**, *12*, 16. [CrossRef]

45. Rush, E.; Puniani, N.; Snowling, N.; Paterson, J. Food security, selection, and healthy eating in a pacific community in auckland new zealand. *Asia Pac. J. Clin. Nutr.* **2007**, *16*, 448–454.
46. Australian Institute of Health and Welfare. *Australia's Health 2018*; AIHW: Canberra, Australia, 2018.
47. Rosenman, R.; Tennekoon, V.; Hill, L.G. Measuring bias in self-reported data. *Int. J. Behav. Healthc. Res.* **2011**, *2*, 320–332. [CrossRef]
48. Grunert, K.G.; Wills, J.M.; Fernández-Celemín, L. Nutrition knowledge, and use and understanding of nutrition information on food labels among consumers in the uk. *Appetite* **2010**, *55*, 177–189. [CrossRef]
49. Mullany, B.; Neault, N.; Tsingine, D.; Powers, J.; Lovato, V.; Clitso, L.; Massey, S.; Talgo, A.; Speakman, K.; Barlow, A. Food insecurity and household eating patterns among vulnerable american-indian families: Associations with caregiver and food consumption characteristics. *Public Health Nutr.* **2013**, *16*, 752–760. [CrossRef]
50. Godrich, S.L.; Davies, C.R.; Darby, J.; Devine, A. What are the determinants of food security among regional and remote western australian children? *Aust. New Zealand J. Public Health* **2017**, *41*, 172–177. [CrossRef]
51. Pollard, C.; Nyaradi, A.; Lester, M.; Sauer, K. Understanding food security issues in remote western australian indigenous communities. *Health Promot. J. Aust.* **2014**, *25*, 83–89. [CrossRef]
52. Bussey, C. Food security and traditional foods in remote aboriginal communities: A review of the literature. *Aust. Indig. Health Bulletin.* **2013**, *13*, 1–10.

nutrients

MDPI

Article

The Food Literacy Action Logic Model: A Tertiary Education Sector Innovative Strategy to Support the Charitable Food Sectors Need for Food Literacy Training

Tanya Lawlis [1,*], Ros Sambell [2], Amanda Douglas-Watson [2], Sarah Belton [1] and Amanda Devine [2]

1 Discipline Nutrition and Dietetics, University of Canberra, Canberra, ACT 2601, Australia; sarah.belton@live.com.au

2 School of Medical and Health Sciences, Edith Cowan University, Joondalup, Perth WA 6027, Australia; r.sambell@ecu.edu.au (R.S.); amanda.douglas-watson@hotmail.com (A.D.-W.); a.devine@ecu.edu.au (A.D.)

* Correspondence: Tanya.Lawlis@canberra.edu.au

Received: 12 March 2019; Accepted: 9 April 2019; Published: 12 April 2019

Abstract: Food literacy is seen as a key component in improving the increasing levels of food insecurity. While responsibility for providing training falls on the charitable service organizations, they may not have the capacity to adequately reach those in need. This paper proposes a tertiary education - (university or higher education) led model to support the food literacy training needs of the food charity sector. A cross-sectional study comprised of online surveys and discussions investigated food services offered by Western Australia (WA) and Australian Capital Territory (ACT) agencies, food literacy training needs for staff, volunteers and clients, and challenges to delivering food literacy training programs. Purposive sampling was used, and ACT and WA charitable service originations (survey: ACT n = 23, WA n = 32; interviews: ACT n = 3, WA n = 2) were invited to participate. Findings suggest organizations had limited financial and human resources to address the gap in food literacy training. Nutrition, food budgeting, and food safety education was delivered to paid staff only with limited capacity for knowledge transfer to clients. The Food Literacy Action Logic Model, underpinned by a tertiary education engagement strategy, is proposed to support and build capacity for organizations to address training gaps and extend the reach of food literacy to this under-resourced sector.

Keywords: charitable food sector; food insecurity; food literacy; nutrition education; training; tertiary education

1. Introduction

Australia is ranked as the 15th most food-secure country in the world [1]. The prevalence of food insecurity amongst the Australian population is estimated to be 4% [2]. Within Australia, the most vulnerable to food insecurity include: Aboriginal and Torres Strait Islander People; people experiencing homelessness, culturally and linguistically diverse groups; elderly; disabled people; young people; and low-income earners [3–5]. The prevalence of food insecurity has been reported to be as high as 71% among newly arrived refugees [2,3,6], and national data suggests one in five Aboriginal and Torres Strait Islander households ran out of food and had not been able to afford to buy more in the previous 12 months [7]. Food insecurity in youth has been associated with poor mental health, particularly hyperactivity/inattention, and can manifest into depression and suicide [8,9] and, in adults, has been is associated with poorer self-reported health status [10].

Food insecurity is defined as the "*limited or uncertain availability of nutritionally adequate and safe foods or limited or uncertain ability to acquire acceptable foods in socially acceptable ways*" [11]. The food insecurity spectrum ranges from being mildly food insecure, whereby there are challenges to accessing adequate food or being able to cook food, to experiencing hunger and malnutrition [12]. A primary reason for food insecurity is poverty [13], however, other environmental factors including organizational, community, and government structures may impede food security [14]. The resultant increase in individual risk against the four pillars of food security, food access, availability, utilization, and stability [14,15], is seen especially in vulnerable groups. Furthermore, there is much evidence in relation to the link between food insecure individuals and chronic disease [16–19].

Improving an individuals' food literacy has been identified as one strategy to improve food insecurity [15,16,20–22] and build resilience to cope with being food insecure [23]. Food literacy is defined as the relative ability to understand the nature of food, its importance, and understand how to use information about food for better health outcomes [24]. The key aspects of food literacy include food access, planning and management, selection, cooking, eating, and nutrition [24]. Research suggests that poor food literacy is a barrier for nutritious food access, wherein individuals with limited nutrition knowledge and skills are more likely to purchase ultra-processed foods [24,25], and have reduced individual creativity in meal preparation and awareness of health benefits of food [26]. An Australian food charity organization [27] reported that food literacy interventions have positively impacted those from low socio-economic demographics, with participation in multiple nutrition education interventions identified as a key component to reducing food insecurity [15].

Community service organizations are often the first point of call for those seeking assistance, and through their many programs, provide access to food and food literacy programs [28]. Despite the availability of food literacy courses and resources for organizations' staff, volunteers, and clients in Australia [29–31], not all of these groups receive training, thus limiting knowledge transfer of food literacy. From a knowledge brokerage perspective, food literacy programs delivered by a familiar community service agency has the potential to provide a safe learning environment; and previous research has demonstrated improved nutrition skills, food choices, preparation, and cooking skills thus reducing the risk of chronic diseases [26]. Therefore the aim of this study was to identify the food services offered by agencies in Western Australia (WA) and Australian Capital Territory (ACT) regions; scope the needs of food literacy training for staff, volunteers, and clients from a staff perspective; investigate challenges of food rescue organizations engagement with existing food literacy training programs; and propose a tertiary education (university or higher education) led model to support the food literacy training needs of the food charity sector.

2. Materials and Methods

2.1. Study Design

A cross-sectional design comprising an online survey to community service agencies and discussions with Chief Executive Officers or Managers from five key food rescue organizations (WA (n = 2) and ACT (n = 3)) was used for the study. Community service agencies that provide programs within the Perth metropolitan area of WA and within Canberra, ACT, were surveyed to scope the current delivery of food literacy programs and training for staff and volunteers and the needs of clients from the staff perspective. Organizations in WA and ACT were randomly selected, based on organization type (emergency relief provider, food rescue organization, charitable food pantry, and providers of services to those who are homeless), were invited to participate in the discussion. The purpose of the discussions was to (1) expand the survey findings; (2) provide differences in context between jurisdictions; and (3) determine challenges to food literacy training and delivery from the organizational perspective. The concept of food literacy was outlined by the interviewer to the interviewees of the food rescue organizations. As discussions were informal and explorative in nature, the conversation flowed freely around the topic area of food literacy, which encompassed nutrition literacy. The Edith Cowan University Human Research Ethics Committee (12509) approved the study, and a reciprocal agreement was provided by the University of Canberra Human Research

Ethics Committee. Informed consent was obtained from participants prior to completing the survey and discussions.

2.2. Recruitment of Agencies

Purposive sampling was undertaken to conduct this study. Community service organizations that provided community food programs were identified using publicly identifiable information (WA n = 112; ACT n = 56). Where an email address was publicly available, an initial email invitation to participate and an online survey link was sent (n = 99, WA; n = 50, ACT). Agencies without this information were contacted by telephone and asked to participate and provided the link or completed the survey with the contact over the phone (n = 13, WA; n = 6, ACT). To improve survey completion, organizations were reconducted at fortnightly intervals between November 2015–February 2016 (WA) and May–July 2016 (ACT).

2.3. Survey Development

An investigator-generated 23 item survey was designed to scope the range of primary services provided, demographics of clients, types of food and food services offered, use of food literacy programs, food literacy training needs of staff, volunteers, and needs of clients from the staff perspective. All closed items had nominal or ordinal response categories. The survey was developed by the researchers from (Removed for blinding). Content and face validity of the survey was conducted prior to administration in this study by key experts from three independent WA food rescue organizations and community service agencies. The final survey was administered online through Qualtrics LLC, Provo, Utah [32], a copy of which can be obtained from the authors.

2.4. Data Analysis

Quantitative data were analyzed using SPSS, Version 21 (IBM Corporation, Chicago, IL, USA). Basic descriptive and frequency analyses were conducted. Transcripts were coded using the thematic analysis process, as outlined by Braun and Clarke [33]. Initial coding of the data identified a consistent alignment of codes across the transcripts with the four pillars of food security: Availability, access, utilization, and stability [14]. These themes also aligned with the aims of the project, in particular aim 2, and informed the development of the model, aim 3. Codes that did not align with the four pillars were not identified during the coding. The coding process was conducted by author R.S. and reviewed by authors T.L. and A.D.

3. Results

3.1. Respondent Demographics

Community service organization Chief Executive Officers or Managers (n = 55) completed the online survey with a response rate of 29% (n = 32) for WA and 41% (n = 23) for ACT. Organizations provided more than one primary service to a range of client groups (Table 1), however, in both ACT and WA, the most reported primary service was, "welfare/homelessness service" (ACT 43% n = 10; WA 59% n = 19). There was greater variation between the proportion and types of client groups serviced by the organizations between ACT and WA, such that the primary client group in the ACT included "low income" (n = 20, 87%) and "Aboriginal and/or Torres Strait Islander people" (n = 14, 61%), whereas, both of these groups were equally reported as the main client group in WA (n = 26, 81%). The "homeless" (n = 23, 72%) and "asylum seekers, migrants or refugees" (n = 19, 59%) groups were also reported as key recipients in WA.

Table 1. Demographic comparison between Western Australia (WA) and Australian Capital Territory (ACT) charitable organizations.

Category	ACT (*n*)	WA (*n*)	Total (*n*)
	23	32	55
Number of Paid Staff (approx.)	55	117	172
Number of People Volunteering (approx.)	166	628	894
Clients Attending and Receiving Food (approx.)	1100	1400	2500
Primary Services Provided by Organisations			
Disability Services	0	1	1
Welfare/Homelessness Services	10	19	29
Health Organisation	1	1	2
Sport/Social and Community Programs	1	4	5
Food Program	7	6	13
Other programs not listed	4	2	6
Mental Health	2	0	2
Alcohol, Drugs and Rehabilitation	1	0	1
Domestic Violence	0	1	1
Client groups			
Aboriginal and Torres Strait Islander People	14	26	40
Asylum Seekers, Migrants or Refugees	6	19	25
Homeless	12	23	35
Low Income	20	26	46
Clients Other than those listed	10	5	15
Individuals with a Disability	1	1	2
Individuals with Mental Health Conditions	2	0	2
Individuals with Alcohol and Drug Problems	2	0	2
Family Specific Focus	4	2	6

Forty-two percent of organizations offered case management services to their clients (ACT 30% $n = 7$; WA 50% $n = 16$). Of these, 87% ($n = 20/23$) included a food literacy program within the case management structure. Programs were either conducted on one occasion (Total $n = 5$; WA $n = 5$) or once a week for several weeks (Total $n = 15$; ACT $n = 7$; WA $n = 8$). Despite 58% of organizations not providing case management and nutrition services to their clients, 60% of total survey respondents ($n = 33/55$) indicated they had access to an onsite kitchen: 18% had access to a domestic size kitchen (Total $n = 10$; 13% ACT $n = 3$; WA 22% $n = 7$) and 42% had access to a commercial kitchen (Total $n = 23$; ACT 52% $n = 12$; WA 34% $n = 11$).

The community service organizations in ACT and WA provided a variety of food services and foods (Total $n = 19$; ACT $n = 9$; WA $n = 10$) to approximately 2500 clients per week (ACT $n = 1100$; WA $n = 1400$, Table 1). The primary food services offered included prepared food (Total $n = 41$; ACT $n = 15$; WA $n = 19$), emergency relief parcels (Total $n = 31$; ACT $n = 11$; WA $n = 20$) and food pantries (Total $n = 19$; ACT $n = 9$; WA $n = 10$). Food provision included fruit (Total $n = 23$; ACT $n = 11$; WA $n = 12$), hot and cold beverages (Total $n = 20$; ACT $n = 10$; WA $n = 10$), snacks (Total $n = 16$; ACT $n = 9$; WA $n = 7$), sandwiches (Total $n = 15$; ACT $n = 10$; WA $n = 5$) and hot meals (Total $n = 15$; ACT $n = 10$; WA $n = 5$).

3.2. Food Literacy Training

The scope of the food literacy training programs listed in the survey were food safety and handling, food budgeting, nutrition and cooking. Food safety and handling was the primary training delivered to paid staff and a priority area in both ACT and WA for volunteers. Similarly, centers in ACT ($n = 7/23$) and WA ($n = 8/32$) organizations, provided some training in food budgeting, nutrition, and cooking for clients. Face-to-face or online training was delivered by a variety of educational providers or provided from within the organization.

Organizations budgeted between $ 0 and $ 5000 per annum (pa) for food literacy training for staff; on average, ACT and WA reported $ 1100 pa and $ 400 pa respectively. The budget reduced considerably for ACT and WA volunteers ($ 400 pa vs. $ 100 pa respectively) and clients ($ 36 pa vs. $ 20 pa, respectively). Reflective of the reported budgets, 32–38% of organizations did not provide any food literacy training for paid staff, and 50–65% did not provide training for volunteers and clients.

3.3. *Main Challenges in Conducting Food Literacy Programs*

The primary challenges experienced by the community service organizations, from the staff perspective when running food literacy programs for clients were similar between ACT and WA. This included inadequacies in client's nutrition knowledge (ACT n = 10 (40%); WA n = 15 (60%)), motivation to prepare healthy food (ACT n = 9 (39%); WA n = 14 (61%)); and skills (ACT n = 9 (50%); WA n = 9 (50%)). Organizational challenges in WA included lack of access to food for clients (n = 9), time (n = 9) and insufficient funding to supplement the food supplied for programs (n = 9). ACT lacked kitchen access and equipment (n = 6).

With unlimited time, facilities and budget, the three priority areas for training staff and volunteers were similar between ACT and WA. For staff, basic nutrition education was prioritized in both jurisdictions; WA prioritized food budgeting (n = 14); ACT prioritized food safety (n = 10). Priorities for WA and ACT volunteers were nutrition education (n = 12) and food safety (n = 12) and for clients, basic nutrition education (n = 16) and food budgeting (n = 16) respectively.

3.4. *Key Organisation Views*

Discussions with Chief Executive Officers or Managers from five key organizations supplemented the survey data and highlighted the role that organizations, agencies, and institutions including universities can play to improve food literacy and reduce food insecurity. Transcripts were coded against the four pillars of food security [14]: Availability, access, utilization and stability. The potential roles are outlined in relation to these pillars below.

3.4.1. Availability

Organizations reported relying on food donations to provide fruit and vegetables and other foods for use in food literacy programs. Program sustainability was affected by the amount of food required beyond donations. Organizations indicated they would benefit from collaborative funding opportunities, thus providing consistent food availability at their services.

3.4.2. Access

Adequate access is fundamental to an individual's food security status. The organizations' ability to support knowledge transfer around access through food literacy programs was proposed to support food security. The programs needed to include the who–who delivers the program; the level–appropriate program tailoring for clients; and, the where–resources to deliver program, location, and access to kitchen facilities, to ensure stability and client engagement. Further discussions highlighted that the delivery of the food literacy programs was critical and required expertise in food and nutrition, pedagogy, cooking skills, and target relevance:

"From what we found that people are saying to us 'we don't want celebrity chefs teaching us how to cook'. It frightens those people that are vulnerable."

"I would say that they (the person running the program) have to be confident at cooking. Again it is about being able to throw things in, being able to be a bit flamboyant with the way they are doing it. Other than just by the book. I think it has to have a bit of flexibility in it for it to suit."

It was suggested that without consideration of these factors, utilization of food literacy programs and food supplied would be reduced, thus lessening the client and organizational impact on food security.

"When people are living in cars, how do they cook? The little stove, doing a bit of camp cooking."

"That is the problem with the end user, the person getting the box of food. They are often people with very limited–they might be homeless or be in a hostel–ability to actually choose and prepare food for themselves.

Their circumstances are that they get what they can and its often soup kitchen or prepared by a charity and given straight to them."

Similar to survey responses, human resources, staff and volunteer turnover, and limited space and facilities to conduct food literacy programs were identified as challenges. Funding in particular was found to be the biggest challenge to overcome.

"Sustainable funding to keep the ball rolling. That's our biggest issue and particularly in those high need areas where there is no money ... for human resources to keep the program running. This is important to inspire and motivate."

3.4.3. Utilization

Food literacy education provides an opportunity to upskill staff, volunteers, and clients to priorities nutrient-rich food consumption. The content and tools of food literacy programs should embed contextualized and well-evidenced information incorporating simple and robust recipes with common and inexpensive ingredients.

"We think we have to measure everything, and I think that sometimes frightens people ... When you take the measurement out it also takes the likelihood of it being wrong which can put people off. The fear of it not being as it should be ... What I think you need to do is really pare it back. It has got to be simple. I cook like that I don't measure anything. Teach people to do it by taste."

"Another thing we found was that some of the barriers to producing this information were the client's knowledge. Maybe some of the programs that are out there are too high a level for those clients."

3.4.4. Stability

Food insecurity and subsequent nutrition insecurity can be outcomes of unstable food supply or lack of infrastructure to provide adequate food and/or training to empower individuals to overcome their food security status. The potential of training programs to build food literacy skills in clients could, in turn, go some way in offering a pathway to a more stable food supply. The organizations, however, had concerns given their limited capacity to provide food literacy programs themselves:

" ... ... What I think we need to be thinking about in this instance is how we cannot just roll this out in Perth metropolitan area, but HOW can we roll it out into the regional centers."

A tertiary education partnership model, which relies on student engagement, a flexible framework with relevant, authentic teaching, and learning structures were discussed with each of the key organizations to address the limited capacity and extend their reach of food literacy training. While the proposal of a partnership model was looked upon favorably, an organization stated that:

"As long as you've got a framework (within this model)–this is your outcome, how you get there might be determined by your clients on the day."

All organizations agreed that a model requires buy-in from stakeholders within community service and food rescue organizations and potential partnerships with other commercial businesses or sectors outside the charitable food sector to be sustainable and successful:

"It is an ownership as well. People like to be involved but they like to own it as well. They would own it by financially contributing."

4. Discussion

This study highlights the challenges experienced by the charitable food sector to improve food security through the provision of food literacy programs. Despite the varying geographical locations, similar findings across the jurisdictions (WA, ACT) were evident, including the fact that the primary services being offered were welfare/homeless services and for low income and Aboriginal and/or Torres Strait Islander peoples. While the amount of funding provided by ACT and WA organizations on food literacy training differed, limited financial support was evident, suggesting other options for food literacy training need to be considered. The priority focus for the training of staff, volunteers, and clients was food safety and handling. Nutrition and food budgeting were prioritized, but lack of funding and facilities limited actual delivery. External organizations provided food literacy training, resulting in additional costs for the organizations, thus limiting uptake and reach.

To provide sustainable programs, charitable food organizations acknowledged that partnerships with business, education, and health sectors were required. Engaging support was difficult due to changing external interests, poor funding models, and the absence of a logical framework to drive the process. Analysis of the survey findings and discussions supported the formulation of a Food Literacy Action Logic Model (Figure 1). This model outlines how the tertiary education sector can partner with the community service and food rescue organizations to provide sustainable food literacy training, foster skill development, and extend reach.

The Food Literacy Action Logic Model is premised upon the four pillars of food security: Availability, access, utilization, and stability [14,15]; and, incorporates the Socio-Ecological Model (SEM) of Health Promotion [34]. The SEM provides a framework to understand the complex and multifaceted interactions within the social system [34]. Accepted globally, the SEM is used to develop and evaluate nutrition, social and health programs [35] and analyze the importance of health/disease related decisions [36]. The SEM has five hierarchical levels: Individual, Interpersonal, Organizational, Community, and Policy/Enabling environments [34]. To achieve food security for the individual, community, and population, it is essential that all four pillars are supported and encompass all SEM levels.

The Food Literacy Action Logic Model guides the tertiary education sector in supporting all four pillars of food security. Engagement with the community services sector supports relationships between stakeholders at all levels of the SEM framework [34]. For example, "Policy/Enabling environments" includes partnerships with national, state, territory and local governments and food industry to improve funding and resources to ensure sustainable food supply and programs. Partnerships between food rescue organizations, food and non-food businesses, and the tertiary sector are needed to increase funding opportunities to improve the sustainability of food literacy programs. In turn, partnerships at the community and organization levels foster trusting environments, thus improving client's access to food and knowledgeable trainers are likely to reduce attrition from programs [37]. The pillar of utilization of food is enhanced by a multi-strategy approach to food literacy education, as demonstrated by the Food Literacy Action Logic Model [37].

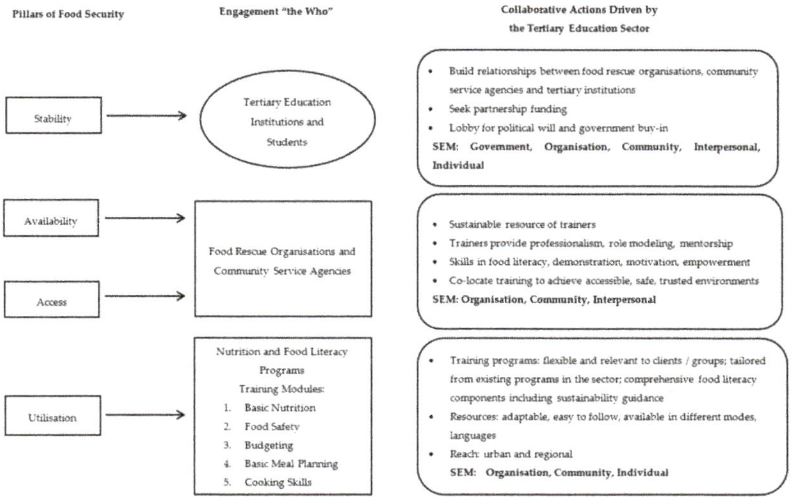

Figure 1. Food Action Logic Model: A schematic representation of collaborative actions driven by the tertiary education sector to address engagement with food rescue and community service organization's to improve food security via a food literacy education model. SEM: Socio-ecological Model.

Limitations

Despite a low response rate, the similarity in responses within each jurisdiction may imply a representative sample albeit from purposive sampling from a comprehensive publicly available database. Survey responses, including the training needs of clients, were based upon the staff perspective only. Discussions with the sector were informal and explorative in nature to determine the needs of the sector to build models for support.

5. Conclusions

Food literacy is one of the many strategies used to address food insecurity. A sustainable model showcasing collaboration with the tertiary education sector and the charitable food sector has been proposed to engage a sustainable student workforce to deliver food literacy training to staff and volunteers in order to improve knowledge transfer to clients. The delivery of flexible, relevant, and authentic food literacy programs tailored for regional and urban environments and contextualized for the client groups will contribute to greater food utilization and social skills for the client with an aim to improve short and long-term health.

Author Contributions: Conceptualization, T.L., R.S. and A.D.; methodology, T.L., R.S., A.D.-W., S.B., and A.D.; software, T.L., R.S., A.D.-W. and S.B.; validation, T.L. and R.S.; formal analysis, T.L., R.S., A.D.-W. and S.B.; investigation, T.L., R.S., A.D.-W., S.B., and A.D.; resources, T.L, R.S. and A.D.; data curation, T.L, R.S. and A.D.; writing—original draft preparation, T.L., R.S., A.D.-W. and S.B.; writing—review and editing, T.L, R.S., and A.D.; visualization, A.D.; project administration, R.S.; funding acquisition, T.L, R.S. and A.D.

Funding: This research was supported by (university name removed for blinding) Collaborative Enhancement Scheme and the (university name removed for blinding) Health Research Institute Grant.

Acknowledgments: The researchers would like to thank the charitable organizations located in Perth, Western Australian and the Australian Capital Territory for participating in this research.

Conflicts of Interest: The authors declare no conflict of interest.

References

1. The Economist Intelligence Unit. *Global Food Index. An Annual Measure of the State of Global Food Insecurity*; The Economist Intelligence Unit: London, UK, 2013.
2. Australian Bureau of Statistics. Australian Health Survey: First Results, 2011–2012. Cat no.4364.0.55.001. Canberra: Australian Bureau of Statistics; 2012. Available online: http://www.abs.gov.au/ausstats/abs@.nsf/Lookup/by%20Subject/4727.0.55.005~{}2012-13~{}Main%20Features~{}Food%20Security~{}36 (accessed on 2 February 2016).
3. Gallegos, D.; Ellies, P.; Wright, J. Still there's no food! Food insecurity in a refugee population in Perth, Western Australia. *Nutr. Diet.* **2008**, *65*, 78–83. [CrossRef]
4. Nolan, M.; Rikard-Bell, G.; Mohsin, M.; Williams, M. Food insecurity in three socially disadvantaged localities in Sydney, Australia. *Health Promot. J. Austr.* **2006**, *17*, 247–254. [CrossRef] [PubMed]
5. Booth, S.; Smith, A. Food security and poverty in Australia—Challenges for dietitians. *Nutr. Diet.* **2001**, *58*, 150–156.
6. Friel, S. Climate change, food insecurity and chronic diseases: Sustainable and healthy policy opportunities for Australia. *NSW Public Health Bull.* **2010**, *21*, 5–6. [CrossRef] [PubMed]
7. Australian Bureau of Statistics. Australian Aboriginal and Torres Strait Islander Health Survey: Nutrition Results-Food and Nutrients, 2012–2013. Cat no.4727 Canberra.2015. Available online: http://www.abs.gov.au/ausstats/abs@.nsf/Lookup/by%20Subject/4727.0.55.005~{}2012-13~{}Main%20Features~{}Food%20Security~{}36 (accessed on 16 February 2016).
8. Melchior, M.; Chastang, J.-F.; Falissard, B.; Galéra, C.; Tremblay, R.E.; Côté, S.M.; Boivin, M. Food insecurity and children's mental health: A prospective birth cohort study. *PLoS ONE* **2012**, *7*, e52615. [CrossRef]
9. McIntyre, L.; Williams, J.V.A.; Lavorato, D.H. Depression and suicide ideation in late adolescence and early adulthood are an outcome of child hunger. *J. Affect Disord.* **2013**, *150*, 123–129. [CrossRef] [PubMed]
10. Stuff, J.E.; Casey, P.H.; Szeto, K.L.; Gossett, J.M.; Robbins, J.M.; Simpson, P.M.; Connell, C.; Bogle, M.L. Household food insecurity is associated with adult health status. *J. Nutr.* **2004**, *134*, 2330–2335. [CrossRef]

11. Radimer, K. Measurement of hoursehold security in the USA and other industrialised countries. *Public Health Nutr.* **2002**, *5*, 859–864. [CrossRef] [PubMed]
12. Ballard, T.J.; Kepple, A.W.; Cafiero, C. *The Food Insecurity Experience Scale: Development of a Global Standard for Monitoring Hunger Worldwide*; Food and Agricultural Organisation: Rome, Italy, 2013.
13. Social Policy Research Centre. *Poverty in Australia 2016*; Australian Council of Social Service Inc.: Strawberry Hills, NSW, Australia, 2016.
14. Food and Agriculture Organisation of the United Nations. Policy Brief: Food Security Geneva: Food and Agriculture Organisation of the United Nations; 2006. Available online: http://www.fao.org/forestry/13128-0e6f36f27e0091055bec28ebe830f46b3.pdf (accessed on 15 August 2015).
15. Innes-Hughes, C.; Bowers, K.; King, L.; Chapman, K.; Eden, B. *Food Security: The What, How, Why and Where to Food Security in NSW*; Discussion Paper; Heart Foundation NSW and Cancer Council NSW: Sydney, Australia, 2010.
16. Stuff, J.E.; Casey, P.H.; Connell, C.L.; Champagne, C.M.; Gossett, J.M.; Harsha, D.; McCabe-Sellers, B.; Robbins, J.M.; Simpson, P.M.; Szeto, K.L.; et al. Household food insecurity and obesity, chronic disease, and chronic disease risk factors. *J. Hunger Environ. Nutr.* **2007**, *1*, 43–62. [CrossRef]
17. Seligman, H.K.; Laraia, B.A.; Kushel, M.B. Food insecurity is associated with chronic disease among low-income NHANES participants. *J. Nutr.* **2010**, *140*, 304–310. [CrossRef] [PubMed]
18. Laraia, B.A. Food insecurity and chronic disease. *Adv. Nutr.* **2013**, *4*, 203–212. [CrossRef]
19. Franklin, B.; Jones, A.; Love, D.; Puckett, S.; Macklin, J.; White-Means, S. Exploring mediators of food insecurity and obesity: A review of recent literature. *J. Community Health* **2012**, *37*, 253–264. [CrossRef] [PubMed]
20. Waterlander, W.; de Boer, M.; Schuit, A.; Seidell, J.; Steenhuis, I. Price discounts significantly enhance fruit ad vegetable purchases when combined with nutrition education: A randomised controlled supermarket trial. *Am. J. Clin. Nutr.* **2013**, *97*, 886–895. [CrossRef]
21. Leung, C.; Cluggish, S.; Villamor, E.; Catalano, P.; Willett, W.; Rimm, E. Few changes in food security and dietary intake from short-term participants in the supplemental nutrition assistance program among low-income Massachusetts adults. *J. Nutr. Educ. Behav.* **2014**, *46*, 68–74. [CrossRef] [PubMed]
22. Miller, C.; Branscum, P. The effect of a recessionary economy on food choice: Implications for nutrition education. *J. Nutr. Educ. Behav.* **2012**, *44*, 100–106. [CrossRef] [PubMed]
23. Butcher, L.; Chester, M.; Aberle, L.; Bobongie, V.J.; Godrich, S.L.; Milligan, R.; et al. Foodbank of Western Australia's healthy food for all. *Brit. Food J.* **2014**, *116*, 1490–1505. [CrossRef]
24. Vidgen, H.A.; Gallegos, D. Defining food literacy and its components. *Appetite* **2014**, *76*, 50–59. [CrossRef]
25. Bowyer, S.; Caraher, M.; Eilbert, K.; Carr-Hill, R. Shopping for food: Lessons from a London borough. *Brit. Food J.* **2011**, *11*, 452–474. [CrossRef]
26. Desjardins, E. *"Making Something Out of Nothing", Food Literacy among Youth, Young Pregnant Women and Young Parents Who Are at Risk for Poor Health*; Word Processing Plus: Toronto, ON, Canada, 2013.
27. FoodBank Australia. *Fighting Hunger in Australia: Foodbank Hunger Report 2016*; Foodbank Australia: Sydney, Australia, 2016.
28. Belton, S.; Jamieson, M.; Lawlis, T. Despite challenges food relief is a conduit to developing relationships, trust and enabling client food security and specialised support: A case study. *J. Hunger Environ. Nutr.* **2019**. [CrossRef]
29. OzHarvest. NEST-Nutrition Education Sustenance Training Sydney, Australia: OzHarvest; 2017. Available online: http://www.ozharvest.org/what-we-do/nest-nutrition-education/ (accessed on 22 August 2017).
30. Foodbank Australia. Healthy Food for all Perth, Western Australia: Food Bank Australia; 2017. Available online: http://www.healthyfoodforall.com.au/food-sensations/ (accessed on 22 August 2017).
31. Australian Red Cross. FoodREDi Education Programs 2017. Available online: https://www.redcross.org.au/about-us/how-we-help/food-security/foodredi-education-programs (accessed on 16 February 2018).
32. Qualtrics LLC. Qualtrics: Online Survey Software and Insight Platform 2013. Available online: https://www.qualtrics.com (accessed on 6 March 2016).
33. Braun, V.; Clarke, V. Using thematic analysis in psychology. *Qual. Res. Psychol.* **2006**, *3*, 77–101. [CrossRef]

34. McLeroy, K.R.; Bibeau, D.; Steckler, A.; Glanz, K. An ecological perspective on health promotion programs. *Health Educ. Quart.* **1988**, *15*, 351–377. [CrossRef]
35. Gregson, J.; Foerster, S.B.; Orr, R.; Jones, L.; Benedict, J.; Clarke, B.; Hersey, J.; Lewis, J.; Zotz, K. System, environmental and policy changes: using the social-ecological model as a framework for evaluating nutrition education and social marketing programs with low-income audiences. *J. Nutr. Educ.* **2001**, *33*, S4–S15. [CrossRef]
36. Kumar, S.; Quinn, S.C.; Kim, K.H.; Musa, D.M.; Hillyard, K.M.; Freimuth, V.S. The social ecological model as a framework for determinants of 2009 H1Niinfluenza vaccine uptake in the US. *Health Educ. Behav.* **2012**, *39*, 229–243. [CrossRef] [PubMed]
37. Barbour, L.; Ho, M.; Davidson, Z.; Palermo, C. Challenges and opportunities for measuring the impact of a nutrition programme amongst young people at risk of food insecurity: A pilot study. *Nutr. Bull.* **2016**, *41*, 122–129. [CrossRef]

MDPI
St. Alban-Anlage 66
4052 Basel
Switzerland
Tel. +41 61 683 77 34
Fax +41 61 302 89 18
www.mdpi.com

Nutrients Editorial Office
E-mail: nutrients@mdpi.com
www.mdpi.com/journal/nutrients

www.ingramcontent.com/pod-product-compliance
Lightning Source LLC
Chambersburg PA
CBHW051724210326
41597CB00032B/5601
* 9 7 8 3 0 3 9 2 1 1 2 0 3 *